Intestinal Failure
and Rehabilitation
A Clinical Guide

CRC Series in Modern Nutrition Science

Series Editor
Stacey J. Bell
Ideasphere, Inc.
Grand Rapids, Michigan

Phytopharmaceuticals in Cancer Chemoprevention
Edited by Debasis Bagchi and Harry Preuss

Handbook of Minerals as Nutritional Supplements
Robert A. DiSilvestro

Intestinal Failure and Rehabilitation: A Clinical Guide
Edited by Laura E. Matarese, Ezra Steiger,
and Douglas L. Seidner

CRC Series in Modern Nutrition Science

Intestinal Failure and Rehabilitation
A Clinical Guide

EDITED BY
Laura E. Matarese
Ezra Steiger
Douglas L. Seidner

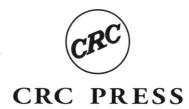

CRC PRESS

Boca Raton   London   New York   Washington, D.C.

Library of Congress Cataloging-in-Publication Data

Intestinal failure and rehabilitation : a clinical guide / edited by Laura E. Matarese,
Ezra Steiger, and Douglas L. Seidner.
     p. ; cm. – (Modern nutrition science; 3)
    Includes bibliographical references and index.
    ISBN 0-8493-1803-3 (alk. paper)
    1. Malabsorption syndromes.
    [DNLM: 1. Malabsorption Syndromes–therapy. 2. Nutrition Therapy. WI 500 I633
2005] I. Matarese, Laura E. II. Steiger, Ezra. III. Seidner, Douglas L. IV. Title. V. Series.

RC862.M3I534 2005
616.3′99—dc22   2004051939

Visit the CRC Press Web site at www.crcpress.com

Series Preface

When I was asked to serve as the series editor of *Modern Nutrition Science*, I jumped at the opportunity. I have worked in the field of nutrition for 30 years as both a researcher and as a dietitian. This role gave me the opportunity to select expert colleagues, many of whom are key thought leaders in the field, to be volume editors for the individual books in the series. I am happy to report that in each case, my first choice for book editor accepted the job.

The books in this series are geared for two audiences: nutritional scientists and healthcare professionals such as dietitians, physicians, nurses, and pharmacists. Each book contains chapters that are scholarly, extensive scientific reviews covering their topics in a comprehensive way. My hope is that these volumes will stimulate new topics of research for nutritional scientists. Busy healthcare practitioners will also use the books as sound resources when providing clinical care.

Many patients today are using alternative therapies to manage their diseases. Keeping up with this evolving field is often difficult. Moreover, especially in the area of dietary supplements, the science behind the perceived benefits is lacking.

The books in this series are written with a definitive structure to the chapters so that specific information is easily found, without having to read the entire chapter. For example, if a patient with breast cancer asks about the use of selenium, one can easily find cancer and efficacious doses without reading the entire chapter.

As Ms. Matarese and Drs. Steiger and Seidner aptly point out in their Preface, successful treatments for patients with short bowel syndrome have only recently become available. Many of these advances were conceived and perfected by this team. For the past 20 years, I have known these investigators at the Cleveland Clinic and their work regarding all aspects of nutrition support. However, when specifically thinking of who could best produce a book on short bowel syndrome management, this group, in my mind, is the best in the country. These editors have contributed scientifically sound chapters on the latest cutting edge techniques for the clinical management of these patients. In addition, they were able to get leading-edge contributors for the remaining chapters. For example, Drs. Grant and Jeejeebhoy pioneered the field of gastrointestinal nutrition. Drs. Byrne and Zeigler spent many years with Dr. Douglas Wilmore studying the effect of glutamine and other nutrients on gut health in these compromised patients. Dr. Howard has spent a career optimizing home feeding of patients without proper bowel function.

When I started working in the field of nutrition support nearly 30 years ago, I never imagined that it would be possible to successfully feed patients with such limited bowel function. I am pleased for the patients with this condition that such advances have occurred. By reading this book, clinicians caring for the nutritional management of these patients will learn from the experts about the latest techniques as well as the scientific support behind these recommendations.

Stacey J. Bell, Ph.D.
Series Editior

Preface

Prior to the introduction of Parenteral Nutrition by Dr. Dudrick and his colleagues at the Hospital of the University of Pennsylvania in the 1960s, patients with short bowel syndrome and intestinal failure would often die of progressive malnutrition and its associated morbidities. The introduction of parenteral nutrition support has given the patient with short bowel syndrome the time needed to achieve maximal intestinal rehabilitation and has allowed these patients to survive until more effective treatment of intestinal failure could be developed. The pioneering work of Drs. Byrne and Wilmore in the 1990s has focused our attention on novel techniques that can be used to enhance intestinal adaptation and absorption. These techniques include modification of diet, special nutrients, oral rehydration solutions, and growth factors. Newer surgical techniques can also be applied for the prevention and treatment of intestinal failure, and the evolving success of intestinal transplantation has given hope for a "cure" of intestinal failure in selected patients. This book brings together an expert group of clinicians to help us understand current information regarding the prevention, diagnosis, care, and management of patients with intestinal failure. The editors of this book are grateful for the many contributions made by these clinicians toward more effective management of patients with intestinal failure. This book is dedicated to our patients and all those who have worked in this field since the pioneering work of Dr. Dudrick and his colleagues.

Laura E. Matarese, M.S., R.D., L.D., F.A.D.A., C.N.S.D.

Ezra Steiger, M.D., F.A.C.S., C.N.S.P.

Douglas L. Seidner, M.D., F.A.C.G., C.N.S.P.

Editor

Laura E. Matarese, M.S., R.D., L.D., F.A.D.A., C.N.S.D., was born and raised in New Haven, Connecticut. She attended Ohio Dominican University, where she received a Bachelor's degree in Food and Nutrition and an Associate's degree in Chemistry. She completed her dietetic internship at the Veterans Administration Medical Center in Cleveland, Ohio, and obtained her Master's degree in Nutrition Science from Case Western Reserve University. She is currently a Ph.D. student at the University of Medicine and Dentistry of New Jersey. She is the author of 150 books, chapters, manuscripts, abstracts, CDs, and videos. She has lectured extensively, both nationally and internationally, and has held numerous positions within the American Dietetic Association and the American Society for Parenteral and Enteral Nutrition. She is a charter Fellow of the American Dietetic Association. She is the recipient of numerous awards, including the American Dietetic Association Foundation Award for Excellence in the Practice of Clinical Nutrition, the American Society for Parenteral and Enteral Nutrition Award for Distinguished Achievement in Nutrition Support Dietetics, and the Dietitians in Nutrition Support Distinguished Service Award. In 1997 she received the Case Western Reserve University Alumna of the Year award, and in 1999 she received the American Dietetic Association Medallion Award for her pioneering work in nutrition support. Laura Matarese is the director of Nutrition Intestinal Rehabilitation at the Cleveland Clinic Foundation. She is responsible for the overall development, direction, and implementation of the nutrition intestinal rehabilitation program. Her research interests include body composition and mucosal adaptation.

Ezra Steiger, M.D., F.A.C.S., C.N.S.P., was born and raised in Cleveland, Ohio. He attended Ohio State University, where he received a B.A. in 1962 and an M.D. in 1966. He did his internship and residency at The Hospital of The University of Pennsylvania from 1966 to 1973, and was an NIH training Fellow in the Harrison Department of Surgical Research during that time. He worked with Drs. Dudrick, Wilmore, Vars, and Rhoads to help develop the art and science of parenteral nutrition, or intravenous hyperalimentation as it was called initially. He was the first to develop the intravenously nourished rat model that is extensively used in parenteral nutrition research today. He served at the Keesler Air Force base in Biloxi, Mississippi, from 1973 to 1975 and was honorably discharged as a Lieutenant Colonel. He came to the Cleveland Clinic Foundation as a Staff Surgeon in General Surgery in 1975, where he started and directed its Nutrition Support Team and its Home Parenteral Nutrition Program. He also served as the vice chairman of General Surgery. He was elected president of the following organizations: the Cleveland Surgical Society, the Ohio State Chapter of the American College of Surgeons, the American Society of

Parenteral and Enteral Nutrition (ASPEN), and the Medical Staff of the Cleveland Clinic Foundation. He served or serves on the following boards: the Board of Governors of the American College of Surgeons, the Oley Foundation, the Board of Trustees of Cleveland Clinic Foundation, and the National Board of Nutrition Support Certification. He has over 150 publications in the scientific literature, mostly dealing with the field of parenteral nutrition in the hospital and at home. Although retired from his surgical practice, Dr. Steiger continues his nutrition support practice at the Cleveland Clinic, caring for patients in the hospital and at home while serving as co-director of the Nutrition Support and Vascular Access Department at the Cleveland Clinic Foundation, and as head of the Intestinal Rehabilitation Program there.

Douglas L. Seidner, M.D., F.A.C.G., C.N.S.P., is originally from East Islip, New York. He received his Bachelor's of Science at the State University of New York at Albany in 1979 and his Medical Degree at the State University of New York at Upstate Medical Center in Syracuse in 1983. He completed an internship and residency in Internal Medicine at the New England Deaconess Hospital at Harvard Medical School and stayed on to complete a fellowship in Nutrition and Metabolism under the direction of Drs. Bruce Bistrian and George Blackburn. This was followed by a fellowship in Gastroenterology at the George Washington University School of Medicine and Health Care Sciences. Dr. Seidner came to the Cleveland Clinic Foundation as a Staff Gastroenterologist in the Departments of Gastroenterology and General Surgery in 1991. He is currently the Director of the Nutrition Support Team, the Chairman of the Nutrition Services Committee and a member of the Intestinal Rehabilitation Program and the Center for Inflammatory Bowel Disease. He is a Fellow of the American College of Gastroenterology and a member of the American Society for Parenteral Nutrition (ASPEN), the American Society for Clinical Nutrition (ASCN), the American Gastroenterological Association, and the American Society for Gastrointestinal Endoscopy. He serves on ASPEN's committee on patient care standards and ASCN's committee on physician education. He has published more than 100 journal articles, abstracts, and book chapters. His research interests include nutritional management of inflammatory bowel disease, intestinal adaptation in short bowel syndrome, and techniques for enteral and parenteral nutrition.

Contributor List

Kareem Abu-Elmagd, M.D., Ph.D., F.A.C.S.
University of Pittsburgh Medical Center
Pittsburgh, Pennsylvania

Christopher C. Ashley, M.D., M.P.H.
Albany Medical College
Albany, New York

Geoffrey Bond, M.D.
University of Pittsburgh School of
Medicine
Pittsburgh, Pennsylvania

Andrew Bragalone, R.Ph., M.B.A.
The Cleveland Clinic Foundation
Cleveland, Ohio

Alan L. Buchman, M.D., M.S.P.H.
Northwestern University
Chicago, Illinois

Theresa A. Byrne, D.Sc., R.D., L.D.N., C.N.S.D.
Nutritional Restart Center
Wellesley, Massachusetts

Charlene W. Compher, Ph.D., R.D., F.A.D.A., C.N.S.D.
University of Pennsylvania School of
Nursing
Philadelphia, Pennsylvania

Darwin L. Conwell, M.D.
The Cleveland Clinic Foundation
Cleveland, Ohio

Guilherme Costa, M.D.
University of Pittsburgh School of
Medicine
Pittsburgh, Pennsylvania

Suzanne Cox, R.D., L.D.N., C.N.S.D.
Nutritional Restart Center
Wellesley, Massachusetts

Victor Fazio, M.B., M.S., F.R.A.C.S., F.A.C.S., F.R.C.S.
The Cleveland Clinic Foundation
Cleveland, Ohio

Erin M. Fennelly, R.D., C.N.S.D.
Georgetown University Transplant
Institute
Washington, D.C.

Concepción Fernández-Estívariz, M.D.
Emory University School of
Medicine
Atlanta, Georgia

John P. Grant, M.D.
Duke University Medical Center
Durham, North Carolina

Cynthia Hamilton, M.S., R.D., L.D., C.N.S.D.
The Cleveland Clinic Foundation
Cleveland, Ohio

Lyn Howard, M.B., F.R.C.P.
Albany Medical College
Albany, New York

Kishore R. Iyer, M.B.B.S., F.R.C.S.
Children's Memorial Hospital
Chicago, Illinois

Khursheed N. Jeejeebhoy, M.D.,
   Ph.D., F.R.C.S.
St. Michael's Hospital
Toronto, Ontario, Canada

Hossam M. Kandil, M.D., Ph.D.
University of Pittsburgh
Pittsburgh, Pennsylvania

Maria N. Karimbakas, R.D., L.D.N.,
   C.N.S.D.
Nutritional Restart Center
Wellesley, Massachusetts

Stuart S. Kaufman, M.D.
Children's National Medical Center and
   Georgetown University Transplant
   Institute
Washington, D.C.

Darlene G. Kelly, M.D., Ph.D.
Mayo Clinic
Rochester, Minnesota

Lorraine M. Leader, M.D.
Emory University School of
   Medicine
Atlanta, Georgia

Menghua Luo, M.D.
Emory University
Atlanta, Georgia

Laura E. Matarese, M.S., R.D., L.D.,
   F.A.D.A., C.N.S.D.
The Cleveland Clinic Foundation
Cleveland, Ohio

George Mazariegos, M.D.
University of Pittsburgh School of
   Medicine
Pittsburgh, Pennsylvania

David C. Metz, M.D.
University of Pennsylvania School of
   Medicine
Philadelphia, Pennsylvania

Stephen J. D. O'Keefe, M.D., M.Sc.,
   F.R.C.P.
University of Pittsburgh
Pittsburgh, Pennsylvania

Neha Parekh, M.S., R.D., L.D.,
   C.N.S.D.
The Cleveland Clinic Foundation
Cleveland, Ohio

Dhanasekaran Ramasamy, M.D.
The Cleveland Clinic Foundation
Cleveland, Ohio

Jorge Reyes, M.D.
University of Pittsburgh School of
   Medicine
Pittsburgh, Pennsylvania

Margaret E. Richard, R.N., M.S.,
   M.S.N., C.P.N.P.
Children's Memorial Hospital
Chicago, Illinois

James S. Scolapio, M.D.
Mayo Clinic
Jacksonville, Florida

Douglas L. Seidner, M.D., F.A.C.G.,
   C.N.S.P.
The Cleveland Clinic Foundation
Cleveland, Ohio

Rex A. Speerhas, R.Ph., C.D.E.,
   B.C.N.S.P.
The Cleveland Clinic Foundation
Cleveland, Ohio

Tyler Stevens, M.D.
The Cleveland Clinic Foundation
Cleveland, Ohio

Ezra Steiger, M.D., F.A.C.S., C.N.S.P.
The Cleveland Clinic Foundation
Cleveland, Ohio

Junqiang Tian, M.D.
Emory University School of Medicine
Atlanta, Georgia

Elizabeth V. Tucker
Oley Foundation for Home Parenteral
  and Enteral Nutrition
Lakeville, Minnesota

Andrew Ukleja, M.D.
Cleveland Clinic Florida
Weston, Florida

Jon A. Vanderhoof, M.D.
University of Nebraska Medical Center
Omaha, Nebraska

Susan Wagner, R.Ph.
The Cleveland Clinic Foundation
Cleveland, Ohio

Naohiro Washizawa, M.D.
Toho University School of Medicine
Tokyo, Japan

Rebecca A. Weseman, R.D., C.N.S.D., L.M.N.T.
University of Nebraska Medical Center
Omaha, Nebraska

Douglas W. Wilmore, M.D.
Harvard Medical School
Boston, Massachusetts

Rosemary J. Young, R.N., M.S.
University of Nebraska Medical Center
Omaha, Nebraska

Thomas R. Ziegler, M.D.
Emory University School of Medicine
Atlanta, Georgia

Massarat Zutshi, M.D.
The Cleveland Clinic Foundation
Cleveland, Ohio

Table of Contents

The Evolution of Care of Patients with Intestinal Failure

Douglas W. Wilmore

Remarkable developments in medical care have occurred over the past half century, and the improvements in the treatment of patients with intestinal failure characterize this extraordinary evolution in enhanced patient outcome. Up until the 1960s and early 1970s, patients who sustained a massive infarction of the small bowel often went unresected at the time of laparotomy, because no nutritional supportive therapy was available for their care in the postoperative period. These individuals would succumb within days to overwhelming sepsis from their necrotic bowel. Patients with severe inflammatory bowel disease or extensive intra-abdominal adhesions would often undergo multiple operations over time but would gradually lose weight, live the life of a debilitated individual (e.g., an "intestinal cripple"), and eventually die of complications associated with yet another operation or of the consequences of severe malnutrition. Over the past 30 years, all of this has changed.

The first major breakthrough was the development of total parenteral nutrition (PN). While intravenous support using a variety of nutrients had been provided throughout the mid-twentieth century, it was not until 1968 that a report described a relatively safe, reliable, long-term method of total intravenous feeding to support a patient with intestinal insufficiency.[1] The infusion of a hypertonic nutrient solution through a central venous catheter to a baby with intestinal atresia and the short bowel syndrome allowed delivery of all necessary nutrients over months and demonstrated that normal growth and development could be achieved by supplying nutrients solely by the intravenous route. The dedicated central line coupled with a system of catheter care ensure relative safety of the infusion site, and the hypertonic solution provided adequate macro and micronutrients in physiologic fluid volumes. While this system was subsequently utilized extensively in the preoperative preparation and postoperative support of patients who could not take or be adequately sustained by enteral feedings, it was not until the 1970s that necessity dictated the extended use of this technique in the home.[2]

Following a normal pregnancy and delivery, a Canadian mother sustained a small bowel infarction, requiring massive intestinal resection. Because of her age and previous good health, she did well following the bowel resection, and was maintained in the hospital on PN. As months passed, it became apparent that hospitalization was both an economically and socially untenable situation for this patient —- both mother and child needed to be in their home. A courageous decision was made by the patient's physicians to send this individual home on parenteral nutrition. A home care program was organized to provide education for the patient on the practical aspects of infusion of the nutritional solutions and catheter care. Appropriately formulated intravenous nutrient solutions were made available to her at home in a timely manner, and nursing and medical support were provided while the patient lived in her environment and cared for her child. The patient did extremely well, and this demonstration set the stage for the development of a home care delivery system throughout North America: such a system would provide nutrition support (and eventually other medical therapies) to patients with intestinal failure outside the hospital setting.

PN was frequently used as a transition therapy for those individuals whose bowel could adapt with time following intestinal resection. Ultimately they would be sustained entirely by enteral feedings and live near-normal lives following bowel compensation.[3] However, in the early 1980s a small group of patients emerged who were dependent on PN for their lifetime. These individuals had extremely short segments of a small bowel or had dysfunctional intestinal remnants that contained pathologic mucosal tissue. It became apparent that unless another intervention was utilized these patients would eventually suffer life-threatening complications from their PN. The initial solution to this problem was intestinal transplantation.

Until this time small bowel transplantation had been attempted by many but was generally unsuccessful. However, achievements made in the field of kidney transplantation and the growing success of both liver and pancreatic transplants focused surgeons on the problems associated with small intestinal grafts. Liver failure was occasionally observed in patients (especially children) with short bowel who were maintained on long-term PN. These individuals could be salvaged by liver transplantation, but combined liver-bowel grafts were proposed as a way to achieve more complete rehabilitation.[4] The major problem associated with intestinal transplantation was the transfer to the host of a large mass of foreign immunological tissue that is contained within the wall and mesentery of the intestine. Through improved immunosuppressive regimens, intestinal transplantation has evolved to the point that isolated small bowel grafts are slowly becoming a recognized method of therapy in a highly selected group of patients,[5] although graft rejection still remains a problem.

The intestinal tract is able to adapt with time following resection; that is, the small and large bowel improves its absorptive function per unit length. The pathways involved in this adaptive response are only now being appreciated, but they include the up-regulation by endogenous growth factors and nutrients that optimize these compensatory effects. Byrne and associates were the first to explore the potential of this new knowledge as a therapeutic approach to patients with short bowel. They administered growth hormone (GH) and the trophic amino acid glutamine to PN-dependent patients with the intestinal failure receiving an individualized, optimal enteral diet. After just four weeks of treatment, approximately 60% of this group could be weaned from intravenous support, and at three years the sustained remission rate was greater than 40%.[6] Others have confirmed the effects of GH on enhancing intestinal absorption,[7] although not all investigators[8,9] have consistently observed these results. More recently, the outcome of a large prospective randomized double-blinded trial revealed the positive effects of GH on weaning patients from PN, but it also confirmed the significant additive effects of oral glutamine administration on weaning when given with GH and an appropriate diet.[10]

Investigations that focus on the effects of a variety of growth factors and nutrients on the bowel have transformed this field of intestinal rehabilitation into an exciting and dynamic area of study. Additional and potentially more effective treatment regimens will almost certainly emerge for use in the rehabilitation of patients with bowel disease. It is important to realize that the clinician now has three options available for the treatment and rehabilitation of the patient with intestinal failure: 1) parenteral support over the short term until intestinal adaptation occurs, 2) intestinal rehabilitation utilizing appropriate nutrients and growth factors to enhance adaptation and/or minimize the time required for PN-associated intestinal compensation, and 3) intestinal transplantation or other bowel-lengthening operations for those individuals who cannot adapt after utilizing the first two options. It is important to assess the risks and benefits of each approach and utilize the most appropriate and cost-effective therapy for a specific patient with intestinal failure. Information is only now being generated to determine the patient's perceptions concerning the benefits of these various forms of therapy,[11] and decision-aiding algorithms have also been proposed to facilitate appropriate therapeutic choices in the patient's care plan.[12]

The treatment of intestinal failure over the past half-century is reflective of the great advances that have been made in medical care in many other areas. We have moved from observing a catastrophic outcome in patients with intestinal failure, to a situation where we now have a variety of options available for the treatment of these individuals. Our task at present is to determine the best and most cost-effective approach in the care and rehabilitation of patients with intestinal insufficiency.

This new volume, edited and written by world authorities in the field of care of patients with intestinal failure, does much to improve our understanding in this area and aids in the important goal of returning these individuals to a more normal and productive life.

REFERENCES

1. Wilmore, D.W. and Dudrick, S.J., Growth and development of an infant receiving all nutrients exclusively by vein, *JAMA*, 203, 860, 1968.
2. Jeejeebhoy, K.N., Wohrab, W.J., Langer, B., Phillips, M.J., Kuksis, A., and Anderson, G.H., Total parenteral nutrition at home for 23 months, without complications, and with good rehabilitation. A study of technical and metabolic features, *Gastroenterol.*, 65, 811, 1973.
3. Goutebel, M.C., Aubert, B.S., Colette, C., Astre, C., Monnier, L.H., and Joyeux, H., Intestinal adaptation in patients with short bowel syndrome, *Dig. Dis. Sci.*, 34, 709, 1989.
4. Starzel, T.E., Todo, S., Tzakis, A., and Murase, N., Multivisceral and intestinal transplantation, *Transplant Proc.*, 24, 1217, 1992.
5. Fishbein, T., Florman, S., Gondolesi, G., Schiano, T., LeLeiko, N., Tschernia, A., and Kaufman, S., Intestinal transplantation before and after the introduction of sirolimus, *Trans.* 73, 1538, 2002.

6. Byrne, T.A., Morrissey, T.B., Nattakon, T.V., Ziegler, T.R., and Wilmore, D.W., A new treatment for patients with short-bowel syndrome: growth hormone, glutamine, and a modified diet, *Ann. Surg.* 222, 243, 1995.

7. Seguy, D., Vahedi, K., Kapel, N., Souberbielle, J-C, and Messing, B., Low-dose growth hormone in adult home parenteral nutrition dependent short bowel syndrome patients: a positive study, *Gastroenterology,* 124, 293, 2003.

8. Szkudlarek, J., Jeppesen, P.B., and Mortensen, P.B., Effect of high dose growth hormone with glutamine and no change in diet on intestinal absorption in short bowel patients: a randomised, double blind, crossover, placebo controlled study, *Gut*, 47, 199, 2000.

9. Scolapio, J.S., Camilleri, M., Fleming, C.R., Oenning, L.V., Burton, D.D., Sebo, T.L., Batts, K.P., and Kelly, D.G., Effect of growth hormone, glutamine, and diet on adaptation in short-bowel syndrome: a randomized, controlled study, *Gastroenterol.,* 113, 1074, 1997.

10. Byrne, T.A., Lautz, D., and Iyre, K. et al., Recombinant human growth hormone (rhGH) reduces parenteral nutrition (PN) requirements in patients with the short bowel syndrome: a prospective, randomized, double-blinded, placebo-controlled study, *J. Parent. Enteral Nutr.*, 27, S17, 2003.

11. Rovera, G.M., Anderson, S., Camelio, N., Pfister, D., Byrne, T.A., and Wilmore, D.W., Enhancing outcome in patients receiving long term TPN, *Clin. Nutr.*, 19, 2, 2000.

12. Wilmore, D.W., Growth factors and nutrients in the short bowel syndrome, *J. Parenter. Enteral Nutr.*, 23, S117, 1999.

1 Anatomy and Physiology of the Gastrointestinal Tract

John P. Grant

CONTENTS

The gastrointestinal tract performs three primary functions in human metabolism: digestion, absorption, and protection. Digestion is a process by which large molecules in the diet are broken down into smaller ones that are acceptable to the enterocytes for absorption. Absorption is a process by which luminal contents enter the mucosal epithelial cells, are transported to the basement membrane, and eventually delivered to the portal vein or lymphatics. In its protective function, the gut serves as a barrier to the entry of luminal pathogens and toxins into the body. To perform these tasks the gastrointestinal tract consumes a considerable amount of energy, accounting for approximately 25% of whole body energy expenditure.

THE OROPHARYNX

Within the oropharynx food is mechanically broken down by the process of chewing. With eating, the background 25-ml-per-hour secretion of saliva can increase up to 300 ml per hour. Alpha-amylases within the saliva degrade starch during chewing and swallowing, although its action ceases in the stomach as it is deactivated by gastric acid. Mucus within the mouth covers food and indeed follows some food into the colon. During passage of food through the gastrointestinal tract, this mucus can attach to mucosal surfaces and form a protective barrier. Saliva also contains specific antimicrobial proteins like lysozyme, lactoferrin, lactoperoxidase, IgA, and nitric oxide, donating substances such as nitrates. Unfortunately many common medications inhibit secretion of saliva, including anticholinergics, analgesics, anti-spasmodics, antidiarrheals, antidepressants, antihistamines, antihypertensives, antip-sychotics, and diuretics. Finally, the natural oral bacterial flora function to defend against bacterial overgrowth and inflammation. Saliva can be stimulated by pilo-carpine 5 mg by mouth three times a day and by cevimeline hydrochloride 30 mg by mouth three times a day.

THE ESOPHAGUS

The esophagus transports food to the stomach. During this transport, lipase secreted from the pharyngeal mucosa hydrolyzes some of the triglycerides to diglycerides and fatty acids.

THE STOMACH

The stomach has four major sections: the gastroesophageal junction, fundus, antrum, and pylorus that leads to the duodenal bulb and small intestines (Figure 1.1). Gastric mucosa consists of crypt cells that mature to surface epithelia cells along deep glands. Mixed within the maturing epithelia cells are pepsinogen-secreting zymogen cells, hydrochloric acid–secreting parietal cells, and mucous cells.

Hydrochloric acid is secreted from parietal cells, which destroys most bacteria ingested with a meal, acting as a barrier to bacterial overgrowth in the proximal small bowel. In addition, the gastric acid denatures protein. Pepsinogen, secreted from zymogen or chief cells, is converted to the active form pepsin, which begins proteolysis. The mucus cells secrete mucin and bicarbonate that form a protective layer over the gastric mucosa, preventing acid and pepsin digestion (Figure 1.2).

The stomach stores, mixes, and grinds food to form an emulsion. To achieve optimal digestion and absorption of nutrients, the speed of movement of food through the gastrointestinal tract is carefully regulated. Gastric emptying, the first point of control for meal passage, is regulated by the load of the meal, the length of intestinal exposure to the nutrients, and the phase of the meal. In general, the larger the meal, the higher the fat content, and the lower the liquid content, the slower the emptying.[1–3]

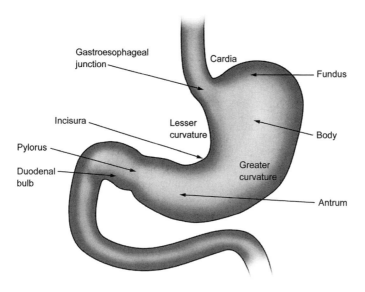

FIGURE 1.1 Gross anatomy of the stomach

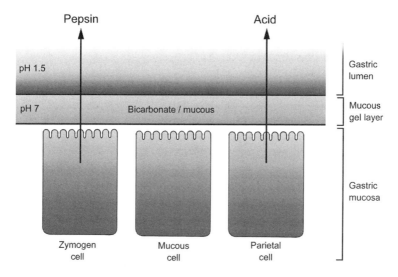

FIGURE 1.2 Secretion of mucin and bicarbonate forms a protective layer over the gastric mucosa, preventing acid and pepsin digestion.

THE SMALL INTESTINE

The small intestine is composed of three distinct segments: duodenum, jejunum, and ileum. Its total length is variable, although it averages around 16 feet. The duodenum is approximately 10 inches long and averages 2 inches in diameter.

The jejunum is approximately 2/5th of the length of the rest of the small bowel. It measures 1.5 in diameter at its beginning and tapers to 1.25 in near its end. The jejunum is relatively thick and has many blood vessels. The bowel wall is characterized by infoldings called plica circularis that are covered by villus projections, and they in turn by microvilli. This anatomy greatly increases the surface area of the intestinal tract. The final absorptive surface area is about 1.7 million square centimeters. It takes about 800 square centimeters to absorb one kilocalorie (100 to 200 square centimeters per kcal, minimum). The ileum comprises the remaining small bowel to the ileocecal valve. It measures 1.25 in in diameter, is thin-walled, and has large Peyer's patches. The villi are diminutive.

Mucosal cells are generated at the base of the villi, in the crypts (Figure 1.3). Migration to the tips of the villi and maturation of these immature cells is rapid, with the average life span being only 3 days. Digestive enzymes are synthesized as the mucosal cells migrate toward the tip.

The upper gastrointestinal flora consists of less than 10^4 organisms per ml of intestinal fluid, composed predominantly of anaerobic streptococci, aerobic lactobacilli, diphtheroids, and fungi. As the distal ileum is approached, the number of bacteria increase to 10^5 to 10^8 per ml of intestinal fluid, with the appearance of gram-negative coliforms and anaerobic Bacteroides species.

The small intestine is a major organ for nutrient absorption. Ingested food is broken down by secreted digestive juices and absorbed along the small bowel, with specific substrates absorbed at selected sites. Once food enters the small intestine, transit is regulated by a number of neural and humoral factors. A fat-induced jejunal brake is dependent on the accelerating effect of cholecystokinin and the slowing

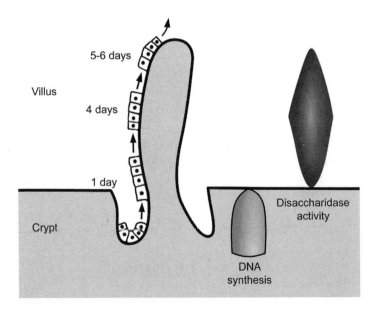

FIGURE 1.3 Maturation and migration of cells lining the small bowel

effect of a peripherally located opioid pathway, and appears to be mediated by the peptide tyrosine tyrosine (peptide YY).[4,5] Intestinal transit is also slowed by a high protein load, with intact whey soy protein slowing transit significantly more than hydrolyzed protein.[6] In addition, low-residue feeding formulas accelerate transit while high-fiber formulas profoundly slow transit.[7] Finally, distention of the right colon by chyme from the ileum results in ileal relaxation and delay of further chyme emptying into the colon.[8]

THE COLON

The colon frames the abdomen, beginning with the ascending colon in the right lower quadrant, transverse colon across the upper abdomen, descending colon down the left side of the abdomen, and ending with the sigmoid colon and rectum (Figure 1.4). The colon is considered an "organ within an organ" in that colonic microflora

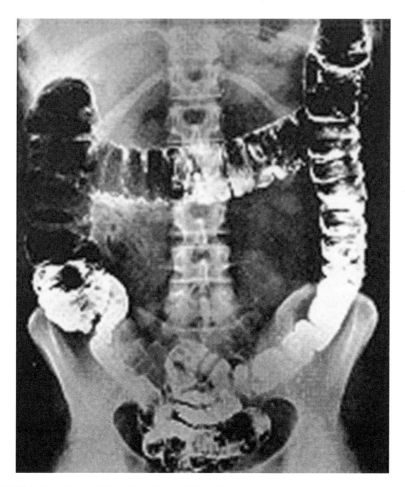

FIGURE 1.4 Outline of the colon depicted by a barium enema

ferment nonabsorbed nutrients and soluble fiber to a form the colonic mucosa can absorb, along with water and electrolytes. As the ileocecal valve is crossed, there is a marked increase in the number and variety of microorganisms, with anaerobes predominating. Colonic bacterial polysaccharidase degradation of dietary fiber and undigested starch results in short-chain fatty acids. These short-chain fatty acids are either used for energy by the colonic bacteria or are absorbed by the colonic epithelium. Once absorbed, short-chain fatty acids have several physiologic effects, including enhanced sodium absorption by the colon, increased colonocyte proliferation, enhanced colonic blood flow, stimulation of the autonomic nervous system, and increased gastrointestinal hormone production. Most important, short-chain fatty acids are the preferred metabolic fuel of the colonic mucosa, providing up to 70% of the daily energy supply.[9]

THE GALT SYSTEM

GALT stands for gut-associated lymphoid tissue, which includes intraepithelial lymphocytes (IEL), lamina propria lymphoid tissue (LPL), Peyer's patches, and mesenteric lymph nodes (Figure 1.5). The intraepithelial lymphocytes are the first to recognize foreign antigens and begin the communication with the rest of the immune system. The Lamina propria lymphoid tissue is the source for IgA. Peyer's patches process antigens from the intraepithelial lymphocytes and transmit information to the mesenteric lymph nodes. The GALT system is responsible for reacting to harmful foreign antigens (e.g., bacterial or viral pathogens) but must not react to

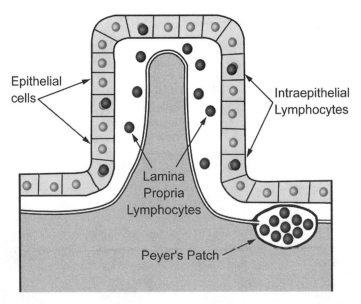

FIGURE 1.5 The gut-associated lymphatic system consists of intraepithelial lymphocytes, lamina propria lymphocytes, Peyer's patches, and mesenteric lymph nodes.

nonthreatening antigens that might result in a chronic inflammatory condition. Both intravenous feeding and starvation result in significant suppression of the GALT with reduction in IgA secretion and increased gut permeability.[10,11] Furthermore, bowel rest is thought to reduce intraluminal bacterial nutrients, resulting in an adaptive response of bacteria to increase adherence to the intestinal wall as a source of nutrients.[12] The adherence is usually associated with cellular injury or even bacterial penetration and an adverse host response.

Several substances have been found to stimulate GALT and help maintain its immune function during intravenous nutrition or bowel rest. Glutamine is an important respiratory fuel for the gastrointestinal tract and also is an important fuel for proliferating cells such as lymphoid tissue. Supplementation of intravenous nutrition with 2% L-glutamine (or glycyl-L-glutamine) was found by Li et al. to reduce atrophy of the small and large bowel during parenteral nutrition in experimental animals; with a decrease in bacterial translocation; maintenance of normal intestinal permeability; preservation of total cell yield from Peyer's patches, intraepithelial space, and the lamina propria; with a normal CD4/CD8 ratio within the laminal propria; and normal intestinal IgA secretion.[13] A second substance that has been studied is Bombesin. Bombesin is a tetradecapeptide analogous to gastrin-releasing peptide in the human. Experimental work in animals has shown Bombesin supplementation of intravenous nutrition maintains normal GALT cell mass, normal CD4/CD8 ratios within the lamina propria, and normal IgA levels within the intestine and the respiratory tract.[14]

In all studies, however, oral or tube enteral nutrition, with either standard or specialized formula products, is the most efficient in maintaining a normal GALT cell mass and function, with normal CD4/CD8 ratios in the lamina propria, and normal quantity of functional IgA within the intestine and the respiratory tracts.

NUTRIENT ABSORPTION

The sites of absorption for various nutrients are depicted in Figure 1.6.

Water: Approximately 9 liters per day of fluid reaches the small intestine, of which about 1.5 liters is dietary in origin. Normally the small bowel absorbs about 7 liters per day, mainly in the jejunum, while the colon absorbs 1 to 1.5 liters per day. However the water-absorptive capacity of the human intestine may reach up to 15 to 20 liters per day in certain conditions.[15] The bulk of water absorption in the small bowel occurs within the first 100 cm of the jejunum and is the result of net solute transport. Several substrates are known to enhance water absorption. Glucose, maltose, and galactose all are strongly related to water absorption with maximum rates of absorption taking place from isotonic solutions containing approximately 56 mM glucose. Fructose is relatively ineffective. Water absorption by the small bowel may also be enhanced by adding sodium chloride, as passive absorption follows absorption of solids.[16] Clinically, high sodium enteral diets enhance water resorption whereas low-sodium

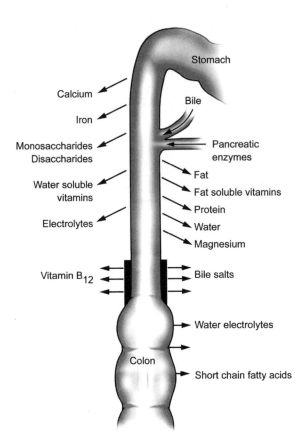

FIGURE 1.6 Major sites of nutrient absorption along the gastrointestinal tract

diets predispose to diarrhea. Finally, the neutral amino acid, leucine, stimulates jejunal absorption of water as well as the dipeptide glycyl-L-alanine and a mixture of glycine and alanine.

Water absorption in the ileum and colon is not linked to solute transport as it is in the jejunum, but is the result of the double ion-exchange process (sodium exchanged for hydrogen, and chloride exchanged for bicarbonate), resulting in loss of osmotically active solute in the lumen, with consequent bulk flow of water out of the lumen.

Sodium and chloride: Sodium absorption is directly coupled to absorption of organic solutes such as glucose, amino acids, water-soluble vitamins, and bile salts (Figure 1.7). Once inside the cell, sodium is extruded against chemical and electrical gradients via a basolateral membrane-associated sodium-potassium-ATPase. Chloride passively follows absorption of sodium. In the colon, there is a neutral sodium chloride transport mechanism where sodium is exchanged for hydrogen and chloride is exchanged for bicarbonate (Figure 1.8).

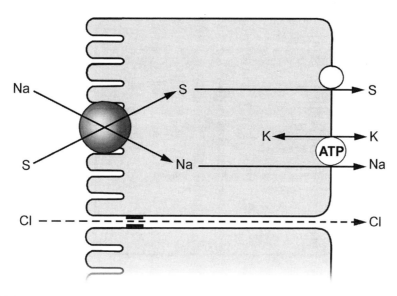

FIGURE 1.7 Sodium absorption by the small intestine is directly coupled with absorption of organic solutes.

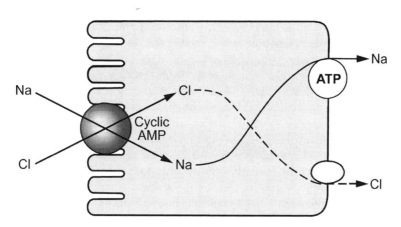

FIGURE 1.8 Sodium absorption by the colon is by a neutral transport mechanism. Sodium is exchanged for hydrogen ion and chloride is exchanged for bicarbonate ion.

Potassium: Overall potassium movement is a result of solvent drag throughout the small bowel and is potential dependent. Potassium is actively secreted in the main colon while the rectosigmoid colon has active potassium absorption, which is exchanged for hydrogen ion.

Calcium: The recommended daily oral intake of calcium is 30 to 40 mEq, of which only 5% to 40% is absorbed. Calcium absorption is passive throughout the entire small intestine.[17] The passive mechanism predominates

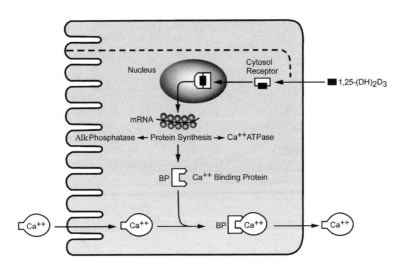

FIGURE 1.9 Active absorption of calcium by the small intestine

at concentrations of calcium greater than 10 mmol per liter. Active absorption of calcium occurs primarily in the duodenum below 10 mmol per liter; active transport occurs with 1,25 dihydroxyvitamin D3, as depicted in Figure 1.9.

Magnesium: Magnesium is primarily absorbed in the distal small bowel. In addition, some magnesium is absorbed in the colon by passive diffusion.

Copper: Daily oral copper requirements have been estimated to be 30 µg/kg, of which 30% to 80% is thought to be absorbed, mainly in the stomach and proximal duodenum.[18,19] Absorption is an active process that requires energy and involves absorption of complexes of copper and amino acids. Copper is excreted in the bile, with urinary losses being < 1% to 2% of dietary intake.

Zinc: An average oral diet contains 10 to 15 mg zinc, of which 1 to 2 mg is absorbed primarily from the upper small intestine. Zinc absorption is thought to be regulated, in part, by the amount of zinc intake, the intake of other elements and dietary components, and mucosal cell zinc concentrations.[20] The major excretory route for zinc is via the feces by a poorly understood mechanism.[21] Pancreatic secretions appear to have high concentrations of zinc.[22] Sweat contains approximately 1 mg zinc per liter. Normal urinary zinc ranges from 300 to 700 µg/24 hours.[23]

Absorption of zinc in the jejunum occurs by binding to a ligand in the lumen that transports it to the mucosa. At the mucosal surfaces it is transferred to a binding site and then transferred by an active process requiring energy, oxygen, and sodium. Absorption of zinc is stimulated by glucose. The major loss of zinc is in the feces. During intravenous nutrition it is suggested to give:[24] 2 mg Zn + 17.1 mg Zn/kg stool lost + 12.2 mg Zn/kg of gastric/duodenal/or jejunal fluid lost.

Iron: The average diet contains 16 to 18 mg iron per day. In the stomach much of the iron released from food is bound to a number of mucins and macromolecular substances forming high-molecular-weight complexes. Additional iron is made unavailable by neutralization — ferric ions undergo increasing polymerization forming colloidal gels as the pH rises toward neutrality and finally form a precipitate of ferric hydroxide. This does not happen to the same extent with ferrous ions, and therefore ferrous ions are more available for absorption. Due to these two processes, only 5% to 10% of iron in the diet is absorbed.

Although the whole small intestine has the capacity to absorb iron, most is absorbed in the duodenum and proximal jejunum. At the brush border, ferrous ions are oxidized to ferric and transported by proposed brush border carrier proteins, presumably regulated by the body's need for iron. At pharmacologic doses passive diffusion occurs. At normal concentrations, iron enters the mucosal cell, either in an ionic form or bound to a nonprotein substance of low molecular weight by a process that is energy-dependent.[25] The iron complex diffuses directly to the vascular border, where it is transferred across the membrane into the plasma by a process requiring oxidative energy. This latter process appears to be the rate-limiting step.[26] In the plasma; iron is transported bound to a protein called transferrin, or siderophilin, which is synthesized in the liver. Iron is cleared from the plasma with a half-life of approximately 60 to 120 minutes, either taken up by erythroid precursors of the bone marrow or deposited in storage complexes.

CARBOHYDRATE

The average diet contains approximately 312 g carbohydrate, representing about 1250 kcal. Sixty percent is starch, 30% sucrose, and 10% lactose, fructose, and glycogen. Carbohydrates are primarily absorbed in the duodenum and proximal jejunum, with 75% absorbed in the first 70 cm of the small bowel. Carbohydrate intolerance is nearly always related to a defect in intestinal surface digestion of a polysaccharide or disaccharide.

Glucose uptake in the small intestine and transport to the bloodstream in the adult is regulated rapidly and reversibly by the amount of glucose in the diet. The increase in uptake is believed to be due to increases in both brush border and basement membrane transport proteins. This enhanced handling of glucose is also seen with intravenous glucose infusion. Fructose uptake and transport is likewise stimulated by an increase of fructose in the diet, but is also stimulated by the addition of glucose or alanine to the diet.

There are three distinct phases of carbohydrate absorption (Figure 1.10):[27]

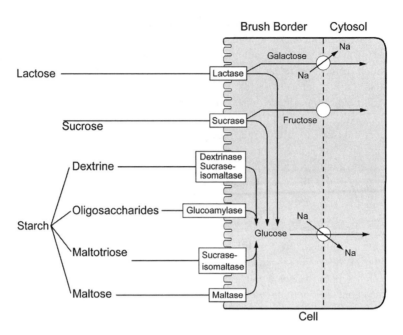

FIGURE 1.10 Carbohydrate processing in the intestinal lumen and at the brush border

Luminal phase: Within the lumen the alpha 1-4 glucosidic bonds of starch are cleaved by salivary and pancreatic alpha amylases, yielding alpha-limit dextrines, maltotriose, and maltose, along with sucrose and lactose.

Brush-Border phase: At the brush border the glycosidases maltase and lactase hydrolyzed the alpha limit dextrans to the monosaccharides: glucose, galactose, and fructose.

Cellular phase: Glucose and other carbohydrates are transported across the plasma membrane by two classes of transport proteins (Figure 1.11). The first is the sodium/glucose cotransporter system (SGLT1), which is an energy-dependent sodium-linked system that transports glucose and galactose against concentration gradients. The second transporter is the facilitative glucose transporter gene family, which mediates the bidirectional, energy-independent, stereo-specific transfer of glucose and other sugars across cell membranes. Within the enterocyte, GLUT5 predominates and transports fructose. Glucose and galactose, as well as fructose most likely, exit the cell at the basement membrane into the blood stream by passive diffusion through GLUT2.

FIBER

Fiber is a nonstarch carbohydrate of plant origin that escapes enzymatic digestion in the small intestine. There are two types of fiber: cellulosic and noncellulosic.

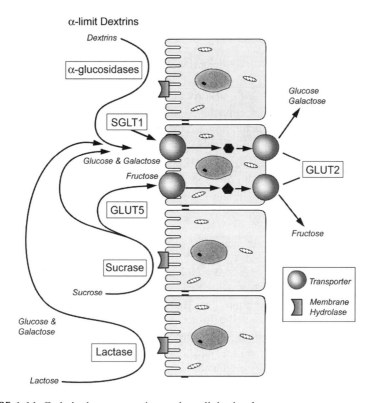

FIGURE 1.11 Carbohydrate processing at the cellular level

Cellulosic fiber: This fiber is high molecular weight nonsoluble fiber such as cellulose and wheat bran. Cellulosic fiber contributes to fecal mass and water content, and reduces the mean stool transit time.

Noncellulosic fiber: This is soluble fiber such as hemicelluloses, pectin, gums, and mucilages. The noncellulosic fiber can contribute to colonic nutrition as it is degraded rapidly by anaerobic microflora of the cecum and colon (fermentation) to give short-chain fatty acids — acetate, propionate, and n-butyrate. Thus noncellulosic fiber enhances colonic blood flow, serves as a fuel for the colonocyte (70%), increases colonocyte proliferation, enhances sodium absorption, and preserves to colonic mucosal barrier.[28]

FAT

Approximately 40% of the calories of a standard diet in the U.S. are provided by fat (from 100 to 180 g/day). Dietary lipids are a major source of energy and provide the essential fatty acids, fat-soluble vitamins, and cholesterol to the body. Ninety-five percent of the fat is in the form of long-chain triacylglycerols. Saturated fatty acids account for approximately 37%, oleic acid 40%, and linoleic acid about 12%

of the total. The majority of triglycerides contain long chain fatty acids of 16 to 18 carbons. A few dietary triglycerides contain medium chain fatty acids of 8 to 12 carbons.

The absorption of fat is very efficient, with 95% of up to 500 grams of ingested fat absorbed. Over 80% of dietary lipids are absorbed within the first 60 cm of the small bowel. The first step in fat absorption is an increase in its surface area by dispersing fat globules as an emulsion. Emulsification is enhanced by cooking, grinding, and chewing. Within the stomach the emulsion is completed by intragastric mixing and the effect of gastric lipase, which helps to create and stabilize the emulsion by generating free fatty acids from triglycerides.

When the emulsion enters the small bowel, it is covered by a monolayer of phospholipids, fatty acid, free cholesterol, and denatured protein (Figure 1.12).[29] The large oil/water surface makes an ideal substrate for pancreatic colipase-dependent lipase, which is only active at oil/water interfaces. This pancreatic lipase digests the emulsion lipids to two free fatty acids and one 2-monoglycerides. Lipolysis continues to reduce the size of the emulsion particles until the hydrolytic products are in excess. These particles bud off as liquid crystals and multilayered liposomes. In the presence of bile salts, these quickly form small unilamellar vesicles that further interact with bile salt micelles to form mixed bile salt micelles. These lipid-saturated micelles diffuse easily across the unstirred water layer and deliver dietary lipid to the apical membrane of the enterocytes. The free fatty acids and monoglycerides are absorbed in the proximal small bowel, probably through action of a specific transport protein, and the bile salts pass on within the intestine to be absorbed in the terminal ileum. Medium-chain triglycerides are significantly more water-soluble and may be absorbed intact with direct transport into the portal system as free fatty acids.

Within the enterocyte, free fatty acids and monoglycerides are transported by two fatty acid-binding proteins to the cytoplasmic face of the endoplasmic reticulum where they are re-esterified to triglycerides by surface enzymes. These new triglycerides are encased as chylomicrons and transferred to the basal membrane and from

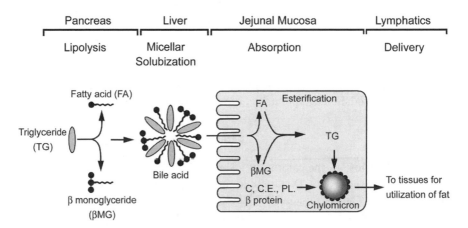

FIGURE 1.12 Complex process of lipid absorption

there into the lymphatic system. In the periphery the chylomicron triglycerides are quickly metabolized, mostly in adipose tissue and muscle, generating chylomicron remnants and ultimately high-density lipoprotein. When metabolized in the liver, much of it may be exported as very low-density lipoprotein.

PROTEIN

In the U.S., the standard diet contains approximately 80 g of protein, or 11% to 14% of the total caloric intake. The protein derives from animal and vegetable sources. It is primarily absorbed in the duodenum and proximal jejunum, yet some does pass into and is absorbed by the colon. Digestion and absorption occurs in three phases (Figure 1.13):

Luminal gastric digestion: Within the stomach protein is denatured by acid secretion, which then renders proteins susceptible to protein lysis by pepsin. Pepsin protein lysis results in large soluble oligonucleotides, peptones, and some single amino acids.[30]

Luminal duodenal phase: Three pancreatic endopeptidases and two pancreatic exopeptidases reduce oligopeptides to free amino acids and di- and tripeptides.

Luminal enterocyte phase: Enterocyte brush border membrane hydrolase to produce amino acids, dipeptides, and tripeptides. There are four major sodium-dependent, group-specific, active transport systems: one for neutral

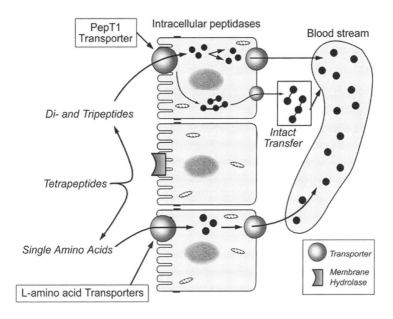

FIGURE 1.13 Protein absorption

amino acids; one for glycine, proline, and hydroxyproline; one for dibasic amino acids and cystine; and one for dicarboxylic amino acids.[31] There is a hydrogen dependent di- and tripeptide transport system (PepT1 Transporter). This transport system can be interfered by cephalosporin antibiotics, which share the same system. Amino acids absorbed by either route the flux from the basolateral membrane via transporters whose kinetic characteristics are sensitive to circulating amino acid concentrations. The mucosal uptake of peptides has an important role in protein absorption. Absorption of alpha-amino nitrogen is greater during perfusion of di- and tripeptides. Yet di- and tripeptides have less effect on sodium and water uptake than free amino acids or complex proteins and can result in diarrhea. Although of theoretical advantage, enteral products containing peptides versus intact protein or free amino acids show little experimental data to support their advantage. Any advantage would be more apparent with increased protein loads, as during cyclical feedings.

MALABSORPTION

Malabsorption may be defined as impaired absorption of fat, carbohydrate, protein, vitamins, electrolytes, minerals, or water. Clinical symptoms of malabsorption include unexplained weight loss, steatorrhea, diarrhea, anemia, tetany, bone pain, pathologic fractures, bleeding, dermatitis, neuropathy, glossitis, and edema. Normal stool patterns range from 3 per week to 3 per day with considerable range and fluid lost. The average water content in 24 hours of stool is 100 ml with 4 mEq of sodium 9 mEq of potassium 2 mEq chloride and no bicarbonate. Normal stool frequency varies widely from as few stools as 3 per week to as many as 3 per day. Diarrhea has been defined as a stool weight > 200 to 500 g per 24 hours.

Various tests are available to help diagnose the presence of malabsorption:

1. **Screening tests:** These tests detect only the more clinically significant degrees of malabsorption.
   a. Gross inspection of the stool: With steatorrhea, the stool is bulky, sticky, and foul smelling, and tends to float.
   b. Microscopic examination of the stool: Increased fat by Sudan II staining suggests impaired fat absorption. Increased numbers of striated muscle fibers suggests impaired protein digestion.
   c. Determination of fat content of a random stool collection: With steatorrhea, fat content of a random 24-hour stool sample may be 25 or more grams.
   d. Determination of protein content of a random stool: More than 3 gm per day protein in a random 24-hour stool is abnormal.
   e. Serum carotene concentration: Carotene is poorly absorbed in the presence of steatorrhea. If dietary intake is adequate, low serum carotene concentrations strongly suggest fat malabsorption.
   f. D-xylose absorption: D-xylose is not metabolized, being excreted unaltered in the urine. This property makes it useful as a test for carbohydrate

absorption. Normally 5 g or more of d-xylose are excreted in the urine within the first 5 hours after oral ingestion of 25 gm. Improved sensitivity has been reported when only 5 g of d-xylose is given orally and blood xylose concentrations at 1 hour are corrected to a constant body surface area.[32]

g. Radiological examination: Radiological examination is useful in evaluating intestinal transit time and motility. In addition, careful studies can identify abnormalities, including fistulas, strictures, mucosal diseases such as Crohn's disease, diverticula, and cancer.

2. **Intake-output balance tests:** Balance tests are more sensitive than screening tests and identify milder degrees of malabsorption.

a. Fat balance: A quantitative measurement of fat in a timed 3- to 5-day stool collection can be compared to measured fat intake (usually 100 g fat per day). With malabsorption, more than 6 g fat per 24 hours (or more than 5% of the measured ingested fat) will pass unabsorbed in the stool.

b. Radioactive tracer tests: A ^{14}C-triolein breath test can evaluate intestinal absorption of neutral fats.[33] ^{13}C-Trioctanion, a stable nonradioactive isotope, has also been used in quantitating fat malabsorption through measurement of 2-hour $^{13}CO_2$ respiratory excretion in a breath test.[34] These tests depend not only on normal absorption but also on normal fat metabolism. Measurement of the stool content of intravenously administered ^{131}I-albumin, ^{51}Cr-albumin, and ^{67}Cu-ceruloplasmin can identify patients with protein-losing enteropathies.

3. **Tests for malabsorption of specific nutrients**

a. Lactose tolerance test: Abnormal absorption of lactose occurs with deficiency of the brush border enzyme lactase as well as in many disorders of the small intestine. Of various tests the most common is the hydrogen breath test. Improved accuracy can be obtained by prolonging the test to 4 hours with simultaneous measurement of the orocecal transit time.[35]

b. Schilling test: Abnormal absorption of vitamin B_{12} occurs in the absence of intrinsic factor and in dysfunction of the terminal ileum.

c. Other radioactive compounds: Radioisotopic methodologies are available for identification of iron, calcium, various amino acids, folic acid, pyridoxine, and vitamin D malabsorption, as well as nearly any other compound that can be labeled with a radioisotope. Bile salt malabsorption can be estimated quite accurately by administration of ^{75}SeHCAT, a taurine conjugate of selenahomocholic acid.[36]

4. **Small bowel biopsy:** Peroral small bowel biopsy has been helpful in diagnosing various mucosal diseases, such as celiac disease, tropical sprue, and Whipple's disease.

SUMMARY

This chapter has presented an overview of the anatomy and physiology of the gastrointestinal tract. An understanding of nutrient digestion and absorption is necessary to anticipate the metabolic consequences of the short bowel syndrome, begin initial metabolic resuscitation, and plan for eventual intestinal rehabilitation.

REFERENCES

1. Lin, H.C. et al., Inhibition of gastric emptying by glucose depends on length of intestine exposed to nutrient, *Am. J. Physiol.*, 256, G404, 1989.
2. Lin, H.C. et al., Inhibition of gastric emptying by sodium oleate depends on length of intestine exposed to nutrient, *Am. J. Physiol.*, 259, G1031, 1990.
3. Lin, H.C. et al., Gastric emptying of solid food is most potently inhibited by carbohydrate in the canine distal ileum, *Gastroenterology*, 102, 793, 1992.
4. Lin, H.C., Zaidel, O., and Hum, S., Intestinal transit of fat depends on accelerating effect of cholecystokinin and slowing effect of an opioid pathway, *Dig. Dis. Sci.*, 47, 2217, 2002.
5. Lin, H.C. et al., Fat-induced ileal brake in the dog depends on peptide YY. *Gastroenterology*, 110, 1491, 1996.
6. Zhao, X.T. et al., Intestinal transit and protein absorption depend on load and degree of hydrolysis of soy protein (Abstr), *Gastroenterology*, 110, A849, 1996.
7. Lin, H.C. et al., Fiber-supplemented enteral formula slows intestinal transit by intensifying inhibitory feedback from the distal gut, *Am. J. Clin. Nutr.*, 65, 1840, 1997.
8. Shafik, A., Shafik, A.A., and Ahmed, I., Effect of colonic distention of ileal motor activity with evidence of coloileal reflex, *J. Gastrointest. Surg.*, 7, 701, 2003.
9. Roediger, W.E.W., Role of anaerobic bacteria in the metabolic welfare of the colonic mucosa in man, *Gut*, 21, 793, 1980.
10. Li, J. et al., Effects of parenteral and enteral nutrition on gut-associated lymphoid tissue, *J. Trauma*, 39, 44, 1995.
11. King, B.K., Li, J., and Kudsk, K.A., A temporal study of TPN-induced changes in gut-associated lymphoid tissue and mucosal immunity, Arch. Surg., 132, 1303, 1997.
12. Mekalanos, J.J., Minireview: Environmental singles controlling expression of virulence determinants in bacteria, *J. Bacteriol.*, 174, 1, 1992.
13. Li, J. et al., Effect of glutamine-enriched total parenteral nutrition on small intestinal gut-associated lymphoid tissue and upper respiratory tract immunity, *Surgery*, 121, 542, 1997.
14. Li, J. et al., Effects of parenteral and enteral nutrition on gut-associated lymphoid tissue, *J. Trauma*, 39, 44, 1995.
15. Love, A.H.G., Mitchell, T.G., and Phillips, R.A., Water and sodium absorption in the human intestine, *J. Physiol. (London)*, 195, 133, 1968.
16. Sladen, G.E. and Dawson, A.M., Interrelationships between the absorption of glucose, sodium and water by the normal human jejunum, *Clin. Sci.*, 36, 119, 1969.
17. Bronner, F., Mechanisms and functional aspects of intestinal calcium absorption, *J. Exp. Zoolog. Part A Comp. Exp. Biol.*, 300, 47, 2003.
18. Cartwright, G.E. and Wintrobe, M.M., Copper metabolism in normal subjects, *Am. J. Clin. Nutr.*, 14, 114. 1964.
19. Dunlap, W.M., James, G.W. III, and Hume, D.M., Anemia and neutropenia caused by copper deficiency, *Ann. Intern. Med.*, 80, 470, 1974.

20. Evans, G.W., Grace, C.I., and Hahn, C., Homeostatic regulation of zinc absorption in the rat, *Proc. Soc. Exp. Biol. Med.*, 143, 723, 1973.
21. Cotzias, G.C., Borg, D.C., and Selleck, B., Specificity of zinc pathway through the body: Turnover of Zn-65 in the mouse, *Am. J. Physiol.*, 202, 359, 1962.
22. Sullivan, J.F., O'Grady, J., and Lankford, H.G., The zinc content of pancreatic secretion, *Gastroenterology*, 48, 438, 1965.
23. Walker, B.E. et al., Plasma and urinary zinc in patients with malabsorption syndromes or hepatic cirrhosis, *Gut*, 14, 943, 1973.
24. Wolman, S.L. et al., Zinc in total parenteral nutrition: Requirements and metabolic effects, *Gastroenterology*, 76, 458, 1979.
25. Cox, T.M. and Peters, T.J., Uptake of iron by duodenal biopsy specimens from patients with iron-deficiency anaemia and primary haemochromatosis, *Lancet*, 1(8056), 123, 1978.
26. Dowdle, E.B., Schachter, D., and Schenker, H., Active transport of Fe-59 by everted segments of rat duodenum, *Am. J. Physiol.*, 198, 609, 1960.
27. Wright, E.M., Martin, M.G., and Turk, E., Intestinal absorption in health and disease-sugars, *Best Pract. Res. Clin. Gastroenterol.*, 17, 943, 2003.
28. Souba, W.W., Scott, T.E., and Wilmore, D.W., Intestinal consumption of intravenously administered fuels, *J.P.E.N. J. Parenter. Enteral Nutr.*, 9, 18, 1985.
29. Rommel, K., Bohmer, R., *Lipid Absorption: Biochemical and Clinical Aspects.* University Park Press, Baltimore, 1976.
30. Whitecross, D.P. et al., The pepsinogens of human gastric mucosa, *Gut*, 14, 850, 1973.
31. Matthews, D.M., Intestinal absorption of peptides, *Phys. Rev.*, 55, 537, 1975.
32. Haeney, M.R. et al., Evaluation of xylose absorption as measured in blood and urine: a one-hour blood xylose screening test in malabsorption, *Gastroenterology*, 75, 393, 1978.
33. Butler, R.N. et al., Clinical evaluation of the 14C triolein breath test: a critical analysis, *Aust. N. Z. J. Med.*, 14, 111, 1984.
34. Watkins, J.B. et al., 13C-trioctanoin: a nonradioactive breath test to detect fat malabsorption, *J. Lab. Clin. Med.*, 90, 422, 1977.
35. Brummer, R.J., Karibe, M., and Stockbrugger, R.W., Lactose malabsorption. Optimalization of investigational methods, *Scand. J. Gastroenterol. Suppl.*, 200, 65, 1993.
36. Preece, J.D., Davies, I.H., and Wilkinson, S.P., Use of the SeHCAT test in the investigation of diarrhoea, *Postgrad. Med. J.*, 68, 272, 1992.

2 The Etiology and Mechanism of Intestinal Failure

Khursheed N. Jeejeebhoy

CONTENTS

The gastrointestinal tract is designed to act as a single unit from the stomach to the colon. Therefore, in order to understand the factors that contribute to intestinal failure it is necessary to identify the role of each of the components in aiding the digestion and absorption of food and in the maintenance of the nutritional status of the host. In this chapter the etiological factors will be considered both from a mechanistic point of view and from the diseases that contribute to the development of intestinal failure. In the literature, *intestinal failure* and *short bowel* are used interchangeably. In practice, while loss of small bowel is the major cause of intestinal failure, there are situations in which the gastrointestinal tract fails to nourish the individual adequately because of a combination of the loss of intestinal, gastric, and pancreatic function. In this chapter the more practical definition of intestinal failure will be used as defined here:

> **Definition:** Intestinal failure occurs when gastrointestinal function is inadequate to maintain the nutrition and hydration of the individual without supplements given orally or intravenously (Table 2.1). In this context it is important to recognize that intestinal failure is a composite of intestinal insufficiency with or without contributing gastric and pancreatic insufficiency. In the presence of normal gastric and pancreatic function, a greater degree of intestinal loss has to occur before there is intestinal failure. In contrast, if there is gastric or pancreatic disease, a lesser degree over intestinal loss can cause failure. Furthermore, major resections of the stomach and pancreas can cause severe malabsorption and effectively behave clinically like "intestinal failure" without loss of intestinal function.

PHYSIOLOGICAL CONSIDERATIONS

STOMACH

The rate of gastric emptying regulates the progress of the meal through the small bowel. In turn the rate of gastric emptying is dependent on the consistency of the meal. Gastric emptying of liquids depends on osmolarity and that of digestible solids on the particle size. Furthermore, intestinal contents entering the distal intestine inhibit gastric emptying.[1]

SMALL BOWEL

Small bowel motility is three times slower in the ileum than in the jejunum.[2] In addition, the ileocecal valve may slow transit.[3] The adult small bowel receives about 5–6 liters of endogenous secretions and 2–3 liters of exogenous fluids per day. It reabsorbs most of this volume in the small bowel. The amount reabsorbed in the small intestine depends on the nature of the meal.[4] With a meat and salad meal, most of the fluid is absorbed in the jejunum, whereas with a milk and doughnut meal less was absorbed proximally and more flows distally. In addition, the absorptive processes are different in the jejunum as compared with the ileum. These differences depend partly on the nature of the electrolyte transport processes and

---

TABLE 2.1
Causes of Intestinal Failure

1. Intestinal resection
   a. Ileal resection
   b. Ileocolic resection
   c. End jejunostomy
2. Mucosal disease
   a. Celiac disease
   b. Whipple's disease
   c. Lymphoma
   d. Ulcerative jejunoileitis
   e. Abetalipoproteinemia
3. Small bowel disease
   a. Dysmotility
   b. Radiation injury and chemotherapy
   c. Inflammatory bowel disease
   d. Neoplasms
   e. Autoimmune disease
   f. Infection, e.g., HIV
4. Gut bypass
   a. Intestinal fistulae
   b. Surgical bypass
5. Maldigestion
   a. Gastric resection
   b. Pancreatic resection

---

partly on the permeability of the intercellular junctions. Water absorption is a passive process resulting from the active transport of nutrients and electrolytes. The transport of sodium creates an electrochemical gradient and also drives the uptake of carbohydrates and amino acids across the intestinal mucosa. In addition, in the ileum there is neutral sodium chloride absorption. However, the net absorption depends not only on these processes but on the extent of back diffusion of the transported material back into the intestinal lumen through "leaky" intercellular junctions. In the jejunum these junctions are very leaky and thus jejunal contents are always isotonic (Figure 2.1). Fluid absorption in this region of the bowel is very inefficient when compared with the ileum. It has been estimated that the efficiency of water absorption is 44% and 70% of the ingested load in the jejunum and ileum respectively. For sodium the corresponding estimates are 13% and 72%.[5] Hence the ileum is important in the conservation of fluid and electrolytes (Figure 2.2).

COLON

The colon has the slowest transit, varying between 24 and 150 hours. The intercellular junctions are the tightest in this part of the bowel, and the efficiency of water and salt absorption in the colon exceeds 90%.[5] In addition, carbohydrate is fermented in the colon to short-chain fatty acids (SCFAs), which have two important actions.

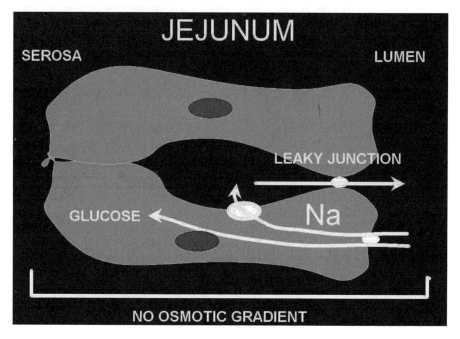

FIGURE 2.1 Architecture of the Jejunal mucosa showing the open paracellular junctions

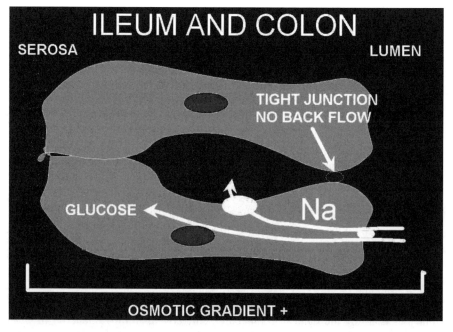

FIGURE 2.2 Architecture of the ileo-colonic mucosa showing impermeable paracellular junctions

First, SCFAs enhance salt and water absorption.[6] Second, the energy content of malabsorbed carbohydrates is salvaged by being absorbed as SCFAs. Our recent data suggest that in short bowel patients this salvage may be greater than in normal patients.[7] Thus, the colon becomes an important organ for fluid and electrolyte conservation and for the salvage of malabsorbed energy substrates in short bowel patients.

UNIQUE FUNCTIONS OF THE ILEUM

The ileum uniquely absorbs vitamin B_{12} and bile salts. Bile salts are essential for the efficient absorption of fats and fat-soluble vitamins. Normally the demand for bile salts imposed by fat absorption cannot be met by synthesis alone. The need for bile salts is met only by ileal resorption of bile salts, which are then recycled into the intestine. With ileal resection the loss of bile salts increases and is not met by an increase in synthesis. The bile salt pool is depleted and fat absorption is reduced. In addition, loss of bile salts into the colon reduces the ability of the colon to reabsorb salt and water, resulting in increased diarrhea. In the colon bile salts are also dehydroxylated to deoxy bile salts, which induce colonic water secretion.

EFFECTS OF INTESTINAL RESECTION

GASTRIC AND INTESTINAL SECRETION AND MOTILITY

Gastric hypersecretion occurs after small bowel resection. While there is concomitant hypergastrinemia, it is not clear whether the two are related. On the other hand, hypersecretion may reduce nutrient absorption by inactivating pancreatic enzymes. Hence, reducing acid secretion improves absorption in short bowel patients.[8] Furthermore, hypersecretion can cause nausea, reflux, and hemorrhage from severe esophageal ulceration, which may require proton pump inhibitors for control.[9]

Gastric motility is enhanced following small bowel resection.[10] While proximal resection does not increase the rate of intestinal transit, ileal resection significantly accelerates intestinal transit.[10,11] In this situation the colon aids in slowing intestinal transit so that in short bowel patients without colons, a marker fed by mouth was completely excreted in a few hours.[12]

ABSORPTION OF FLUID AND ELECTROLYTES

The effect of intestinal resection depends on the extent and site of resection. Proximal resection results in no bowel disturbance because the ileum and colon absorb the increased fluid and electrolyte load efficiently. The remaining ileum continues to absorb bile salts, and thus, there is little reaching the colon to impede salt and water resorption. In contrast, when the ileum is resected the colon receives a much larger load of fluid and electrolytes and also receives bile salts, which reduce its ability to absorb salt and water, resulting in diarrhea. In addition, if the colon is resected the ability to maintain fluid and electrolyte homeostasis is severely impaired.[13]

ABSORPTION OF NUTRIENTS

Absorption of nutrients occurs throughout the small bowel, and the removal of the jejunum alone results in the ileum taking over most of the lost function and with no malabsorption.[14] In contrast, even a loss of a 100 cm of ileum causes steatorrhea.[15] The degree of malabsorption increases with the length of resection and the variety of nutrients malabsorbed increases.[16,17] Balance studies of energy absorption showed that the absorption of fat and carbohydrate were equally reduced to between 50% and 75% of intake.[18] However, nitrogen absorption was reduced to a lesser extent than that of carbohydrate and fat, namely to 81% of intake. In short bowel patients, Ladefoged et al.[17] found that the degree of calcium, magnesium, zinc, and phosphorus absorption was reduced but did not correlate with the remaining length of bowel, and they recommended that in these patients parenteral supplementation be mandatory. Our studies showed similar reduction in absorption, but only half required parenteral replacement. The data taken as a whole suggest that it is easier to meet needs for energy and nitrogen by increasing oral intake than the needs for electrolytes and divalent ions. A review of the literature prior to the availability of parenteral nutrition shows that resections up to 33% result in no malnutrition and those up to 50% could be tolerated without special aids; however, those in excess of 75% require nutrition support to avoid severe malnutrition.[19]

ADAPTATION OF THE INTESTINE

Following resection, the remaining small bowel hypertrophies and increases absorptive function.[20,21] This process enhances the ability of the remaining bowel to recover the lost function and is thus an important compensatory process. The factors that influence this adaptation are complex and are discussed next, as are the effects of parenteral nutrition (PN).

Eating exposes the gastrointestinal tract to a unique set of stimuli, which does not occur when it is kept constantly empty, a process called bowel rest. The advent of PN resulted in the ability to rest the bowel for short or long periods of time without causing malnutrition, a situation that had not been possible previously. This process nourished the body but excluded the gut from nutrient and hormonal stimuli that occur during the ingestion of an oral diet. The advent of defined formula diets (DFD) without residue and diets composed of monomers, such as glucose instead of polymeric starch, modified the stimuli received by the gut when exposed to a normal diet. It should also be recognized that since nutrients are absorbed progressively along the length of the bowel, the jejunum is exposed to a higher concentration of nutrients than the ileum. Resection of the proximal bowel results in the ileum receiving more nutrients. Resection of the ileum, on the other hand, does not alter the jejunal nutrient load but may reduce stimuli from hormones released by the ileum.

Effect of Excluding Food from the Bowel Lumen

Hypoplasia of the mucosa is the most obvious change in experimental animals, when food is excluded from the lumen. At the same time body composition can be simultaneously maintained by the use of PN.[22]

In growing or neonatal animals, PN and bowel rest will maintain normal body growth but will result in reduced bowel length, and gastric and pancreatic hypoplasia.[23,24,25] Despite the occurrence of mucosal hypoplasia, the development of disaccharidase enzymes and glucose transport is accelerated and mucosal levels of these enzymes increased in neonatal animals receiving PN.[24,25] Hypoplasia occurred mainly in the proximal small bowel and is less evident distally.[26] In addition, PN and bowel rest increased intestinal permeability[27] and altered the response to endotoxin.[28] These dramatic effects of withdrawing food by mouth and giving PN in animals is not as pronounced in humans. A month of PN does not cause atrophy; it is only after several months of being nil per os (NPO) that villus atrophy occurs in humans.[29]

The nature of the feed influences the degree of hypoplasia. Refined liquid feed causes relative hypoplasia as compared with a solid diet.[23]

Factors Influencing Bowel Atrophy

In general it appears that the decreased digestive and absorptive activities of the mucosa during bowel rest are the major reasons for hypoplasia. This concept is supported by the fact that simply increasing the tonicity of the bowel contents results in an increase of the mucosal mass.[30] Absorption of amino acids results in a nonspecific increase of mucosal function and mass.[31] Finally, disaccharide hydrolysis followed by absorption stimulates mucosal growth to a greater extent than equivalent monosaccharide absorption.[32]

SCFAs that are produced by fermentation in the colon were shown to prevent or reduce mucosal atrophy in animals receiving PN and bowel rest, even when given parenterally.[33] Dietary fiber is the main source of colonic fermentable substrate for SCFAs production. Therefore, fiber in the diet aids the maintenance of mucosal mass. For the same reasons, DFDs are not quite as good as a solid diet in this regard. Glutamine is a nutrient for the bowel mucosa, and the supplementation of PN with glutamine preserves gastric and colonic mass in PN-fed animals but does not preserve small bowel mucosal height.[34]

Does Bowel Rest Induce Gut Atrophy in Man?

In the rat, bowel rest with PN causes atrophy in days[35] but in man even after 21 days of bowel rest with PN there is no change in gut hormone production after a meal,[36] nor is there any histological atrophy.[29] In children bowel rest caused atrophy only when prolonged beyond 9 months.[29] However, there is a reduction in the size of the microvilli and a fall in brush border enzyme activity.[37]

In summary, animal data suggest that when the bowel is not used, it atrophies. Mucosal atrophy is due to a combination of the lack of functional stimulation and the absence of hormonal, biliary, and pancreatic secretion. The only convincing trophic factors are SCFAs and their precursor, dietary fiber and glutamine. In addition, there some evidence for the role of vitamin A, zinc, and glutathione as being weaker trophic factors.[38]

IMPLICATIONS FOR MANAGEMENT OF SHORT BOWEL SYNDROME

JEJUNAL RESECTION WITH INTACT ILEUM AND COLON

Patients in this category can be fed orally immediately and rarely have any problems. The conventional approach is to give clear fluids and then a fluid diet with nutrients, then soft followed by regular food. There is no evidence this approach is beneficial. Patients can take fluids and solids in small quantities as soon as they can pass gas and feel hungry. The process of refeeding after resection is given in detail in the next section, "Practical Considerations."

ILEAL RESECTION OF LESS THAN 100 CM WITH COLON LARGELY INTACT

Patients in this category have so-called bile salt–induced diarrhea, and are best helped by the administration of 4 g of cholestyramine three times a day to bind bile salts left unabsorbed by the resected ileum. Vitamin B_{12} absorption should be measured and if low should be injected intramuscularly in doses of 100 to 200 µg per month.

ILEAL RESECTION OF MORE THAN 100 TO 200 CM WITH COLON LARGELY INTACT

This group of patients has little difficulty in maintaining nutrition with an oral diet, but has fatty acid diarrhea. For such a patient, fat restriction is mandatory. With the larger resection, the bile salt pool is depleted and cholestyramine is no longer beneficial. Parenteral vitamin B_{12} replacement is required.

RESECTION IN EXCESS OF 200 CM OF SMALL BOWEL AND LESSER RESECTION WITH ASSOCIATED COLECTOMY

Patients of this class require the graduated adaptation program described in the next section titled "Practical Considerations."

RESECTION LEAVING LESS THAN 60 CM SMALL BOWEL OR ONLY DUODENUM: MASSIVE BOWEL RESECTION

Patients in this category need parenteral nutrition (PN) indefinitely. However, many patients even in this category may show a surprising degree of adaptation and require less parenteral nutrition and benefit from orally absorbed nutrients. The indication to reduce parenteral nutrition is weight gain beyond the desired limit and the fact that reduced infusion does not cause electrolyte imbalance and dehydration.

PRACTICAL CONSIDERATIONS

CONTROL OF DIARRHEA

Diarrhea is due to a combination of increased secretions, increased motility, and osmotic stimulation of water secretion due to malabsorption of luminal contents. Initially diarrhea is controlled by keeping the patient NPO to reduce any osmotic component. Gastric hypersecretion can be controlled by the continuous infusion of appropriate doses of intravenous proton pump inhibitors. In addition, loperamide can be used to slow gastric and intestinal transit. If loperamide does not work, then codeine or diphenoxylate may be tried.

INTRAVENOUS FLUIDS

In the immediate postoperative period, all patients will require intravenous fluids and electrolytes to replace losses. Sodium and potassium chloride as well as magnesium are the most important ions to be replaced, and plasma levels of these ions should be monitored frequently. Fluid is infused according to measured losses and to maintain an adequate urine output. The infusion is tapered as oral intake is increased.

ORAL FEEDING

The next consideration is to determine the nature of oral feeds. In patients who have more than 100 cm of remaining jejunum, refeeding should be progressive with a view ultimately to feeding a normal oral diet. In patients with less than 100 cm of jejunum as the only small bowel remaining, dietary intake and fluids cause increased fluid loss.[39] By contrast, in patients who have little small bowel left, the initial target should be small volume isotonic feeds containing a glucose-electrolyte content similar to the oral rehydration solution. The composition of this solution should be glucose 100 mmol/L with sodium chloride 60 mmol/L, sodium citrate 60 mmol/L. It has been shown that fluid absorption improves with increasing sodium concentration. In addition, to provide sufficient sodium to absorb dietary carbohydrate it is necessary to ingest 10–15 g of sodium chloride as tablets with meals. Such a regimen avoids osmotic stimulation of secretion and yet stimulates the bowel to absorb, thus promoting adaptation. Progressive feeding should be attempted with the following plan. The same carbohydrate-electrolyte feeds as above should be started. A mixture of a similar composition has been shown to be well absorbed by patients with massive resection who have previously been dependent on intravenous fluids. The diet should be lactose-free since lactase levels in such patients are reduced. Vitamin B_{12} absorption should be measured, and if subnormal, injections of 100 to 200 micrograms per month should be started.

Early observations had suggested that low fat diets are beneficial. The theory behind this concept was that malabsorbed long-chain fatty acids (LCT) can cause colonic water secretion. However, soluble carbohydrates are also malabsorbed with a very short bowel and using a controlled crossover design in two studies[10,16] we showed that a high-fat diet was comparable to a high-carbohydrate diet in regard to total fluid, energy, nitrogen, sodium, potassium, and divalent ion absorption. We therefore recommend a low lactose diet containing high calories from both fat and carbohydrate and a high nitrogen intake. In adults who require about 30 kcal/kg/day, we aim to increase intake gradually to about 60 kcal/kg/day to provide sufficient absorbed calories despite malabsorption. The rationale for this approach is discussed by Woolf et al.[12] Supplements of potassium, magnesium, and zinc are given while monitoring serum levels. In particular potassium as gluconate may be added to a concentration of 12 mmol/L in the carbohydrate-electrolyte fluid. In addition we have found that magnesium heptogluconate is especially useful as a supplement to correct hypomagnesemia without causing diarrhea. It is possible to add 30 mmol of magnesium per liter of glucose-electrolyte mixture and sipped over the day.

PARENTERAL NUTRITION

In patients with less than 100 cm of remaining jejunum and in those with a combined small bowel and colon resection, parenteral nutrition is lifesaving. It is started in such patients within a few days of the resection, and initially 32 kcal/kg of a mixed energy substrate and 1 g/kg amino acids is infused with sodium 150–200 mM, potassium 60–100 mM, calcium 9–11 mM, magnesium 7–15 mM, and zinc 70–100 micromoles per day. Among trace elements zinc is the most important as we have found large losses in patients with a high endogenous output of intestinal fluids. Oral feeds are simultaneously started and attempts are made to reduce parenteral feeding as oral feeds are increased. It will become apparent whether the patient needs parenteral feeding on a long-term basis. If that is the case, then the patient should be started on a program of home parenteral nutrition (HPN). We have found that as the bowel adapts over months, and even years, the patient requires less parenteral feeding, and ultimately about 30% of our patients initially requiring HPN can be weaned off HPN by using up to 2 liters of oral rehydration solution, high calorie diet, and supplements of potassium, magnesium, calcium, fat soluble vitamins, and zinc. They are monitored regularly until the weight is stable and they are electrolyte balanced. Hypomagnesemia is particularly a serious problem in these patients. Ingestion of magnesium salts orally enhances diarrhea and therefore it often becomes difficult to use magnesium supplements orally. The author has successfully used magnesium heptogluconate for this purpose. This preparation is available as a palatable liquid, which is added to the electrolyte supplement in quantities of 30 mM per day. If this approach is not successful, then magnesium sulfate is infused through an indwelling catheter in doses of 12 mM 1 to 3 times a week to supplement the oral intake.

Vitamin supplementation needs a comment. These patients can absorb water soluble vitamins but have difficulty absorbing fat-soluble vitamins. They require large doses of vitamin A, D, and E to maintain normal levels. Also, pills often pass out whole in these patients, hence liquid preparations have to be used. We recommend the measurement of these vitamin levels and supplementation with aqueous preparations of vitamin A and E (Aqasol A and E) and 1,25 dihydroxy-vitamin D in doses that normalize the plasma levels. Normalization may not be possible with oral vitamins in some individuals, especially vitamin E levels.

In some patients an oral diet will maintain weight and body composition, but these patients need intravenous fluids and electrolytes to maintain hydration and normal levels of electrolytes, especially magnesium. Short bowel patients may not be able to maintain normal weight and body composition in addition to requiring intravenous fluids and electrolytes for hydration. These patients need full parenteral nutrition containing protein, energy, electrolytes, vitamins, and trace elements.

SUMMARY

Appreciation of the function of the different segments of the gastrointestinal tract in promoting absorption and motility allows a rational understanding of the effects of intestinal resection and disease. In particular the jejunum has a high capacity for absorption but cannot concentrate its contents and salvage fluid from the lumen. The ileum and colon can concentrate their contents and salvage fluid from the lumen. In addition, the ileum recycles bile salts and uniquely absorbs vitamin B_{12}. The colon also can salvage energy from unabsorbed carbohydrate by bacterial fermentation and absorption of the short-chain fatty acid products of fermentation.

On the basis of this information, a rational plan of management can be formulated to maximize absorption of nutrients as well as fluid and electrolytes and to recommend supplements.

REFERENCES

1. Malagelada, J.-R., Gastric, pancreatic and biliary response to a meal. In *Physiology of the Gastrointestinal Tract.* 1st ed, Johnson, L.R., Ed. Raven Press, New York, 1981.
2. Summers, R.W., Kent, T.H., and Osborne, J.W., Effects of drugs, ileal obstruction and irradiation on rat gastrointestinal propulsion, *Gastroenterology*, 59, 731, 1970.
3. Ricotta, J. et al., Construction of an ileocecal valve and its role in massive resection of the small intestine, *Surg. Gynecol. Obstet.* 152, 310, 1981.
4. Fordtran, J.S. and Locklear T.W., Ionic constituents and osmolality of gastric and small-intestinal fluids after eating, *Am. J. Dig. Dis.* 11, 503, 1966.
5. Powell, D.W., Intestinal water and electrolyte transport. In *Physiology of the Gastrointestinal Tract*, 2nd ed., Johnson, L.R., Ed., Raven Press, New York, 1987.
6. Binder, H.J. and Mehta, P., Short-chain fatty acids stimulate active sodium and chloride absorption in vitro in the rat distal colon, *Gastroenterology* 96, 989, 1989.
7. Royall, D., Wolever, T.M.S, and Jeejeebhoy, K.N., Clinical significance of colonic fermentation, *Am. J. Gastroenterol.* 85, 1307, 1990.
8. Cortot, A., Fleming, C.R., and Malagelada, J.R., Improved nutrient absorption after cimetidine in short-bowel syndrome with gastric hypersecretion, *N. Engl. J. Med.*, 300, 79, 1979.
9. Tang, S.-J. et al., The novel use of an intravenous proton pump inhibitor in a patient with short bowel syndrome, *J. Clin. Gastroenterol.* 34, 62, 2002.

10. Nylander, G., Gastric evacuation and propulsive intestinal motility following resection of the small intestine in the rat, *Acta. Chir. Scand.* 133, 131, 1967.

11. Reynell, P.C. and Spray, G.H., Small intestinal function in the rat after massive resections, *Gastroenterology* 31, 361, 1956.

12. Woolf, G.M. et al., Diet for patients with a short bowel: High fat or high carbohydrate? *Gastroenterology* 84, 823, 1983.

13. Cummings, J.H., James, W.P.T., and Wiggins, H.S., Role of the colon in ileal-resection diarrhea, *Lancet* I, 344, 1973.

14. Booth, C.C., Aldis, D., and Read, A.E., Studies on the site of fat absorption. 2. Fat balances after resection of varying amounts of small intestine in man, *Gut* 2,168, 1961.

15. Hoffman, A.F. and Poley, J.R., Role of bile acid malabsorption in the pathogenesis of diarrhea and steatorrhea in patients with ileal resection. I. Response to cholestyramine or replacement of dietary long-chain triglycerides by medium-chain triglycerides, *Gastroenterology* 62, 918, 1972.

16. Hylander, E., Ladefoged, K., and Jarnum, S., Nitrogen absorption following small intestinal resection. *Scand. J. Gastroenterol.* 15, 853, 1980.

17. Ladefoged, K., Nicolaidou, P., and Jarnum, S., Calcium, phosphorus, magnesium, zinc and nitrogen balance in patients with severe short bowel syndrome, *Am. J. Clin. Nutr.* 33, 2137, 1980.

18. Woolf, G.M., Miller, C., Kurian, R., and Jeejeebhoy, K.N., Nutritional absorption in short bowel syndrome: evaluation of fluid, calorie, and divalent cation requirements, *Dig. Dis. Sci.* 32, 8, 1987.

19. Haymond, H.E., Massive resection of the small intestine: analysis of 257 collected cases, *Surg. Gynecol. Obstet.* 61, 693, 1953.

20. Flint, J.M., The effect of extensive resection of the small intestine. *Johns Hopkins Med. J.* 23, 127, 1912.

21. Althausen, T.L. et al., Digestion and absorption after massive resection of small intestine; recovery of absorptive function as shown by intestinal absorption tests in 2 patients and consideration of compensatory mechanisms, *Gastroenterology* 16, 126, 1950.

22. Lo, C.W. and Walker, W.A., Changes in the gastrointestinal tract during enteral or parenteral nutrition, *Nutr. Rev.* 47, 193, 1989.

23. Goldstein, R.M. et al., The effects of total parenteral nutrition on gastrointestinal growth and development, *J. Pediatr. Surg.* 20, 785, 1985.

24. Shulman, R.J., Effect of different total parenteral nutrition fuel mixes on small intestinal growth and differentiation in the infant miniature pig, *Gastroenterology* 95, 85, 1988.

25. Gall, D.G. et al., Effect of parenteral and enteral nutrition on postnatal development of the small intestine and pancreas in the rabbit, *Biol. Neonate* 51, 286, 1987.

26. Morgan, W. et al., Total parenteral nutrition and intestinal development: a neonatal model, *Pediatr. Surg.* 22, 541, 1987.

27. Purandare, S. et al., Increased gut permeability to fluorescin isothiocyanate-dextran after total parenteral nutrition in the rat, *Scand. J. Gastroenterol.* 24, 678, 1989.

28. Fong, Y.M. et al., Total parenteral nutrition and bowel rest modify the metabolic response to endotoxin in humans, *Ann. Surg.* 210, 449, 1989.

29. Jeejeebhoy, K.N., TPN potion or poison. *Am. J. Clin. Nutr.* 74, 160, 2001.

30. Weser, E., Babbitt, J., and Vandeventer, A., Relationship between enteral glucose load and adaptive mucosal growth in the small bowel, *Dig. Dis. Sci.* 30, 675, 1985.

31. Levine, G.M., Nonspecific adaptation of jejunal amino acid uptake in the rat, *Gastroenterology* 91, 49, 1986.

32. Weser, E., Babbit, J., and Vandeventer, A., Intestinal adaptation. Different growth responses to disaccharides compared with monosaccharides in rat small bowel, *Gastroenterology* 91, 521, 1986.
33. Koruda, M.J. et al., Parenteral nutrition supplemented with short-chain fatty acids: effect on the small-bowel mucosa in normal rats, *Am. J. Clin. Nutr.* 51, 685, 1990.
34. Grant, J.P. and Snyder, P.J., Use of L-glutamine in total parenteral nutrition, *J. Surg. Res.* 44, 506, 1988.
35. Hughes, C.A., Prince, A., and Dowling, R.H., Speed of change in pancreatic mass and in intestinal bacteriology of parenterally fed rats, *Clin. Sci.* 59, 329, 1980.
36. Greenberg, G.R. et al., Effect of total parenteral nutrition on gut hormone release in humans, *Gastroenterology* 80, 988, 1981.
37. Gucdon, C., Schmitz, J., Lerebours, E. et al., Decreased brush border hydrolase activities without gross morphologic changes in human intestinal mucosa after prolonged total parenteral nutrition in adults, *Gastroenterology* 90, 373, 1986.
38. Ziegler, T.R. et al., Trophic and cytoprotective nutrition for intestinal adaptation, mucosal repair, and barrier function, *Annu. Rev. Nutr.* 23, 229, 2003.
39. Nightingale, J.M.D. et al., Jejunal efflux in short bowel syndrome, *Lancet* 336, 765, 1990.

3 Diarrhea in Short Bowel Syndrome

Stuart S. Kaufman and Erin M. Fennelly

CONTENTS

The normally functioning gastrointestinal tract provides adequate fluid, electrolytes, macronutrients, and micronutrients in the appropriate hunger mechanisms and nutrient supply. The basis for water absorption is passive flow along concentration gradients established by active particle transport along the length of the stomach, small bowel, and colon. Macronutrient assimilation is highly efficient, occurring for the most part in the upper small intestine. Efficient macronutrient digestion and assimilation requires dispersion in water secreted from the upper GI tract, also in response to active particle transport. In most situations in patients with intestinal failure, diarrhea results when loss of intestinal absorptive capacity is high, specifically in excess of gut secretory capacity. The impact of gut loss is a function both of the region as well as the amount of loss because different regions of the GI tract vary in their capacity for solute and water absorption

0-8493-1803-3/05/$0.00+$1.50
© 2005 by CRC Press LLC

NORMAL ALIMENTARY TRACT-STRUCTURE AND FUNCTION

The small bowel is about 250 cm long in the full-term newborn infant. Subsequent growth is highly variable, as small bowel length increases to approximately 400–750 cm by adulthood.[1,2] Because solid foods must be liquefied for digestion and assimilation, the upper digestive tract secretes approximately 8,000 mL of fluid into the gut lumen daily under the stimulus of food, accompanied by a variable quantity of dietary water.[3] Contributions to lumen fluid are as noted in Table 3.1. Although most regions of the gut secrete and absorb fluid simultaneously, the balance favors absorption in most of the jejunum and ileum (6,500 mL) and colon (1,000–1,500 mL), resulting in only about 200 mL of fecal water loss daily.[3] It is axiomatic that the magnitude of diarrhea following intestinal resection is determined by the location as well amount of gut loss, or, more accurately, the type and quantity of *remnant* bowel, given the considerable variation in normal small bowel length.[4] Resection of 400 cm of jejunoileum may result in profound increases in stool volume and nutrient malabsorption when original small bowel length is only 450 cm. Conversely, the same amount of resection may have little or no effect in persons with native small bowel length of 500 cm or more.

MECHANISMS OF NORMAL WATER AND SOLUTE BALANCE IN THE GASTROINTESTINAL TRACT

Water moves into and out of gut mucosa epithelial cells down concentration gradients established by a concurrent flow of electrically neutral dietary solutes such as simple sugars and charged molecules.[5] Water flow in the stomach is primarily secretory, that is, directed into the lumen. The major driving force for gastric secretion is the active transport of hydrogen ion (H^+) out of parietal cells into the lumen in exchange for potassium cation (K^+) by the gastric acid pump, $H^+ - K^+$ ATPase, on the plasma membrane.[6,7] Negatively charged bicarbonate (HCO_3^-), which is generated simultaneous with formation of H^+, moves into the plasma in exchange for chloride (Cl^-), which then follows its gradient into the lumen to maintain electrical neutrality. Stimulation of acid secretion with enteral nutrition increases gastric fluid volume, while histamine$_2$ receptor antagonists and proton pump inhibitors reduce H^+ secretion and gastric fluid production.

TABLE 3.1
Components of Alimentary Tract Fluid (per day)

Saliva	500 mL
Gastric juice	2000 mL
Bile	1500 mL
Pancreatic fluid	1000 mL
Duodenal fluid	3000 mL

The primary driving force for particle movement in small intestinal epithelial cells, or enterocytes, is the active, energy-consuming transport of sodium cations (Na^+) out of cells along their basal cell surface coupled to inwardly directed movement of K^+ into the enterocytes. This active flux of sodium and potassium is accomplished via the plasma membrane pump, $Na^+ - K^+$ ATPase.[5] As sodium egress quantitatively exceeds potassium ingress, both an outward to inward sodium gradient and a net negative intracellular electrical charge are established. The enterocyte electrochemical gradient maintained by $Na^+ - K^+$ ATPase is utilized to establish other solute gradients that can drive water either into or out of the cells based on the directions of the gradients.

The luminal surface of the small bowel is organized into a dense carpet of tongue-like protrusions or villi (singular = *villus*) that are in continuity with underlying glandular crypts. Crypt enterocytes are primarily secretory, while villus enterocytes are primarily absorptive. Absorption and secretion also vary depending on the region of the alimentary tract; net water flux in the duodenum is directed toward the lumen, while in most of the jejunum, ileum, and colon, the balance favors absorption.[8] In crypt enterocytes, net secretion occurs because of the high density of plasma membrane carrier proteins present on the basal enterocyte surface that direct the passive influx of Na^+ (and K^+) coupled with Cl^-, which maintains electrical neutrality.[8] Cl^-, the intra-enterocyte concentration of which is high, then passes down its gradient into the bowel lumen, bringing water into the lumen along this gradient (Figure 3.1). In contrast, the absorptive character of villus enterocytes is made possible by a high density of plasma membrane carrier proteins on the luminal surface, quantitatively the most important of which brings Na^+ in to the cell in conjunction with glucose (or galactose) in exchange for H^+. H^+ egress into the gut lumen provides the driving force for expulsion of negatively charged bicarbonate ion via another membrane carrier, which is electrically balanced by uptake of Cl^-; the net result is uptake of NaCl in a 2:1 proportion with glucose (Figure 3.2). Villus enterocytes take up additional particles using numerous other luminal plasma membrane carriers, and water passively follows. Among these carriers are those coupling passive influx of Na^+ with fructose and amino acids down the Na^+ gradient established by $Na^+ - K^+$ ATPase.[8]

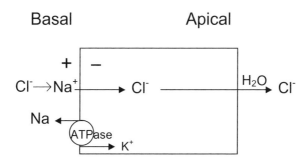

FIGURE 3.1 Schema of electrolyte and secondary water flux in the crypt enterocyte

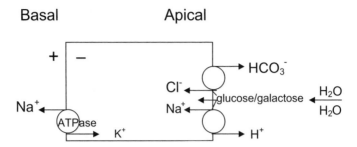

FIGURE 3.2 Schema of electrolyte and secondary water flux in the villus enterocyte

Any pathological process that selectively involves villi as compared to crypts may alter the balance between secretion and absorption in the region involved. Thus, enteric viral infections, which typically injure villus enterocytes, produce diarrhea in part by permitting unopposed electrolyte and fluid secretion from crypt enterocytes.[9] Ingested solutes that are absorbed poorly, including magnesium cations or lactose in lactase-deficient persons, diminish the osmotic gradient for water absorption in the jejunum and ileum, and thereby tend to increase fecal fluid loss. Similarly, reduction in surface area following massive resection of the jejunum or ileum reduces the surface area for absorption of numerous dietary molecules and the products of their luminal break down, including monosaccharides, amino acids, and fatty acids. Should the increased solute and water load presented to the colon exceed its absorptive capacity, a corresponding increase in liquid stool output will result.

Solutes absorbed by colonic mucosa include Na^+ and Cl^- that are exchanged with K+ and HCO_3^-.[3] Additionally, short chain fatty acids are passively transported in the colon, providing impetus for absorption of additional lumen water.[10-12] Short chain fatty acids are produced by bacterial fermentation of complex starches and soluble fibers not absorbed in the small bowel.[13] They are assimilated both in unionized and ionized (negatively charged) form, the latter in exchange for HCO_3^-, which represents another source of alkali loss into the colon lumen (Figure 3.3). The quantity of short chain fatty acids produced and absorbed in the colon, mainly

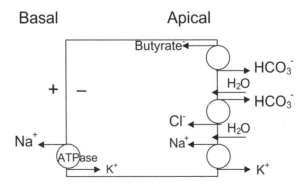

FIGURE 3.3 Schema of electrolyte and secondary water flux in the colonocyte

butyric acid and also proprionic and acetic acid, are substantial, delivering up to 1,100 extra calories daily that would otherwise be lost in stools.[13] Similarly, there exists some capacity for uptake of medium chain fatty acids, should the diet include medium chain triglycerides not absorbed fully in the small bowel. In contrast, the colon is impermeable to long chain fatty acids.

FUNCTIONAL CONSEQUENCES OF INTESTINAL RESECTION

PROXIMAL INTESTINAL LOSS

The intact small intestine possesses substantial digestive reserve; most macronutrients are assimilated within the first 200 cm.[14] If this region is completely resected, the remaining distal small bowel is generally adequate for complete macronutrient absorption, resulting in little or no effect on stool volume or consistency. In addition, the stomach also contributes to preservation of macronutrient absorption by remnant small bowel by replacing proximal small bowel secretions required to dilute liquefied solid food. Gastric acid secretion may increase for several months after major intestinal resection in proportion to the magnitude of the resection, possibly because of a parallel reduction in release of enteric hormones such as somatostatin that inhibit acid production.[15] In some patients, gastric hyperacidity may transiently cause malabsorption post-resection by inactivating pancreatic enzymes and precipitating bile acids. However, diarrhea is rarely substantial after proximal intestinal resection, because the intact ileum and colon has sufficient functional reserve to increase fluid uptake three to fivefold.[3]

DISTAL INTESTINAL LOSS

In general, extensive resection of distal small intestine, that is, ileum, has the potential to alter digestion and thereby reduce nutrient, fluid, and electrolyte absorption more than resection of an equivalent length of proximal intestine, that is, jejunum.[1,3] The concept that loss of ileum should significantly impair nutrient assimilation is counterintuitive, given that most macronutrient assimilation normally occurs in the upper third to half of the small bowel. However, the ileum is the only intestinal segment that reabsorbs bile salts actively, and if sufficient ileum is lost, about 100 cm in adults and 50 cm in children, the compensatory increase in hepatic bile salt synthesis will not keep pace with increased fecal bile salt loss.[16] In that case, the proximal intestinal lumen bile salt concentration will be inadequate for efficient lipid emulsification, resulting in fat malabsorption. Colon fluid losses are increased, both because the colon is impermeable to long chain fatty acids, resulting in an additional nonabsorbable osmotic load, and because long chain fatty acids exert a direct stimulatory effect on colonocyte electrolyte secretion.[16] Clinically important losses of K^+ and HCO_3^- are especially notable. Lesser degrees of ileal loss sufficient to produce bile acid malabsorption but not bile acid depletion or fat malabsorption may still increase colon fluid losses and produce diarrhea by the same mechanism.[17] Chronic pancreatitis that eventuates in pancreatic insufficiency occurs in some patients following intestinal resection.[18] Whether pancreatic insufficiency acts in concert with bile acid deficiency to worsen fat malabsorption in a significant number of patients remains conjectural.

Loss of distal small bowel, ileocecal valve, and colon accelerate gastric emptying of liquids and increase proximal small bowel motility directly, thereby shortening total intestinal transit time independent of that resulting from reduction in intestinal length per se.[19] A shorter transit time further reduces total contact between luminal contents and the mucosal surface, adding to the aggregate reduction in nutrient, fluid, and electrolyte assimilation. Hormones normally secreted by the distal ileal and colonic mucosa, including peptide PYY and GLP-1, probably mediate the normal ability of terminal small bowel to slow intestinal transit, referred to as the "ileal brake."[20] However, the relative contributions of the distal ileum, ileocecal valve, and proximal colon in slowing proximal motility remain incompletely defined.

Colon Loss

Under physiological conditions, the colon plays a secondary role in digestion. At most, 20% of complex dietary starch and even less (< 5%) of dietary nitrogen and lipid escape small intestinal absorption.[3] Physiological malabsorption of carbohydrate in the small intestine, including dietary fiber, is followed by colonic bacterial fermentation to bioavailable short chain fatty acids, thereby precluding a potentially major source of osmotically induced fecal water loss as well as promoting nutrient recovery. Although the colon cannot take up long-chain fatty acids, the actual volume of extra fecal solid and water associated with post-resection steatorrhea is usually modest and responsive to dietary fat restriction. The colon absorbs only a small absolute quantity of the fluid reclaimed during digestion, only about 10%–15% of the total. Thus, the impact of colon loss on nutrient and fluid balance is highly dependent on the amount of additional small intestinal loss. Following resection of most of the colon with preservation of the small bowel, shortened transit time fails to cause major nutrient impairment owing to the considerable digestive reserve of the small bowel. Fluid losses increase in association with corresponding loss of sodium and chloride, equivalent to about 75-90 mEq/L. These quantities are not generally sufficient to result in dehydration or electrolyte depletion if compensated with additional intake.

CLINICAL PRESENTATION OF MALABSORPTION AND DIARRHEA FOLLOWING INTESTINAL RESECTION

As the foregoing discussion indicates, both the magnitude and location of intestinal resection determine the severity of diarrhea and, by implication, complexity and difficulty of management. The most extreme situation is the patient left with a terminal enterostomy following small bowel resection, either because all or most of the colon has been removed, or because residual colonic disease contraindicates re-anastomosis. When only duodenum and less than 100 cm of jejunum are present, absorption by the remnant jejunum is inadequate to salvage the volume of fluid secreted by more proximal bowel combined with usual pancreatic, biliary, gastric, and salivary sources.[21, 22] These patients will invariably require IV fluid and electrolyte supplementation.[4] Supplementation by the enteral route alone will almost never restore positive fluid and electrolyte balances, because any quantity of enteral intake will precipitate an even larger amount of enterostomy output.[1] Similarly, antiperistaltic drugs may reduce enterostomy output but will not reestablish positive fluid balance. Fat malabsorption is marked. However, in the absence of a colon, a diet high in fat does not usually provoke mucosal electrolyte secretion,[14] although exceptions to this pattern are reported.[23] In these patients, diets high and low in fat are tolerated equally well, and the former are likely to reduce parenteral calorie requirements. In contrast, no advantage accrues to consumption of a diet rich in complex carbohydrates, since salvage by colonic bacterial fermentation is not available. Consequently, most patients with a terminal enterostomy will require supplemental IV macronutrients in addition to fluid and electrolytes, although the quantity required is relatively less than that of fluid and electrolytes, in light of the high efficiency of macronutrient assimilation by the normal intestinal mucosa.[21] Should the remnant small bowel mucosa be abnormal, for example, when resection is indicated by Crohn's disease or chronic ischemic enteropathy, IV macronutrient requirements will be correspondingly increased.

Patients with a jejunoileal length exceeding about 100–120 cm and a terminal enterostomy usually do not require parenteral nutrient or fluid support, because the additional segment of more distal, absorptive small bowel is usually sufficient to accommodate food-stimulated upper gastrointestinal secretions in addition to the nutrients themselves.[4,21] Quantitatively, the minimum requirement for freedom from parenteral fluid in adults is a positive balance (net absorption) of about 1.4 kg/day.[24] This balance is most likely to be achieved when with a high level of fluid intake containing a high concentration of sodium, 90-120 mEq/L, in order to ensure an optimal extra- to intracellular gradient for sodium, and thereby, water absorption.[1,6] The minimum requirement for assimilation of enteral calories to avoid parenteral feeding is 84% of the basal metabolic rate or aggregate absorption of about one-third of ingested calories.[4,24] Thus, malnutrition will be prevented only if caloric intake is consistently threefold greater than usual expenditures. The rare ability of a patient to subsist without parenteral nutrition while absorbing only 25% of ingested calories implies that a marked alteration in body metabolism occurs in response to severe malabsorption.

Restoration of continuity with some length of colon following intestinal resection, that is, the establishment of a jejunocolostomy, alters the character of an optimal diet.[25] Given the ability of colon to reabsorb both fluid and sodium as well as salvage malabsorbed carbohydrate as short chain fatty acids, less jejunum, only about 60 cm, is required to maintain independence from parenteral fluid or calories. In this circumstance, a diet relatively high in complex carbohydrates is appropriate, as utilization of the colon remnant for nutrient as well as fluid and electrolyte assimilation is maximized. Furthermore, antiperistaltic agents such as loperamide more effectively prolong transit time when the colon is in continuity with small intestine than when it is not.[25] Patients have the greatest chance to avoid intravenous nutrition support following massive small intestinal resection when colon removal is avoided altogether; that is, the patient is left with an intact terminal ileum and ileocecal valve. The major pathophysiological effect of resection is likely to be bile salt malabsorption and, depending on the length of ileum removed, some steatorrhea. However, a high complex carbohydrate diet will compensate for deficient fat absorption and extra fecal water loss resulting therefrom, and only 35 cm of jejunoileum is needed to avoid parenteral nutrition when in continuity with an ileocecal valve and intact colon.[21, 22]

CONCLUSION

The primary question for the patient who has experienced an intestinal resection is whether parenteral nutritional and/or fluid support will be required and, as a corollary, what dietary interventions can be made that maximize function of the remnant bowel. The greatest disability results from massive resection of the small bowel and colon, which leaves the patient with the means of preparing nutrients for assimilation but without the means for accomplishing assimilation itself. The least degree of disability results from loss of the upper intestine with preserved lower small bowel and colon, because the distal bowel is inherently better able to assume functions of the upper intestine than the converse. Understanding the etiology of diarrhea and malabsorption in the patient with an anatomically deficient gastrointestinal tract is facilitated by knowledge of normal mechanisms of fluid and electrolyte transport in the gastrointestinal tract, particularly regional differences in physiology. With this knowledge, prognosis can be realistically assessed, and appropriate long-term interventions carried out.

REFERENCES

1. Lennard-Jones, J.E., Review article: practical management of the short bowel, *Aliment. Pharmacol. Ther.* 5:563-577, 1994.
2. Fitzsimmons, J., Chinn, A., and Shepard, T.H., Normal length of the human fetal gastrointestinal tract, *Pediatr. Path.,* 8:633-641, 1988.
3. Sundaram, A., Koutkia, P., and Apovian, C.M., Nutritional management of short bowel syndrome in adults, *J. Clin. Gastroenterol.,* 34:207-220, 2002.
4. Nightingale, J.M., Management of patients with a short bowel syndrome, *Nutrition,* 15:633-637, 1999.
5. Wright, E.M. and Loo, D.D.F., Coupling between Na^+, sugar, and water transport across the intestine, *Ann. N.Y. Acad. Sci.,* 915:54–66, 2000.
6. Sial, S., Koussayer, T., and Klein, S., Nutritional management of a patient with short-bowel syndrome and large-volume jejunostomy output, *Nutrition,* 10:37–40, 1994.
7. Helander, H.F. and Keeling, D.J., Cell biology of gastric acid secretion, *Baillieres Clin. Gastroenterol.,* 7:1–21, 1993.
8. Holtug, K., Hansen, M.B., and Skadhauge, E., Experimental studies of intestinal ion and water transport, *Scand. J. Gastroenterol. Suppl.,* 216:95–110, 1996.
9. Hamilton, J.R., The pathophysiological basis for viral diarrhea: a progress report, *J. Pediatr. Gastroenterol. Nutr.,* 11:P150–154, 1990.

10. Cummings, J.H., Colonic absorption: the importance of short chain fatty acids in man, *Scand. J. Gastroenterol. Suppl.*, 93:89–99, 1984.
11. Lifschitz, C.H., Carrazza, F.R., Feste, A.S., and Klein, P.D., In vivo study of colonic fermentation of carbohydrate in infants, *J. Pediatr. Gastroenterol. Nutr.*, 20:59–64, 1995.
12. Steed, K.P., Bohemen, E.K., Lamont, G.M., Evans, D.F., Wilson, C.G., and Spiller, R.C., Proximal colonic response and gastrointestinal transit after high and low fat meals, *Dig. Dis. Sci.*, 38:1793–1800, 1993.
13. Nordgaard, I., What's new in the role of colon as a digestive organ in patients with short bowel syndrome? *Nutrition*, 14:468–469, 1998.
14. Jeppesen, P.B. and Mortensen, P.B., Colonic digestion and absorption of energy from carbohydrates and medium-chain fat in small bowel failure, *J. Parenter. Enteral Nutr.*, 23:S101–S105, 1999.
15. Hyman, P.E., Everett, S.L., and Harada, T., Gastric acid hypersecretion in short bowel syndrome in infants: association with extent of resection and enteral feeding, *J. Pediatr. Gastroenterol. Nutr.*, 5:191–197, 1986.
16. Buchman, A.L., Scolapio, J., and Fryer, J., AGA technical review on short bowel syndrome and intestinal transplantation, *Gastroenterology*, 124:1111–1134, 2003.
17. Anderson, C.D. and Heimburger, D.C., Medical management of the difficult patient with short bowel syndrome, *Nutrition*, 9:536–539, 1993.
18. Rovera, G.M., Sigurdsson, L., Reyes, J., Bouch, L.D., Naylor, E.W., and Kocoshis, S.A., Immunoreactive trypsinogen levels in pediatric patients with intestinal failure awaiting intestinal transplantation, *Clin. Transplantation*, 13:395–399, 1999.
19. Tavakkolizadeh, A. and Whang, E.E., Understanding and augmenting human intestinal adaptation: a call for more clinical research, *J. Parenter. Enteral Nutr.*, 26:251–255, 2002.
20. Olesen, M., Gudmand-Høyer, E., Holst, J.J., and Jørgensen, S., Importance of colonic bacterial fermentation in short bowel patients. Small intestinal malabsorption of easily digestible carbohydrate, *Dig. Dis. Sci.*, 44:1914–1923, 1999.
21. Carbonnel, F., Cosnes, J., Chevret, S., Beaugerie, L., Ngô, Y., Malafosse, M., Parc, R., Le Quintrec, Y., and Gendre, J.P., The role of anatomic factors in nutritional autonomy after extensive small bowel resection, *J. Parenter. Enteral Nutr.*, 20:275–280, 1996.
22. Messing, B., Crenn, P., Beau, P., Boutron-Ruault, M.C., Rambaud, J-C., and Matuchansky, C., Long-term survival and parenteral nutrition dependence in adult patients with the short bowel syndrome, *Gastroenterology*, 117:1043––1050, 1999.
23. Higham, S.E. and Read, N.W., Effect of ingestion of fat on ileostomy effluent, *Gut*, 31:435–438, 1990.
24. Jeppesen, P.B. and Mortensen, P.B., Intestinal failure defined by measurements of intestinal energy and wet weight absorption, *Gut*, 46:701–706, 2000.
25. Awouters, F., Megens, A., Verlinden, M., Schuurkes, J., Niemegeers, C., and Janssen, P.A.J., Loperamide. Survey of studies on mechanism of its antidiarrheal activity, *Dig. Dis. Sci.*, 38:977–995, 1993.

4 Abnormalities in Fluid and Electrolyte Absorption in Intestinal Failure

Andrew Ukleja and James S. Scolapio

CONTENTS

Intestinal failure as a result of short bowel syndrome (SBS) encompasses a spectrum of metabolic disturbances.[1] Fluid and electrolyte imbalance is one of the major complications and a cause of morbidity in patients with SBS.[2-3] Fluid and electrolyte abnormalities result clinically in dehydration, diarrhea, and rapid weight loss. Correction of fluid and electrolyte imbalance is especially important immediately after massive bowel resection. The degree of water and electrolyte disturbances is affected by numerous factors, including a more extensive small bowel resection, resection of the ileocecal valve, colon removal, and disease of the remaining intestine. Intestinal resections are followed by a process of compensatory intestinal hypertrophy

0-8493-1803-3/05/$0.00+$1.50

and adaptation with continuous improvement in the ability of the remaining intestine to absorb fluids, electrolytes, and nutrients.[4-6] This chapter focuses on the pathophysiologic effects that an extensive bowel resection has on fluid and electrolyte absorption and correction of these abnormalities after intestinal failure.

NORMAL INTESTINAL FLUID AND ELECTROLYTE TRANSPORT

Under normal circumstances, 99% of fluids and ions presented in the ingested food and gastrointestinal secretions are absorbed. During a 24-hour period, 8 to 10 liters (L) of water enter the proximal small intestine. Typically, about 2 L of water come from ingested food and drinks. The other 7–8 L per day are derived from the endogenous secretions of the gastrointestinal tract: saliva (1 L), gastric juice (2 L), pancreatic secretions (2 L), bile (1–1.5 L) and small bowel secretions (1–2 L). The endogenous secretions provide the necessary pH, salts, aqueous medium, and osmolarity for the efficient digestion of nutrients and co-absorption of fluids and electrolytes. In a normal setting, approximately 600 ml/day of water reaches the colon, and about 100–200 ml/day of water is lost in feces.[7-8]

The intestine has the ability to adjust to a wide range of luminal compositions and volumes. Fluid absorption is dependent on the nature of the ingested meal. The electrolyte composition of the bowel content changes as it progresses down the intestine. For example, in patients with lactose intolerance after massive bowel resection, luminal osmotic load is not dissipated, resulting in net water shift from the blood into the intestine lumen. The intestinal mucosa has the capacity to recognize and respond to alterations in intramural and systemic conditions. Acute changes in serum sodium and water balance will stimulate rapid shift of fluid and electrolytes in the intestine.

Absorption and secretion of water and electrolytes occurs in the two different regions of intestinal mucosa.[9] Villous cells serve as the primary sites for absorption, and crypt cells are the predominant sites for secretion. To provide efficient water and ion absorption and secretion, mucosal transport, capillary flow, lymphatic function, absorption, and filtration must be coordinated. Many luminal, mucosal, motor, and circulatory factors are involved in modulation and regulation of fluid and electrolyte transport. Hormones, neurotransmitters, and paracrine substances involved in the intestinal transport of water and electrolytes are shown in Table 4.1.

Depending on the location of bowel resection, secretion of hormones and peptides will be affected. For example, gastrin-, cholecystokinin (CCK)-, and secretin-producing cells are present in the proximal small bowel, while neurotensin-containing cells are mainly restricted to the ileum. Opioid peptides, including enkephalins, stimulate the absorption of sodium, chloride, and water.

In case of plasma volume expansion, water is shifted into the intestinal lumen by passive filtration. Adrenergic stimulation plays an important role in dehydration and hypovolemia. Volume contraction results in adrenergic stimulation with catecholoamine release.[10-11] The other mechanism in hypovolemia involves stimulation of renin-angiotensin axis.[12] Angiotensin enhances absorption of sodium and water in the jejunum.[13] Aldosterone stimulates water and sodium absorption, potassium

TABLE 4.1
Neurohumoral Mediators Regulating Intestinal Water and Electrolyte Transport [82–88]

Origin	Action	
	Prosecretory	Proabsorptive
Mucosal epithelial cells		
	Gastrin	Somatostatin
	Guanylin	
	Neurotensin	
	Serotonin	
Lamina propria cells		
	Arachidonic acid metabolites	
	Bradykinin	
	Histamine	
	Platelet-activating factor	
Enteric neurons		
	Acetylcholine	Norepinephrine
	Serotonin	Neuropeptide Y
	Substance P	
	VIP	
Blood		
	VIP	Corticosteroids
	Calcitonin	Epinephrine
	Prostaglandins	Mineralocorticoids
	Atrial natriuretic peptides	Angiotensin

secretion in the colon, and to a lesser degree, in the ileum, in response to dehydration. Aldosterone has a similar effect on water and electrolytes transport in the kidneys. Glucocorticoids release enhances absorption of sodium and water, and potassium secretion in the colon.

Intestinal mucosa functions, digestion, and transport are coordinated with changes in bowel motility.[14–15] Normal intestinal motility, that is, mixing and propulsive activity, ensures the proper absorption of water, ions, and nutrients. The relationship between intestinal water and ions transport and intestinal motility is very complex.[16] It has been shown that enteric reflexes coordinate intestinal water and electrolyte secretion with smooth muscle contraction.[17] Slowing of the propulsive motor activity is the major mechanism of action for antidiarrheal agents in short bowel syndrome.

PATHOPHYSIOLOGY OF INTESTINAL FAILURE

This section focuses on mucosal function and effects of bowel resection on electrolyte and fluids movements. The effect of intestinal resection on absorption of fluids and electrolytes will depend on both the extent and the site of resection. Reduction of functional absorptive surface area and rapid transit time of intestinal content are seen after massive resection of the small bowel. This will reduce contact time between luminal nutrients and pancreatic and biliary secretions, limiting fluid and ions absorption contributing to the severity of diarrhea.

STOMACH

Gastric emptying studies have shown that the emptying of fluids from the stomach was faster than normal in patients with a very short length of jejunum ending at a jejunostomy, whereas solids emptying was at a normal rate. These findings were not observed in patients with colon in continuity, even with very short length of residual jejunum.[18]

DUODENUM

Very little net water absorption occurs in the duodenum. The duodenum is highly water-permeable, and very large fluxes of water occur in both directions from bowel lumen to blood and the opposite. As a result of hypertonicity of duodenal content, net water flux occurs from blood to duodenal lumen, thus allowing rapid osmotic equilibration of intestinal content with serum. It has been shown in healthy subjects that food is diluted 2–3 times by salivary, gastric, biliary, and pancreatic secretions when it reaches the distal duodenum.[19] In patients with intestinal failure, distal resections are more common. Thus, duodenal function is typically preserved.

JEJUNUM

A large volume of fluid absorption takes place in the small intestine. The jejunum is more active in absorbing water than the ileum. Water movement in response to an osmotic gradient has been shown to be nine times greater in the jejunum than in the ileum.[19] Water absorption generally results from the passive movement of water across the epithelial membrane in response to osmotic and hydrostatic pressure.[20-21] Ions are the most important contributor to osmotic pressure in the intestinal lumen. In general, jejunal luminal content tends to remain isotonic with plasma because of the relative permeability of the mucosal membrane. The jejunum differs from the ileum and colon in its handling of water and sodium. Sodium absorption in the upper jejunum can take place only against a small concentration gradient, as it is dependent on water movement. It is coupled with the absorption of glucose and some amino acids.[22] Movement of sodium into the lumen occurs when the luminal sodium concentration is low. In a perfusion study, absorption from the intestinal content occurred only if sodium concentration was at least 90 mmol/L, and secretion into the lumen occurred when its concentration was lower.[23] The maximal jejunal absorption of sodium from a bowel occurs when sodium concentration is around 120 mmol/L.[24] Nutrients such as glucose and amino acids promote water and sodium absorption by solvent drag.[25-26] Monovalent ions are absorbed in larger quantities when compared with divalent ions. Sodium absorption is active in the jejunum and occurs at the highest rate compared to other segments of intestine. Na^+ is absorbed along the entire length of the intestine. Na^+ absorption is enhanced by the presence

TABLE 4.2
Transport of Na$^+$, K$^+$, Cl$^-$ and HCO$_3^-$ in the Small and Large Bowels

Segment of Bowel	Sodium	Potassium	Chloride	Bicarbonate
Jejunum	Active absorption	Passive absorption	Absorption	Absorption
Ileum	Active absorption	Passive absorption	Absorption, partly in exchange for HCO$_3^-$	Secretion, partly in exchange for C$^-$
Colon	Active absorption	Net secretion when (K$^+$) concentration in lumen <25 mEq	Absorption, partly in exchange for HCO$_3^-$	Secretion, partly in exchange for Cl$^-$

of glucose, galactose, and neutral amino acids. Na$^+$ crosses the brush border membrane down the electrochemical gradient by the Na$^+$/K$^+$ - ATP-ase. For movement of other electrolytes, see Table 4.2.

Drinking water (or a dilute sodium solution with a concentration of less than 60–90 mmol/L) by a healthy subject results in sodium secretion into the lumen during the passage of the drink through the duodenum and upper jejunum in response to the concentration gradient. Then, secreted sodium is absorbed during the passage through the distal small bowel and colon. In a patient with a jejunostomy, secreted sodium is lost because the sodium concentration of jejunostomy output is remarkably constant at about 90 mmol/L. Thus, patients with a high jejunostomy who drink water (or fluids with low sodium content) literally wash sodium out of their body. Balance studies in patients with a high jejunostomy have shown that drinking isotonic glucose-sodium solutions leads to sodium loss when its concentration was < 60 mmol/L and to sodium absorption when it was 90 mmol/L or more.[27] Patients with a high-output jejunostomy should, therefore, restrict their intake of water and dilute sodium solutions or substitute glucose-electrolyte replacement solutions for them. This is the experimental base for glucose-electrolyte replacement solutions used in short bowel syndrome.[28]

In the proximal small bowel, water absorption follows sodium and nutrient absorption. Most other electrolytes are absorbed by simple diffusion down a concentration gradient.[29] Potassium absorption in the jejunum is exclusively passive, with net flux from lumen to blood. Potassium absorption in the small intestine is a consequence of its enhanced concentration in the lumen due to the absorption of water. Both chloride and bicarbonate are absorbed in large amounts in the jejunum. Chloride is normally absorbed passively and by Na$^+$/Cl$^-$ co-transport. Most of bicarbonate from pancreatic and hepatic secretions is absorbed in the jejunum.[30] (See Table 4.2.)

The proximal small bowel is a site for the release of hormones such as gastric inhibitory peptide (GIP) and vasoactive intestinal peptide (VIP), cholecystokinin, and serotonin.[31–33] Therefore, it is not surprising that gastric hypersecretion is more likely to occur after proximal versus distal intestine resection.[34] Gastric acid damages intestinal mucosa and inactivates digestive enzymes, leading to a reduction of protein and lipid digestion. This stimulates peristalsis and impairs further fluid absorption. A reduction in secretion of CCK and secretin results in reduced gallbladder contraction and pancreatic secretions.

Resections of jejunum are less common than ileal resections. Permanent defect in the absorption macronutrients and electrolytes is rarely seen with jejunectomy and preserved ileum due to the capacity of the ileum to take over all the absorptive functions.

Ileum

The luminal content becomes more concentrated in the ileum because its mucosa has lower permeability than jejunum. Resection of terminal ileum may destroy the ileal brake, resulting in rapid transit of luminal content as well as fluid and electrolyte loss. Ladefoged et al. has shown that intestinal sodium loss and sodium depletion were not related to the length of small bowel resection, indicating that sodium absorption and homeostasis are within wide ranges and they are unaffected by the length of bowel resection.[35] Excessive fecal losses of sodium and water, very high plasma aldosterone levels, and a urinary sodium excretion of less than 5 mmol/24 hours have been shown in patients with small bowel resections and ileostomy.

Sodium/chloride cotransport is the main mechanism for NaCl absorption in the ileum. Sodium is cotransported with bile salts in the terminal ileum. In the distal ileum, chloride absorption depends on HCO_3-dependent chloride absorption. Bicarbonate is usually secreted in the distal small bowel. However, if bicarbonate concentration is high in the ileum, its net absorption occurs. Sodium absorption is exclusively passive in the ileum.[36]

Irreversible loss of bile salts is associated with distal ileum resection more than 100 cm. In the ileum, 90% of conjugated bile salts are absorbed and enter enterohepatic circulation. If the ileum is resected or diseased, bile salts absorption is impaired, resulting in a significant loss of fecal bile salts. Non-absorbed bile acids cause irritation of the colon mucosa, leading to watery diarrhea.[37-38] As a consequence of bile salt depletion, concentration of bile salts in the small bowel lumen will decrease, leading to impairment of fat absorption. Therefore, in patients with colon in continuity, steatorrhea from fat malabsorption due to bile salt depletion aggravates fecal losses of fluid and electrolytes.

Ileocecal Valve

The ileocecal valve prolongs transit time, allowing increased contact time of luminal nutrients with the mucosal surface. This indirectly affects water and electrolytes absorption. In the absence of ileocecal valve, colonic bacteria can reflux into the small bowel, increasing the risk of bacterial overgrowth in the small bowel. This can lead to deconjugation of bile acids that cause chloride secretion by the colonic mucosa and further compromise fluid absorption.

Colon

The main function of the colon is absorption of the fluids entering from the ileum. In an adult, 0.5-1.5 L of fluid is absorbed by the colon each day.[39] The colon has a great capacity for fluid and electrolyte absorption with net maximum for water 5–6 L, 700 mmols of sodium, and 40 mmols of potassium per day.[40-41] In contrast to the small bowel, colon fluid is usually hypertonic (300–400 mOsm/L) to plasma because of the relative impermeability of the colon to water and the continued production of solutes by colonic bacteria.[42-43] Impaired absorption of fluids and electrolytes in the small bowel can overwhelm the absorptive capacity of the colon and lead to severe electrolyte deficiencies.[44] The total amount of sodium and potassium absorption in the colon is lower than in the small intestine.

In the proximal colon, sodium absorption is based on Na^+/Cl^- co-transport. In the distal colon, sodium is absorbed against a large electrochemical gradient via amiloride-sensitive sodium channels and Na^+/Cl^- co-transport. Potassium can be absorbed or secreted depending on its luminal concentration. In the rectosigmoid colon, active potassium absorption takes place predominantly by potassium/hydrogen exchange. In the colon, potassium net secretion is predominant. Moreover, the colon plays an important role in excretion of potassium and bicarbonate. Metabolic acidosis (normal anion gap or hyperchloremic) may arise as a result of excessive bicarbonate loss.

Both bile salts and free fatty acids can alter the ability of the colon to absorb water and sodium. Certain forms of fiber and carbohydrates can be degraded by colonic bacteria into titratible acids, which can increase osmotic load and alter the absorption of water and electrolytes.[45]

The colon has the slowest motility of the intestine, and its absence increases the rate of transit. Preservation of colon is very important after extensive small bowel resection due to not only providing bowel length but also affecting intestinal transit. Fluid losses are less severe with the colon in continuity. Patients with at least half of the colon are able to maintain a normal sodium homeostasis.[35]

The colon continuity is highly desirable. However, its presence may be associated with certain complications.[46] The presence of colon in continuity may result in diarrhea, lactic acidosis, and formation of calcium oxalate renal stones. Deconjugation of bile salts to free bile acids by colonic bacteria stimulates water and electrolyte secretion, causing choleretic diarrhea. Diarrhea may be so severe that colectomy may be required.

Lactase deficiency may develop as a result of small bowel resection, leading to hyperosmolarity of intestinal content. This can impair fluid and electrolyte absorption.[47-48] Unabsorbed carbohydrates, which escaped small intestinal absorption, produce osmotic diarrhea and can rarely cause severe anion-gap metabolic acidosis as a result of conversion of these carbohydrates to D-lactate by lactobacillus bacteria. D-lactic acid accumulates, leading to D-lactic acidosis, characterized by hyperchloremia, an elevated anion gap, and elevated serum and urinary D-lactate.[49] Clinically, patients present with headache, drowsiness, ataxia, blurred vision, and behavioral changes.

Patients with colons in continuity are at risk for oxalate nephrolithiasis and interstitial fibrosis.[46] Hyperoxaluria is frequently present in the patients with ileal resections due to increased oxalate absorption in the colon. Two mechanisms are involved in formation of oxalate renal stones. Fat malabsorption in the short bowel results in calcium binding to lumenal fatty acids first instead of to oxalate. This prevents a formation of insoluble calcium oxalate and allows free oxalate to be absorbed in the colon. The other mechanism involves increased oxalate absorption because of altered colon permeability due to excessive bile salts and fatty acids. Chronic interstitial changes in the kidneys can worsen electrolyte disturbances by leading to salt-losing nephropathies.[50]

CLINICAL CONSEQUENCES OF SEGMENTAL INTESTINAL RESECTION

Fluid and electrolyte losses depend on length of bowel resection and its site. Proximal small bowel resections rarely result in severe diarrhea, because the ileum and colon have a large capacity to absorb excess of fluid and electrolytes. Lactose intolerance and malabsorption of calcium, magnesium, and iron are common complications of proximal resections. If both the colon and ileum are resected, the remaining bowel cannot concentrate the lumenal content, leading to dehydration, hypokalemia, and hypomagnesemia. This is called end-jejunostomy syndrome.

Patients with end-jejunostomy experience severe disturbances in fluid and electrolyte balance because of rapid emptying of liquids and insufficient residual absorptive surface to recover unabsorbed fluid and electrolytes. Patients with only 60–100 cm of intact jejunum tend to have a large stoma output. Unabsorbed fluids may also flush out nutrients and lead to a substantial degree of steatorrhea. Severe sodium depletion associated with hypovolemia and prerenal azotemia is characterized by low plasma volume, low urine sodium, and an elevated plasma level of aldosterone. The most common cause for end-jejunostomy is extensive ileocolectomy for Crohn's disease. Other conditions include mesenteric ischemia, radiation enteritis, diverting jejunostomy for fistula, or anastomotic leak. Common causes of end-ileostomy are colectomy for ulcerative colitis, radiation enteritis, and colon cancer. Ileum is able to compensate for absorptive functions if jejunum is removed. On the other hand, the ileum cannot compensate for the reduced levels of jejunal inhibitory enterohormones, such as GIP and VIP after jejunal resection. During the adaptation phase, which begins with a few weeks after resection and may last 1–2 years, stabilization of fluid and electrolytes is expected. Distal resections induce greater adaptive responses than proximal resections, with ileum having better capacity for adaptation. [51-52]

MANAGEMENT OF FLUID AND ELECTROLYTE LOSSES

Maintaining fluid and electrolyte homeostasis is often difficult in patients who have undergone massive intestinal resection. Aggressive replacement of fluids and electrolytes is necessary to reduce life-threatening sodium depletion and dehydration.

Treatment strategies include parenteral supplements, altering the diet, slowing intestinal transit, and sipping glucose-electrolyte solutions. Extremely poor absorption of water, electrolytes, and all other nutrients is seen during the early postoperative period. Replacement of fluid and electrolytes is the key factor in the early phase of short bowel in order to achieve optimal outcome. In patients with a jejunostomy and output exceeding 3 or 4 L/day, it is difficult to replace this loss with an oral supplement. In patients with high-output jejunostomies, high levels of plasma aldosterone secondary to sodium depletion are suggestive of insufficient parenteral saline infusion. To screen for sodium depletion, sodium concentration in urine should be measured. In difficult cases, the simple balance studies may be of benefit in assessing the absorptive capacity of the residual intestine. The volume of stoma output gives a good estimate of intestinal sodium loss since the concentration in ileostomy effluents varies within a narrow range.

PARENTERAL FLUID AND ELECTROLYTES

Fluid loss from the gastrointestinal tract tends to be the greatest during the first days after a massive bowel resection. Ostomy output can exceed 5 L/day, with sodium losses of 270–360 mmol/day.[35] Severe dehydration may result in hemodynamic instability, hypotension, and renal failure. Intravenous replacement is invariably required initially. Vital signs, intake and output, central venous pressure, and electrolyte measurements should be monitored to evaluate rapid metabolic changes. If acute sodium depletion occurs with pre-renal uremia and hypotension, urgent intravenous replacement with at least 3–4 L of normal saline is needed over 2–3 days before attempting to maintain balance with oral supplements of water and sodium. Patients with urine output less than 1 L/d are at risk of developing renal dysfunction and should receive intravenous fluids. Judicious supplementation of salts and fluids will help to restore sodium homeostasis. A correction of prerenal azotemia, increase in body weight, and increase in renal sodium excretion are seen with restoration of fluid and electrolyte balance.

PARENTERAL NUTRITION

The inability of the bowel to adequately absorb fluids, electrolytes, and nutrients early in the course of intestinal failure requires immediate nutritional support with parenteral nutrition. Parenteral nutrition (PN) can be initiated on the second or third postoperative day, after cardiopulmonary stabilization. Many patients need to infuse the equivalent of 2–3 L of normal saline intravenously each night, with or without nutrients; some patients need parenteral electrolyte and fluid replacement alone and can meet their nutrition needs with oral supplements. Those patients receiving PN require potassium at 60–100 mmol daily as part of the nutrient solution. Patients who need a parenteral electrolyte supplement alone rarely need the addition of potassium.

In patients with a stoma and bowel length less than 100 cm, the stoma output after a meal tends to be greater than that of the meal consumed, due to dilution by exocrine secretions. Thus, there is a net loss of fluid and sodium from the body resulting from this negative intestinal balance.[53] Such patients need parenteral supplements. In patients with a remaining small bowel of 100 cm or less, PN is essential for survival. Patients with less than 50 cm of jejunum will require PN permanently even with functional colon.[54–55] Some of the patients with a jejunostomy and small bowel length less than 100 cm may maintain adequate nutrition with parenteral supplementation of water, electrolytes, and minerals. PN should be tapered gradually with an increasing rate of enteral feeding and decreasing volume of intestinal fluid losses. Initially, the volume of PN should be reduced to 1 L day and then the frequency of PN administration should be reduced to every other day, every third day, etc., until the desired goal is achieved.

ENTERAL FLUIDS AND ORAL REHYDRATION SOLUTIONS

Enteral feeding is always preferred due to the stimulation of adaptation and the prevention of fluctuation in fluid balance. It is essential to start enteral nutrition as soon as possible. A patient with a very short length of bowel and high stoma output may need to stay off enteral nutrition for several weeks after a large resection to avoid further increase in stomal output and fluid loss.[56–57] Patients with extreme short bowel should avoid eating large portions of food or unrestricted foods such as fatty foods, concentrated sweets, sugar (osmotic diarrhea), fiber, and dairy products, such as milk (lactose intolerance) since they may increase fluid losses and stoma output.[58–60]

The patient should be discouraged from drinking plain water if he or she has difficulty maintaining a water and electrolyte balance.

Most patients with a jejunostomy need a supplement of water and sodium to compensate for high stomal losses.[46] Those patients with losses less than 2 L daily can usually compensate with an oral rehydration solution (ORS). In patients with excessive fluid losses, sipping of glucose-electrolyte ORS may be able to reduce stoma loss and improve electrolyte absorption.[61–62] This approach allows for optimal active sodium absorption and subsequent water absorption by solvent drag.[25] ORS should contain at least 90 mMol/L of sodium to improve absorption of water and electrolytes. The optimal sodium concentrations in ORS for maximum sodium absorption have been suggested to be between 90 and 120 mMol. Different formulas are commercially available.[63] (See Table 4.3.) Most common compositions, made up to 1 L with tap water, include: sodium chloride 60 mmol (3.5 g), sodium bicarbonate 30 mmol (2.5 g), glucose 110 mmol (20 g), or sodium chloride 120 mmol (7.0 g), glucose 44 mmol (8.0 g). Sodium bicarbonate can be replaced by sodium citrate to improve palatability and absorption.[64] Replacement of glucose by its polymer does not result in increased sodium absorption.[65] One or two liters of ORS sipped at intervals daily is usually adequate. Camilleri et al. has shown that hypo-osmolar sipping solution can maintain fluid homeostasis in patients with SBS.[66] A high concentration of glucose is not desired because an increase in the osmolarity of fluids will result in impaired water absorption and diarrhea. Sport drinks have suboptimal electrolyte-glucose composition and should not be substituted for ORS

TABLE 4.3
Compositions of Selected Oral Rehydration Solutions

Products	Content					
	Sodium mEq/L	Potassium mEq/L	Chloride mEq/L	Citrate mEq/L	Osmolarity mOsm/L	Glucose g/L
Ceralyte 50	50	20	98	30	<220	40
Ceralyte 70	70	20	98	30	235	40
Ceralyte 90	90	20	98	30	260	40
Equalyte	78	22	68	30	305	25
Pedialyte	45	20	35	30	300	20
Rehydralate	74	19	64	30	305	25
WHO	90	20	80	30	200	20
Washington University	105	0	100	10	250	20

in patients with SBS. Compositions of sport drinks and common beverages for comparison with ORS are shown in Table 4.4.

Another option is to use salt capsules containing 8.5 mmol of sodium (500 mg of NaCl), given with food, since sodium absorption is coupled with glucose and amino-acids. Absorption is equivalent to ORS, but the amount of salt that can be taken in this way is limited by palatability.[65]

The concentration of potassium in jejunostomy fluid is an average 15 mmol/L. Intestinal potassium balance is usually positive unless the length of the small bowel is less than 60 cm.[53] Potassium supplements are rarely needed in patients with a short bowel, maintained on an oral diet.

DRUG THERAPY

Gastric antisecretory drugs have a special place in the initial phase after massive bowel resection. Large fluid losses from a jejunostomy are in part due to the dilution of food by gastric acid secretion. H_2-blockers have been shown to decrease jejunostomy output

TABLE 4.4
Comparison of Content of Selected Sport Drinks and Beverages

Product	Content					
	Sodium mEq/L	Potassium mEq/L	Chloride mEq/L	Base mEq/L	Osmolarity mOsm/L	Glucose g/L
Gatorade	22	3	27	0	333	40
Ceralyte sport	20	5	–	6	250	50
Apple juice	2	35	0	0	690	110
Ginger ale	3	3	0	0	540	55
Chicken broth	250	8	250	0	450	0

and improve the absorption of nutrients and fluids by reducing gastric acid production.[67] An H$_2$-blocker administered daily can decrease PN infusion requirements due to reduced fluid and sodium loss.[68] Omeprazole, a proton pump inhibitor, appears to be effective in this respect as well.[69] Octreotide, an analogue of somatostatin, decreases gastric, biliary, and pancreatic secretion, and it also slows gastrojejunal transit.[70] Octreotide has been shown to increase absorption of sodium, chloride, and water in the ileum and colon. Octreotide reduces jejunostomy volume and sodium loss in patients with negative intestinal balance.[71–72] Only those patients with the high jejunostomy output of more than 3 L daily may find it beneficial. There is no benefit for patients who are in positive intestinal balance. The beneficial effect of loperamide, codeine, and alpha 2-receptor agonist, clonidine has been related to a proabsorptive effect from increasing contact time between luminal fluid and absorptive surface.[73–76] Antidiarrheal drugs such as codeine phosphate or lopermide reduce the output from an ileostomy. Their benefit in patients with a jejunostomy is equivocal.[77–78] Balance studies have shown an important therapeutic effect of antidiarrheal drugs by decreasing fluid and sodium loss.[79–80] Usefulness of these drugs can be assessed by measuring jejunostomy output or stool numbers and daily weight. These drugs should be given about an hour before meals. Bulking agents do not appear to play a role in controlling jejunostomy output. [81] Their role in patients with a short bowel and colon in continuity is unknown. Cholestyramine, an ion-exchange resin, binds bile salts, and it is mainly used in malabsorption of bile salts, causing diarrhea without steatorrhea. Therefore, there is no role for the use of cholestyramine in the patients with an end-jejunostomy. Clinical settings for drug therapy are shown in Table 4.5. The management of diarrhea in SBS is reviewed in the third chapter of this book.

TABLE 4.5
Drugs Used to Slow Intestinal Transit and Reduce Fluid and Electrolyte Losses

Drug	Clinical Setting Stage after Bowel Resection
H-2 receptor blockers	Early phase
Ranitidine	
Famotidine	
Proton pump inhibitors	Early phase
Omeprazole	
Pentoprazole	
Rabeprazole	
Lansoprazole	
Codeine	Early phase/maintenance
Loperamide	Early phase/maintenance
Diphenoxylate/atropine	Early phase/maintenance
Octreotide	Adaptation phase, in high output ileostomy/jejunostomy
Bile acid sequestrants	Ileal resection <100cm, and colon in continuity
Cholestyramine	
Colestipol	

SUMMARY

Fluid and electrolyte homeostasis is critical in patients with intestinal failure. Close monitoring of fluids and electrolytes is important. Understanding basic physiology helps to manage and predict the degree of fluid and electrolyte losses. Balance studies may be helpful in more precise management of difficult patients with intestinal failure.

REFERENCES

1. Weser, E., Fletcher, J.T., and Urban, E., Short bowel syndrome, *Gastroenterology*, 77, 572, 1979.
2. Griffin, G.E. et al., Enteral therapy in the management of massive gut resection complicated by chronic fluid or electrolyte depletion, *Dig. Dis. Sci.*, 27, 902, 1982.
3. Ladefoged, K., Intestinal and renal loss of infused minerals in patients with severe short bowel syndrome, *Am. J. Clin. Nutr.*, 36, 52, 1982.
4. Althausen, T.L. et al., Digestion and absorption after massive resection of the small intestine, Part Two, *Gastroentereology*, 16, 126, 1950.
5. Porus, R.L., Epithelial hyperplasia following massive small bowel resection in man, *Gastroenterology*, 48, 753, 1965.
6. Dowling, R.H. and Booth, C.C., Functional compensation after small bowel resection in man, *Lancet*, 2, 146, 1966.
7. Billich, C.O. and Levitan, R., Effects of sodium concentration and osmolarity on water and electrolyte absorption from the intact human colon, *J. Clin. Invest.*, 48, 1336, 1969.
8. Phillips, S.F. and Giller, J., The contribution of the colon to electrolyte and water conservation in man, *J. Lab. Clin. Med.*, 81, 733, 1973.
9. Field, M., Pathways for ion and water movements across intestine: an overview, in *Intestinal secretion. Proceedings of the Third BSG, SK and F International Workshop*, Turnberg L.A., Ed., Smith, Kline and French, Philadelphia, 1983, ch. 1.
10. Tapper, E.J., Bloom, A.S., and Lewand, D.L., Endogenous norepinephrine release induced by tyramine modulates intestinal ion transport, *Am. J. Physiol.*, 241, G264, 1983.
11. Powell, D.W., Intestinal water and electrolyte transport, in *Physiology of the Gastrointestinal Tract, 2nd ed.*, Johnson, L.R., Ed. Raven Press, New York, 1987, 1267.
12. Levens, N., Control of intestinal absorption by the renin-angiotensin system, *Am. J. Physiol.*, 249, G3, 1985.
13. Levens, N.R., Modulation of jejunal ion and water absorption by endogenous angiotensin after hemorrhage, *Am. J. Physiol.*, 246, G634, 1984.
14. Womack, W.A. et al., Villous motility: relationship to lymph flow and blood flow in the dog jejunum, *Gastroenterology*, 94, 977, 1988.
15. Read, N.W. et al., Relationship between changes in intraluminal pressure and transmural potential difference in the human and canine jejunum *in vivo*, *Gut*, 18, 141, 1977.
16. Read, N.W., The relationship between intestinal motility and intestinal secretion, *Clin. Res. Rev.*, 1 (Suppl. 1), 73, 1981.
17. Sjovall, H., Hagman, I., and Abrahamsson, H., Relationship between interdigestive duodenal motility and fluid transport in humans, *Am. J. Physiol.*, 259, G348, 1990.

18. Nightingale, J.M.D. et al., Disturbed gastric emptying in the short bowel syndrome. Evidence for a "colonic brake," *Gut,* 34, 1171, 1993.

19. Fordtran, J.S. and Locklear, T.W., Ionic constituents and osmolality of gastric and small intestinal fluids after eating, *Am. J. Dig. Dis.,* 11, 503, 1966.

20. Field, M., Rao, M.C., and Chang, E.B., Intestinal water and electrolyte transport and diarrheal disease, *N. Engl. J. Med.,* 321, 800, 1989.

21. Armstrong, W.M., Cellular mechanisms of ion transport in the small intestine, in *Physiology of the Gastrointestinal Tract,* 2nd ed., Johnson, L.R., Ed., Raven Press, New York, 1987, 1251.

22. Fordtran, J.S., Rector, F.C. Jr., and Carter, N.W., The mechanisms of sodium absorption in the human small intestine, *J. Clin. Invest.,* 47, 884, 1968.

23. Spiller, R.C., Jones, B.J.M., and Silk, D.B.A., Jejunal water and electrolyte absorption from two proprietary enteral feeds in man: importance of sodium content, *Gut,* 28, 681, 1987.

24. Sladen, G.E. and Dawson, A.M., Inter-relationships between the absorptions of glucose, sodium and water by the normal human jejunum, *Clin. Sci.,* 36, 119, 1969.

25. Fordtran, J.S., Stimulation of active and passive sodium absorption by sugars in the human jejunum, *J. Clin. Invest.,* 55, 728, 1975.

26. Karasov, W.H. and Diamond, J.M., Adaptive regulation of sugar and amino acid transport by vertebrate intestine, *Am. J. Phisiol.,* 345, G443, 1983.

27. Rodrigues, C.A. et al., What is the ideal sodium concentration of oral rehydration solutions for short bowel patients?, *Clin. Sci.,* 74 (Suppl.18), 69, 1988.

28. Lennard-Jones, J.E., Oral rehydration solutions in short bowel syndrome, *Clin. Therap.,* 12 (Suppl. A), 129, 1990.

29. Turnberg, L. et al., Interrelationships of chloride, bicarbonate, sodium, and hydrogen transport in the human intestine, *J. Clin. Invest.,* 49, 557, 1970.

30. Minhas, B., Sullivan, S.K., and Field, M., Ileal HCO_3 secretion *in vitro.* Effects of Na^+ and Cl^-, *Gastroenterology,* 98, A548, 1990.

31. Schwartz, C.J. et al., Vasoactive intestinal peptide stimulation of adenylate cyclase and active electrolyte secretion in intestinal mucosa, *J. Clin. Invest.,* 54, 536, 1974.

32. Cassuto, J. et al., 5-Hydroxytryptamine and cholera secretion. Physiological and pharmacological studies in cats and rats, *Scand. J. Gastroenterol.,* 17, 695, 1982.

33. Cooke, H.J., Hormones and neurotransmitters regulating intestinal ion transport. in *Current topics in gastroenterology-diarrheal diseases,* Field, M., Ed., Elsevier, New York, 1991, 23.

34. Strause, E., Gerson, E., and Yalow, R.S., Hypersecretion of gastrin associated with the short bowel syndrome, *Gastroenterology,* 166, 175, 1974.

35. Ladefoged, K. and Olgaard K., Sodium homeostasis after small-bowel resection, *Scand. J. Gastroenterol.,* 20, 361, 1985.

36. Gustin, M.C. and Goodman, D.B.P., Isolation of brush border membranes from the rabbit descending colon epithelium. Partial characterization of a unique potassium-activated ATPase, *J. Biol. Chem.,* 256, 10651, 1981.

37. Ladefoged, K., Hessov, I., and Jarnum, S., Nutrition in short bowel syndrome, *Scand. J. Gastroenterol.,* 216 (suppl.), 122, 1996.

38. Vanderhoof, J.A. and Langnas, A.N., Short-bowel syndrome in children and adults, *Gastroenterology,* 113, 1767, 1997.

39. Scolapio, J.S. and Ukleja, A., Short-bowel syndrome, *Curr. Opin. Clin. Nutr. Metab. Care,* 1, 391, 1998.

40. Debongnie, J.C. and Phillips, S.F., Capacity of the human colon to absorb fluid, *Gastroenterology,* 74, 698, 1978.

41. Binder, H.J. and Rawlins, C.L., Electrolyte transport across isolated large intestinal mucosa, *Am. J. Physiol.*, 225, 1232, 1973.

42. Cummings, J.H., James, W.P.T., and Wiggins, H.S., Role of the colon in ileal-resection diarrhoea, *Lancet*, 1, 344–47, 1973.

43. Hylander, E., Ladefoged, K., and Jarnum, S., *Scand. J. Gastroenterol.*, 15, 55, 1980.

44. King, D.R., Does the colon adopt small bowel features in a small bowel environment?, *Aust. N. Z. J. Surg.*, 66, 543, 1996.

45. Mitchell, J.E., Brever, R.I., and Zucherman, L., The colon influences ileal resection diarrhea, *Dig. Dis. Sci.*, 25, 33, 1980.

46. Nightingale, J.M.D. et al., Colonic preservation reduces need for parenteral therapy, increases incidence of renal stones but does not change high prevalence of gall stones in patients with short bowel, *Gut*, 33, 1493, 1992.

47. Marteau, P., Do patients with short-bowel syndrome need a lactose-free diet?, *Nutrition*, 13, 13, 1997.

48. Arrigoni, E. et al., Tolerance and absorption of lactose from milk and yogurt during short bowel syndrome in man, *Am. J. Clin. Nutr.*, 60, 926, 1994.

49. Day, A.S., D-lactic acidosis in short bowel syndrome: a review, *N. X. Med. J.*, 112, 277, 1999.

50. Dobbins, J.W. and Binder, H.J., Effect of bile salts and fatty acids on the colonic absorption of oxalate, *Gastroenterology*, 70, 1096, 1976.

51. Scolapio, J.S. and Fleming, C.R., Short-bowel syndrome, *Gastroenterol. Clin. North Am.*, 27, 467, 1998.

52. Purdum, P.P. and Kirby, D.F., Short bowel syndrome: a review of the role of nutrition support, *JPEN*, 15, 93, 1991.

53. Nightingale, J.M.D. et al., Jejunal efflux in short bowel syndrome, *Lancet*, 336, 765, 1990.

54. Buchman, A.L., The clinical management of short bowel syndrome: steps to avoid parenteral nutrition, *Nutrition*, 13, 907, 1997.

55. Gouttebel, M.C. et al., Total parenteral nutrition needs in different types of short bowel syndrome, *Dig. Dis. Sci.*, 31, 718, 1986.

56. Ukleja, A., Tammela, L.J., Lankisch, M.R. et al., Nutritional support for the patient with short-bowel syndrome, *Curr. Gastroenterol. Rep.*, 1, 331, 1999.

57. Vanderhoof, J.A., Enteral and parenteral nutrition in patients with short-bowel syndrome, *Eur. J. Pediatr. Surg.*, 9, 214, 1999.

58. Woolf, G.M. et al., Diet for patients with a short bowel: high fat or high carbohydrate?, *Gastroenterology*, 84, 823, 1983.

59. Allard, J.P. and Jeejeebhoy, K.N., Nutritional support and therapy in the short bowel syndrome, *Gastroenterol. Clin. North Am.*, 18, 589, 1989.

60. Anderson, H., Isaksson, B., and Sjogren, B., Fat-reduced diet in the symptomatic treatment of small bowel disease, *Gut*, 15, 351, 1997.

61. Hill, G.L. et al., Long term changes in total body water, total exchangeable sodium and total body potassium before and after ileostomy, *Br. J. Surg.*, 62, 524, 1975.

62. Beaugerie, L. et al., Isotonic high-sodium oral rehydration solution for increasing sodium absorption in patients with short bowel syndrome, *Am. J. Clin. Nutr.*, 53, 769, 1991.

63. MacMahon, R.A., The use of the World Health Organization's oral rehydration solution in patients on home parenteral nutrition, *JPEN*, 8(5), 720, 1984.

64. Rolston, D.D.K. et al., Acetate and citrate stimulate water and sodium absorption in the human jejunum, *Digestion*, 34, 101, 1986.

65. Nightingale, J.M.D. et al., Oral salt supplements to compensate for jejunostomy losses: comparison of sodium chloride capsules, glucose electrolyte solution, and glucose polymer electrolyte solution, *Gut*, 33, 759, 1992.

66. Camilleri, M. et al., Balance studies and polymeric glucose solution to optimize therapy after massive intestinal resection, *Mayo. Clin. Proc.*, 67, 755, 1992.

67. Cortot, A., Fleming, C.R., and Malagelada, J.R., Improved nutrient absorption after cimetidine in short-bowel syndrome with gastric hypersection, *N. Engl. J. Med.*, 300, 79, 1979.

68. Jacobsen, O. et al., Effects of cimetidine on jejunostomy effluents in patients with severe short-bowel syndrome, *Scand. J. Gastroenterol.*, 21, 824, 1986.

69. Nightingale, J.M.D. et al., Effect of omeprazole on intestinal output in the short bowel syndrome, *Aliment. Pharmacol. Ther.*, 5, 405, 1991.

70. de Montigny, S. et al., Effect of a long acting analog of somatostatin (SMS 201-995) on water and electrolytes losses, nutrient absorption and gastrointestinal transit in short bowel syndrome, *Gastroenterology*, 100, A519, 1991.

71. Shaffer J.L. et al., Does somatostatin analogue (SMS201-995) reduce high output stoma effluent? A controlled trial, *Gut*, 29, A1432, 1988.

72. Ladefoged, K. et al., Effect of a long acting somatostatin analogue SMS 201-995 on jejunostomy effluents in patients with severe short bowel syndrome, *Gut*, 30, 943, 1989.

73. Theodorou, V. et al., Absorptive and motor components of the antidiarrheal action of loperamide: an *in vivo* study in pigs, *Gut*, 32, 1355, 1991.

74. Schiller, L.R. et al., Mechanism of the antidiarrheal effect of loperamide, *Gastroenterology*, 86, 1475, 1984.

75. Quito, F. and Brown, D., Jejunal proabsorptive actions of selective opiate agonists administered via the cerebral ventricles, *Neuropeptides*, 14, 39, 1989.

76. Schiller, L.R. et al., Studies of the antidiarrheal action of clonidine, Effect on motility and intestinal absorption, *Gastroenterology*, 89, 982, 1985.

77. Schiller, L.R. et al., Studies of the mechanism of the antidiarrheal effect of codeine, *J. Clin. Invest.*, 70, 999, 1982.

78. Burks, T., Mechanisms of opioid antidiarrheal therapy, in *Textbook of Secretory Diarrhea*, Lebenthal, E. and Duffey, M., Eds., Raven Press, New York, 1991, 409.

79. Burleigh, D.E., Loperamide but not morphine has anti-secretory effects in human colon, *in vitro, Eur. J. Pharmacol.*, 202, 277, 1991.

80. Remington, M., Fleming, C.R., and Malagelada, J.R., Inhibition of postprandial pancreatic and biliary secretion by loperamide in patients with short bowel syndrome, *Gut*, 23, 98, 1982.

81. Newton, C.R., Effect of codeine phosphate. Lomotil and isogel on ileostomy function, *Gut*, 19, 377, 1978.

82. Rodrigues, C.A. et al., The effects of octreotide, soy polysaccharide, codeine and loperamide on nutrient, fluid and electrolyte absorption in the short bowel syndrome, *Aliment. Pharmacol. Ther.*, 3, 159, 1989.

83. Ottaway, C.A., Neuroimmunomodulation in the intestinal mucosa, *Gastroenterol. Clin. North Am.*, 20, 511, 1991.

84. Krejs, G.J., Effects of somatostatin infusion on VIP-induced transport changes in the human jejunum, *Peptides*, 5, 271, 1984.

85. Hanglow, A.C., Bienenstock, J., and Perdue, M.H., Effects of platelet-activating factor on ion transport in isolated rat jejunum, *Am. J. Physiol.*, 257, G845, 1989.

86. Kellum, J.M. Jr. and Jaffee, B.M., Release of immunoreactive serotonin following acid perfusion of duodenum, *Ann. Surg.*, 184, 633, 1976.

87. Johnson, L.R., Regulation of gastrointestinal mucosal growth, *Physiol. Rev.,* 68, 456, 1988.
88. Pettersson, G.B. et al., In vitro studies of serotonin release from rat enterochromaffin cells:studies of gut serotonin release, *J. Surg. Res.,* 29, 141, 1980.

5 Metabolic and Nutritional Consequences of Intestinal Failure

Christopher C. Ashley

CONTENTS

Malnutrition is a broad concept referring to a deficit of individual or population nutritional resources relative to nutritional requirements for optimal growth and health. Worldwide, malnutrition is largely the result of socioeconomic factors, and its effects are felt most poignantly by the children of the developing world. The patient with intestinal failure and malnutrition represents an interesting contrast in that the typical patient is usually an adult in the industrialized world. Whatever the particular cause, the consequences of malnutrition are the same. These consequences are the subject of this chapter.

0-8493-1803-3/05/$0.00+$1.50

MALNUTRITION

Traditionally, *kwashiorkor* is a Ghanese term referring to the consequences of weaning a first infant so that a second may take the mother's milk. The first infant would receive a diet replete in calories but low in protein, leading to the observed clinical presentation of stunting, pot belly, anemia, edema, lethargy, skin depigmentation, hair loss or change in color, and wasting of lean body mass. The term *marasmus* is derived from the Greek *marasmos* meaning "to waste away" and has been used to refer to the clinical presentation of children who receive inadequate protein and total calories, resulting in both wasting and stunting without prominent retention of water. These conditions have been studied and described by Graham Hill.[1] Patients suffering from protein calorie malnutrition have been referred to as marasmic when marked deficits of total body fat and protein are present with only a modest increase in extracellular water. In these patients the plasma albumin is normal but acute-phase reactants are depressed. Patients with kwashiorkor, in contrast, are described as hypermetabolic but fat and protein stores are relatively well preserved. Total body water, total extracellular water, and total extracellular water in the lean body mass are all characteristically elevated while serum albumin is depressed. Those with both marasmus and kwashiorkor, or mixed-protein calorie malnutrition, suffer deficits of total body fat and protein with elevated total body water and depression of both serum albumin and acute-phase reactants. In the following discussion of malnutrition, the only distinction that will be made between forms of malnutrition in regard to the presence of protein calorie malnutrition or its absence.

The problems of malnutrition have been well known in the surgical patient since the correlation between malnutrition and poor surgical outcome was first pointed out in 1936 by Studley.[2] In this series of patients, who underwent surgery for peptic ulcer disease, those patients with greater than 20% preoperative weight loss had a postoperative mortality of rate of 33% versus those with less than 20% preoperative weight loss whose mortality rate was 3.5%. This first observation of increased surgical morbidity and mortality in the presence of malnutrition has been replicated by numerous authors over time. Studley's observation is germane to a broader population of patients because malnutrition exerts a number of deleterious effects on human physiology and is a component of many medical disorders. One classic study found 43% of general medical patients met the definition for protein calorie malnutrition by simple laboratory and anthropometric measurements.[3] Our specific knowledge about malnutrition in humans has been limited by the obvious ethical difficulties in conducting controlled trials in human subjects. Much of our understanding of starvation, malnutrition, and intestinal failure is the result of studies of populations of patients with eating disorders, victims of famine, bariatric surgical patients, and those with established intestinal failure. We do know that human physiology is remarkably resilient in the face of malnutrition. In a study of famine in Sudan, subjects were able to recover from body mass indices less than 10 kg/m^2 (18–26 normal range).[4] On the other hand, it should not be forgotten that, despite the existing technologies for specialized nutrition support, extremes of malnutrition eventually progress to the point that recovery becomes impossible. When indicated, nutrition support should be instituted aggressively and, if required for more than a few months in the face of permanent gastrointestinal disease, continued with the conviction that it has become a life-sustaining treatment in the same sense as dialysis in renal failure and mechanical ventilation in respiratory failure.[5]

INTESTINAL FAILURE

The natural consequence of failing to meet the total caloric requirements of the body is weight loss. Generally, this loss occurs gradually (1–2 lbs/wk). More rapid losses usually imply fluid losses and not major changes in lean body mass. A patient who was in robust health previously and whose intestinal function is impaired, whether from short length, inflammation, aperistalsis, or some other cause, will lose fat while lean body mass is preserved. The failure to preserve lean body mass in the face of a short, inflamed, or aperistaltic bowel defines intestinal failure. Weight loss without loss of lean body mass does not carry the same implications as weight loss with wasting of lean body mass. Although alarming to patients, families, and sometimes clinicians, progressive wasting of fat stores alone rarely has a clinical impact on the patient. Making the distinction between simple weight loss and evolving protein calorie malnutrition can be difficult. Identifying those patients who are at high risk for poor outcome due to malnutrition by clinical judgment, anthropometrics, laboratory measure, or functional test is essential to making good use of available techniques of specialized nutrition support to reduce the likelihood of complications in this difficult population.

PREDICTING THE RISK OF INTESTINAL FAILURE AND MALNUTRITION

Malnutrition from intestinal failure is the common end point of a myriad of etiological processes. Intestinal failure either develops abruptly, after a catastrophic insult to the gastrointestinal tract and extensive surgical resection, or over years, as a result of the progression of a chronic gastrointestinal disease. In the former situation, parenteral nutrition (PN) is almost always begun initially during the postoperative period so that close fluid and electrolyte balance can be maintained during a period of potentially difficult hemodynamic management. Ordinarily these patients have abundant nutritional reserves because of their previously normal gastrointestinal tract function. Within a few weeks it is usual for some degree of enteral support to be instituted, and then, over the next several months, strategies are developed to achieve the goal of gradually weaning the patient off PN as autonomous total enteral nutrition is restored. In the second situation, nutrition support is typically instituted in a stepwise fashion as gastrointestinal function becomes more tenuous over time due to the natural history of the underlying disease and/or repeated shortening of gut as a result of necessary surgical treatment of the underlying disease (e.g., in Crohn's disease). The nutritional management of these patients can be complicated because of their depleted nutritional state at baseline. In many cases there is considerable overlap between the two groups.

What conditions need to exist for intestinal failure and malnutrition to ensue? The simplest way in which malnutrition can result from intestinal failure is in an inability to adequately provide calories to meet the individual's basal metabolic requirements as well as those demands that may result from physical activity, inflammatory states, or postsurgical healing. In thinking about whether a patient will be able to meet his or her nutritional requirements, one should review the available data on which patients are at risk for needing total PN. Much work has been done to try to establish an objective means for evaluating intestinal function. Measures of intestinal length (on the antimesenteric border), quantification of nutrient absorption, and estimates of functional enterocyte mass using measures of plasma markers have been tried so that an accurate prediction can be made about the likelihood of needing long-term PN. Some generalizations can be made as a result of this work. The longer the remaining intestine, the better. The presence of a jejuno-ileo anastomosis is preferential to a jejuno-colic anastomosis, which is in turn preferential to an end jejunostomy. One study found that in a Cox regression analysis of 103 short bowel patients, remaining bowel length and the presence of a jejuno-ileal anastomosis correlated with intestinal sufficiency whereas end-jejunostomies were correlated with intestinal failure.[6] The "critical" lengths of remaining small bowel required to avoid permanent dependence upon PN (as determined by radiographic analysis) were >35 cm in patients with jejuno-ileal anastomosis, >60 cm in patients with jejuno-colic anastomosis, and >115 cm in patients with end jejunostomies. These objective measures are helpful in making an initial assessment of likelihood of progression to intestinal failure, but relationships in the gut are complex and not understood completely. The importance of the colon may be due in part to its role in hormonal feedback inhibition of gastric emptying, the so-called "colonic brake" described by Nightingale and colleagues, and to its role in short-chain fatty acid absorption and nitrogen conservation.[7–9]

Another approach to defining a threshold for malnutrition is to determine a level of wet and dry weight absorption necessary to stave off intestinal failure.[10] In one study, 45 patients on home PN were compared with 44 non-home PN patients who had either short bowel syndrome or malabsorption of 2 MJ/day. This latter group was selected intentionally to represent a group of patients who had borderline intestinal failure. In each group, both intake and output of dry weight (calories) and water were carefully recorded. The lower 5% of the confidence interval for the energy absorption in these non-home PN patients was taken as a cutoff for intestinal failure. This was calculated to be approximately 84% of the basal metabolic rate (as determined by the Harris-Benedict equation, see Table 5.1) for these patients, or 4.9 MJ/day.

Wet weight absorption in these patients was 1.4 kg/day. Those patients who were able to remain off PN showed a highly variable level of dry and wet weight absorption; expressed as a percentage of their basal metabolic rates, the ranges were 24%–86% and 23%–95%, respectively. In patients on PN, energy absorption varied from net secretion; in patients with very short guts, to complete absorption; in those with pseudo obstruction and insufficient oral intake. In the non-home PN group patients, if the subset whose absorption rates were under 50% was considered, the most common adaptive response used to avoid PN was hyperphagia. Caloric intake among these patients ranged between 200% and 400% of basal metabolic rate, or

TABLE 5.1
Harris-Benedict Equation

Basal Energy Expenditure =

For men:
  [66 + (13.7 x weight in kg) + (5 x height in cm) – (6.8 x age in years)] x stress factor
For women:
  [655 + (9.6 x weight in kg) + (1.7 x height in cm) – (4.7 x age in years)] x stress factor

Stress factor varies from 0.8 to 2.5 based on level of physiologic stress

---

between 10 and 24 MJ/day and 3 to 7 kg/day of wet weight. In the patient with intestinal failure on PN, nutrients and fluids are provided directly to the systemic circulation so support does not have to be so generous. However, due to the physiologic stress of recent surgeries or inflammatory states due to medical comorbidity (e.g., inflammatory bowel disease) and the possibility of preexisting malnutrition, the calories supplied to these patients are frequently more than would be predicted by the basal metabolic rate and level of patient activity alone. Fluid requirements are also frequently increased due to extraordinary losses from the gastrointestinal tract. The important point here is that the patient with intestinal failure does not necessarily require more calories than would otherwise be necessary. The fact of having a short gut does not create a hypermetabolic state. However, these patients commonly have many other reasons to require considerably more calories and free water than normal persons. The standard recommendation is for between 25 and 35 kcal/kg of lean body weight to be provided and absorbed. To accomplish this enterally in some patients with short bowel syndrome could require four times this amount while parenteral delivery of nutrients in the patient with established intestinal failure might be accomplished with just the recommended amount. Patients who are either malnourished or stressed may require additional calories, but care should be taken since these same groups of patients may not be prepared to utilize all the provided calories safely and have the potential to suffer from either refeeding syndrome or hyperglycemia, respectively.

Using markers of enterocyte metabolism is a relatively novel approach to the old problem of estimating risk of intestinal failure. A number of candidate compounds may eventually be explored but the work of Crenn focused on citrulline.[11] Fifty-seven patients with short gut were evaluated and followed for two years. Thirty-seven of the original patients were fully dependent on PN at the end of the study, and 20 were only transiently dependent. Postabsorptive measures of plasma citrulline were highly correlated with other measures of intestinal capacity — for example, net digestive capacity for protein and fat. More important, plasma citrulline was highly discriminatory between patients who would be permanently dependent on PN and those who would not. A cutoff of 20 micromoles/L of citrulline was studied and found to be 92% sensitive and 90% specific when used to identify patients who would be permanently dependent on PN. The related positive predictive value was 95% and the negative predictive value was 86%. This tool also compared very favorably with alternate measures of the likelihood of intestinal failure used by this group.

CONSEQUENCES OF MALNUTRITION

Whatever the anatomic predisposition, the final determination of the presence of intestinal failure and malnutrition is usually a clinical one. The consequences of malnutrition impact every organ system. In some cases the specific nutritional deficit is clearly understood. In other cases only the specific sign or symptom is recognized while the underlying etiologic mechanism remains obscure. Understanding the various manifestations of malnutrition is essential to recognizing the diagnosis and instituting the most appropriate therapy in a timely fashion.

NEUROPSYCHIATRIC

The neuropsychiatric consequences of malnutrition are well recognized. Foremost among the varied psychological manifestations of malnutrition is depression. Depression and anxiety have been well correlated with indices of disease activity and malnutrition in patients with inflammatory bowel disease.[12] The same correlation is also strong in those with malnutrition as their only identifiable problem.[13] Anorexia is well known to occur in undernourished and hypermetabolic patients with inflammatory bowel disease and to be well correlated with the level of their disease activity.[14] The disinhibited activity of inflammatory cytokines is related directly to the severity of anorexia in these patients. Preliminary data have associated alteration in pineal function with starvation and altered sleep cycles.[15]

PULMONARY

Alteration of ventilatory mechanics is a well-known consequence of undernutrition.[1] Respiratory muscle dysfunction and atrophy no doubt underlie the gross difficulties in weaning, cough, atelectasis, and infection that are encountered in the malnourished patient.[17–19] Not surprisingly, nutrition support has proved important in permitting ventilated patients to meet the metabolic demands of weaning.[20] Overnutrition can precipitate difficulty in ventilatory weaning by raising the respiratory quotient and creating additional work of breathing by raising pCO_2 and so prolonging the weaning process.[21] This latter phenomenon has been addressed by reducing carbohydrate as a proportion of total calories in provided specialized nutritional support.[22] The malnourished state has also been shown to suppress the hypoxic ventilatory drive by 42% as determined by Doekel et al.[23] This data was replicated years later and it was shown that keeping the patient in positive nitrogen balance was not sufficient to prevent suppression of the hypoxic drive, although hypercapneic drive was preserved despite starvation in both studies.[24]

An issue related to impaired ventilatory mechanics is the effect of starvation on skeletal muscle. In protein calorie malnutrition, early effects on muscle may result from cellular energy store (ATP) depletion. Eventually, muscle catabolism begins, which particularly impacts the population of type II skeletal muscle fibers.[16,25] Early improvement in muscular strength has been attributed to the repletion of cellular energy stores (ATP), while restoration of strength to baseline levels is slow and relates to the rate at which muscle bulk and type II fiber populations can be restored. Glycolytic enzyme activity in type II muscle fibers has been proposed as an explanation of wasting in cancer because enzymes are paradoxically not down-regulated.[26] The same activity has implications in insulin sensitivity as it relates to refeeding, where it may explain improvements in insulin sensitivity attributed to nutrition support, and exercise, where muscle metabolism of glucose is improved.[27,28]

CARDIAC

Sudden death has been described in a small cohort of 17 obese patients on prolonged protein-sparing diets (5 months) of 300–400 kcal/day implying arrhythmogenic potential of the malnourished state or diet.[29] Bradycardia and prolonged QT interval are well-described electrocardiographic phenomena associated with anorexia nervosa, as are wasting of ventricular mass, mitral valve prolapse, and pericardial effusion.[30–33] The most serious toxicity of the refeeding syndrome is related to the hypophosphatemia that results from the metabolic reactivation that occurs with the reintroduction of energetic substrate and regeneration of mitochondrial ATP, which results in an intracellular migration of phosphate.[34] Anorectic patients are known to have higher vagal tone than age-matched controls, which may potentiate some of the other known cardiac effects of malnutrition noted above.[35] Malnutrition may result in L-carnitine deficiency, which has been linked to heart failure by several investigators and has been proposed as a therapeutic agent even in the absence of measured deficiency because of its ability to enhance contractility and clear toxic metabolites that can accumulate in the face of ischemia.[36–38]

GASTROINTESTINAL

Starvation states have been shown to impact gut morphology and function.[39,40] Even in the presence of adequate PN, deprivation of enteral nutrition has been demonstrated to result in intestinal villous atrophy and increased mucosal permeability. These changes have been proposed as an etiologic explanation for the hypothesized bacterial translocation that had been used to explain gram negative septicemia that is known to occur in stressed and starved patients.[41] Glutamine was identified by Windmueller and Spaeth as the primary fuel for the enterocyte[42] and has been subsequently studied as a means of reversing the effects of the starved state on the gut with some success,[40] although its precise mechanism remains obscure.[43] Direct evidence of bacterial translocation has not been rigorously proved in humans, but the seriousness of its proposed consequences has generated much enthusiasm for enteral feeding to preserve intestinal integrity.[44] Loss of colonic mucosal integrity can result in a diarrheal state from impaired absorption of water and salt related to a lumenal deficiency of short-chain fatty acids.[45,46] Malnutrition can also result in diarrhea because of related dysmotility and bacterial overgrowth,[47] fat malabsorption from impaired pancreatic function,[48–52] or an increased incidence of symptomatic parasitic infection.[53] Although usually not a cause of diarrhea, gastric acid secretion has also been shown to be impaired in undernourished states.[54]

METABOLIC/ENDOCRINE

Insufficient caloric intake results in the body drawing on existing energy stores to supply the deficit and meet ongoing energy requirements. It is not surprising to find that malnutrition and short-term starvation has resulted in disorders of thermogenesis since energetic reserves may not be readily available in the face of cold stress.[55,56] Muscular and hepatic glycogen stores are the first to be depleted, and these are seldom adequate to provide for more than several hours of use. Fat stores are metabolized next, and this process results in the presence of ketones in the systemic circulation and urine. Protein and fat oxidation that results from the starvation state produces free water and creates an overexpansion of extracellular volume that protein depletion (negative nitrogen balance) and hypoalbuminemia exacerbate whether or not clinical edema is manifest.[16] Hyponatremia may be recognized in these patients, but it nearly always is the result of a primary expansion of the extracellular fluid volume.

BONE DENSITY

Malnutrition and reduced bone mineral density have been clearly correlated in a wide range of clinical entities. The acid-base milieu has been linked to osteoporosis and is particularly relevant in light of starvation ketosis, which is known to create defects in bone remodeling.[57,58] Malabsorption can result in wasting of calcium complexed with fat and deficiency of the fat soluble vitamins (particularly vitamin D, which can lead to osteomalacia)[59] and fatty acids, both of which may impair calcium absorption and promote osteoporosis.[60,61] Global undernutrition may also cause osteoporosis, as in anorexic women whose risk of fracture is known to be increased.[62,63] When anorexics are compared to women with hypothalamic amenorrhea, osteoporosis is most strongly correlated with lean body mass in the former group and with duration of amenorrhea in the latter group, indicating that there may be both nutritional and hormonal factors that influence bone density in women.[64] Another study found that in anorectic patients low lean body mass and duration of amenorrhea correlated best with the degree of observed osteopenia.[65] Animal studies have confirmed the role of both estrogen deficiency and protein calorie malnutrition in the etiology of osteoporosis.[66] Patients with celiac disease are also known to be at high risk for osteoporosis from malabsorption and secondary hyperparathyroidism.[67] In inflammatory bowel disease, risks of fat malabsorption (and associated increased fecal calcium loss), protein calorie malnutrition, and corticosteroid use are combined in one population and are known to be associated with osteoporosis.[68] Malnutrition interferes with bone mineralization on four levels: acid-base milieu, hormonal milieu, specific nutrient deficiencies, and protein calorie malnutrition. The mechanism for protein calorie restriction remains speculative but in animal models has been linked to lowered plasma levels of insulin-like growth factor-I, impaired cortical bone formation, and osteoblast resistance to IGF-I.[69]

Growth Retardation

Intrauterine malnutrition can result in growth retardation and low birth weight.[70] Ongoing malnutrition can cause physical and cognitive developmental delay, and this delay can become irreversible if it is not corrected in a timely fashion.[71] Furthermore, it is becoming clear that the repercussions of early growth delay from protein calorie malnutrition are more far-reaching than previously imagined.[72] The implications of prolonged periods of malnutrition during development and early life are thought to bear upon so-called physiologic switches regulating gene activation that are turned permanently "on" or "off" based on environmental cues. It is this phenomenon that has been used to explain the high prevalence of obese adult children of Danish women who were in their first trimester during the German occupation and starved; presumably "thrifty" gene switches were activated in response to the environment of starvation.[73] This association has also been made between intrauterine malnutrition and adult diabetes and cardiovascular risk.[74,75] More recently malnutrition during the first year of life has been linked to adult hyperglycemia and plasma insulin levels independent of body mass index.[76] The most common manifestation of malnutrition in children is growth delay. In one East African population, an anthropometric survey identified 44% of children as malnourished when compared with National Center for Health Statistics (NCHS) anthropometric standards.[77] This was particularly compelling because only 14% of these children were clinically diagnosed as malnourished because the prominent manifestation of malnutrition in these children was smaller stature alone, making the point that the consequences of malnutrition are not always obvious. Among those children who are malnourished, there is a direct relationship between degree of protein calorie malnutrition and growth stunting by several measures.[78] Furthermore, it is well recognized that sex hormone levels are suppressed in anorectic patients who exhibit growth retardation, puberty delay, infertility, and amenorrhea.[79–82] Various endocrinopathies (hypothalamic-pituitary axis, thyroid, etc.) related to protein calorie malnutrition have been reported and may relate to the growth retardation and developmental delay that is clinically familiar.

Impaired Healing

The observed defects of healing in patients with malnutrition occur either as a result of failure to repair an existing wound or spontaneous development of tissue breakdown. In either instance the usual mechanisms for tissue repair have been impaired. Surgical wounds that heal by primary intention frequently do so without complication, apparently having metabolic priority, but those that heal by secondary intention, open surgical wounds, burns, and decubitus ulcers strongly reflect the nutritional status of the patient, with malnourished patients exhibiting impaired or absent tissue granulation.[83] Indices of wound healing after surgery are not only impaired in the malnourished state[84] but recover with nutrition support, such as total parenteral nutrition. Problems with wound healing can be preempted by preoperative nutrition support.[85] Although preventive preoperative nutrition is preferable, there is some data to support use of postoperative support.[86–87] The relative benefits of enteral versus parenteral support continue to be debated although it is generally agreed that wherever possible enteral feeding should be used since some portion of enterocyte nutrition is derived directly from the lumen of the gut. The degree of patient malnutrition relates directly to risk for the development of pressure sores,[88–90] but the benefits of nutrition support have been relatively difficult to demonstrate in this setting. It is the complications in wound healing in patients with impaired immune response and impaired healing from malnutrition that are more easily shown.[91] A role for zinc in healing of pressure sores, vascular ulcers, and surgical wounds is suggested in the literature as well as for other factors: vitamin A, C, and E but the evidence for improvement of healing in the absence of deficiency is sparse.[92] The principal factor in impaired wound healing is protein calorie malnutrition.

IMPAIRED IMMUNE RESPONSE

Malnutrition can result in a generalized depression of the human immune response. The mechanisms by which this can occur include protein calorie malnutrition and a variety of specific nutrient deficiencies. In general, protein calorie malnutrition has the most clinically significant impact epidemiologically because it is a more widespread problem than specific nutrient deficiencies. B and T lymphocyte function is impaired in protein calorie malnutrition,[93] as is macrophage function,[94] capacity for antigen presentation,[95] antibody affinity,[96] and both secretory immunoglobulin levels[97] and complement activity[98] are diminished. The impact of these effects on host immuno-competence is well studied. Cell mediated and humoral arms of the immune response are impaired, although the former is thought to be more important in failing to protect against infection.[99] Increased rates of infections of the chest, urinary tract, gastrointestinal tract, and sepsis are known.[100–103] Data exist to support that the correction of malnutrition will quickly correct the underlying deficit in immune function.[104]

CONCLUSION

Although fundamental to any discussion of malnutrition, macronutrient deficit is only a part of the story. Fluid and electrolyte disturbances can have immediate life-threatening consequences to the malnourished patient and are discussed in some detail in Chapter 4. Vitamins, minerals, and trace element abnormalities can certainly impact the clinical course of many patients and are covered in Chapter 6. The bedside nutritional assessment can enable a clinician, who is cognizant of each patient's history (vis-à-vis their weight, dietary intake, and GI losses) and anatomy, to antic-ipate the multiorgan system consequences of malnutrition, and is discussed in Chapter 10. Bedside nutritional assessment remains an essential part of every patient's medical management, especially since nutrition support technologies are available widely that can provide total or partial support to at-risk persons. Nevertheless, the clinician's impulse to consider a patient's nutritional status remains the most impor-tant step in correcting and avoiding malnutrition in modern medical practice.

REFERENCES

1. Hill, G.L., Jonathan, E. Rhoads Lecture. Body composition research: Implications for the practice of clinical nutrition, *JPEN*, 16, 197, 1992.
2. Studley, H.O., Percentage of weight loss: A basic indicator of surgical risk in patients with chronic peptic ulcer, *JAMA*, 106, 458, 1936.
3. Bistrian, B.R. et al., Prevalence of malnutrition in general medical patients, *JAMA*, 235, 1567, 1976.
4. Collins, S., The limit of human adaptation to starvation, *Nat. Med.*, 1, 810, 1995.
5. Allison, S.P., Undernutrition, in *Intestinal Failure*, Nightingale, J., Ed., Greenwich Medical Media Ltd., London, 2001, chap. 13.
6. Carbonnel, F. et al., The role of anatomic factors in nutritional autonomy after extensive small bowel resection, *JPEN*, 20, 275, 1996.
7. Nightingale, J.M.D. et al., Colonic preservation reduces need for parenteral therapy, increases incidence of renal stones, but does not change high prevalence of gallstones in patients with a short bowel, *Gut*, 33, 1493, 1992.
8. Jeppesen, P.B. and Mortensen, P.B., The influence of a preserved colon on the absorption of medium chain fat in patients with small bowel resection, *Gut*, 43, 478, 1998.
9. Nordgaard, I., Mortensen, P.B., and Langkilde, A.M., Small intestinal malabsorption and colonic fermentation of resistant starch and resistant peptides to short-chain fatty acids, *Nutrition*, 11, 129, 1995.
10. Jeppesen, P.B. and Mortensen, P.B., Intestinal failure defined by measurements of intestinal energy and wet weight absorption, *Gut*, 46, 701, 2000.
11. Crenn, P. et al., Postabsorptive plasma citrulline concentration is a marker of absorptive enterocyte mass and intestinal failure in humans, *Gastroenterol.*, 119, 1496, 2000.
12. Addolorato, G. et al., Inflammatory bowel disease: A study of the association between anxiety and depression, physical morbidity, and nutritional status, *Scand. J. Gastroenterology*, 32, 1013, 1997.
13. Brozek, J., Bibliographical note on behavioral aspects: On the margin of the 50th anniversary of the Minnesota Starvation-Nutritional Rehabilitation experiment, *Percept. Mot. Skills*, 81, 395, 1995.
14. Bannerman, E. et al., Altered subjective appetite parameters in Crohn's disease patients, *Clin. Nutr.*, 20, 399, 2001.
15. Brown, G.M., Day-night rhythm disturbance, pineal function and human disease, *Horm. Res.*, 37, 105, 1992.
16. Hill, G.L., Jonathan E. Rhoads Lecture. Body composition research: Implications for the practice of clinical nutrition, *JPEN*, 16, 197, 1992.
17. Kelsen, S.G., Ference, M., and Kapoor, S., Effects of prolonged undernutrition on structure and function of the diaphragm, *J. Appl. Physiol.*, 58, 1354, 1985.
18. Arora, N.S. and Rochester, D.F., Respiratory muscle strength and maximal voluntary ventilation in undernourished patients, *Am. Rev. Respir. Dis.*, 126, 5, 1982.
19. Arora, N.S. and Rochester, D.F., Effect of body weight and muscularity on human diaphragm muscle mass, thickness and area, *J. Appl. Physiol.*, 52, 64, 1982.
20. Bassili, H.R. and Deitel, M., Effect of nutritional support on weaning patients off mechanical ventilators, *JPEN*, 5, 161, 1981.
21. DeMeo, M.T., Mobarhan, S., and van De Graaff, W., The hazards of hypercaloric nutritional support in respiratory disease, *Nutr. Rev.*, 49, 112, 1991.

22. al-Saady, N.M., Blackmore, C.M., and Bennett, E.D., High fat, low carbohydrate, enteral feeding lowers PaCO2 and reduces the period of ventilation in artificially ventilated patients, *Intensive Care Med.*, 15, 290, 1989.

23. Doekel, R.C. Jr. et al., Clinical semi-starvation: Depression of hypoxic ventilatory response, *N. Engl. J. Med.*, 295, 358, 1976.

24. Baier, H. and Somani, P., Ventilatory drive in normal man during semistarvation, *Chest*, 85, 222, 1984.

25. Church, J.M., Choong, S.Y., and Hill, G.L., Abnormalities of muscle metabolism and histology in malnourished patients awaiting surgery: Effects of a course of intravenous nutrition, *Br. J. Surg.*, 71, 563, 1984.

26. Church, J.M., Choong, B.Y., and Hill, G.L., Abnormal muscle fructose bisphosphatase activity in malnourished cancer patients, *Cancer*, 58, 2448, 1986.

27. Greenberg, G.R. et al., Effects of total parenteral nutrition on gut hormone release in humans, *Gastroenterology*, 80, 988, 1981.

28. Berger, M. et al., Effect of physical training on glucose tolerance and on glucose metabolism of skeletal muscle in anaesthetized normal rats, *Diabetologia*, 16, 179, 1979.

29. Sours, H.E. et al., Sudden death associated with very low calorie weight reduction regimens, *Am. J. Clin. Nutr.*, 34, 453, 1981.

30. Vanderdonckt, O. et al., The 12-lead electrocardiogram in anorexia nervosa: A report of 2 cases followed by a retrospective study, *J. Electrocardiol.*, 34, 233, 2001.

31. Romano, C. et al., Reduced hemodynamic load and cardiac hypotrophy in patients with anorexia nervosa, *Am. J. Clin. Nutr.*, 77, 308, 2003.

32. Schocken, D.D., Holloway, J.D., and Powers, P.S., Weight loss and the heart. Effects of anorexia nervosa and starvation, *Arch. Intern. Med.*, 149, 877, 1989.

33. Silverman, J.A. and Krongrad, E., Anorexia nervosa: A cause of pericardial effusions? *Pediatr. Cardiol.*, 4, 125, 1983.

34. Marik, P.E. and Bedigian, M.K., Refeeding hypophosphatemia in critically ill patients in an intensive care unit. A prospective study, *Arch. Surg.*, 131, 1043, 1996.

35. Petretta, M. et al., Heart rate variability as a measure of autonomic nervous system function in anorexia nervosa, *Clin. Cardiol.*, 20, 219, 1997.

36. Duran, M. et al., Secondary carnitine deficiency, *J. Clin. Chem. Clin. Biochem.*, 28, 359, 1990.

37. Martin, M.A. et al., Myocardial carnitine and carnitine palmitoyltransferase deficiencies in patients with severe heart failure, *Biochim. Biophys. Acta.*, 1502, 330, 2000.

38. Pauly, D.F. and Pepine, C.J., The role of carnitine in myocardial dysfunction, *Am. J. Kidney Dis.*, 41, S35, 2003.

39. Elia, M. et al., Effect of total starvation and very low calorie diets on intestinal permeability in man, *Clin. Sci. (Lond.)*, 73, 205, 1997.

40. Buchman, A.L. et al., Parenteral nutrition is associated with intestinal morphologic and functional changes in humans, *JPEN*, 19, 453, 1995.

41. Panigrahi, P. et al., Role of glutamine in bacterial transcytosis and epithelial cell injury, *JPEN*, 21, 75, 1997.

42. Windmueller, H.G. and Spaeth, A.E., Identification of ketone bodies and glutamine as the major respiratory fuels *in vivo* for postabsorptive rat small intestine, *J. Biochem. Chem.*, 253, 69, 1978.

43. Reeds, P.J. and Burrin, D.G., Glutamine and the bowel, *J. Nutr.*, 131, 2505S, 2001.

44. Lipman, T.O., Bacterial translocation and enteral nutrition in humans: An outsider looks in, *JPEN*, 19, 156, 1995.

45. Roediger, W.E., Famine, fiber, fatty acids and failed colonic absorption: Does fiber fermentation ameliorate diarrhoea?, *JPEN*, 8, 4, 1994.

46. Roediger, W.E. and Rae, D.A., Trophic effect of short chain fatty acids on the mucosal handling of ions by the defunctioned colon, *Br. J. Surg.* 69, 23, 1982.

47. Guerrant, R.L. et al., Mechanisms and impact of enteric infections, *Adv. Exp. Med. Biol.*, 473, 103, 1999.

48. Winter, T.A. et al., The effect of severe undernutrition, and subsequent refeeding on digestive function in human patients, *Eur. J. Gastroenterol. Hepatol.*, 12, 149, 2000.

49. Chowdhury, P. and Rayford, P.L., Effect of food restriction on plasma cholecystokinin levels and exocrine pancreatic function in rats, *Ann. Clin. Lab. Sci.*, 31, 376, 2001.

50. Fan, B.G., Axelson, J., Sternby, B. et al., Total parenteral nutrition affects the tropic effect of cholecystokinin on the exocrine pancreas, *Scand. J. Gastroenterol.*, 32, 380, 1997.

51. Sauniere, J.F. and Sarles, H., Exocrine pancreatic function and protein-calorie malnutrition in Dakar and Abidjan (West Africa): Silent pancreatic insufficiency, *Am. J. Clin. Nutr.*, 48, 189, 1988.

52. Sauniere, J.F. et al., Exocrine pancreatic function of children from the Ivory Coast compared to French children. Effect of kwashiorkor, *Dig. Dis. Sci.*, 31, 481, 1986.

53. Gendrel, D., Treluyer, J.M., and Richard-Lenoble, D., Parasitic diarrhea in normal and malnourished children, *Fundam. Clin. Pharmacol.*, 17, 189, 2003.

54. Winter, T.A. et al., Impaired pancreatic secretion in severely malnourished patients is a consequence of primary pancreatic dysfunction, *Nutrition*, 17, 230, 2001.

55. Mansell, P.I. et al., Defect in thermoregulation in malnutrition reversed by weight gain. Physiological mechanisms and clinical importance, *Q. J. Med.*, 76, 817, 1990.

56. Fellows, I.W. et al., The effect of undernutrition on thermoregulation in the elderly, *Clin. Sci. (Lond.)*, 69, 525, 1985.

57. Hahn, T.J., Halstead, L.R., and DeVivo, D.C., Disordered mineral metabolism produced by ketogenic diet therapy, *Calcif. Tissue Int.*, 28, 17, 1979.

58. Phelps, K.R. et al., Acidosis-induced osteomalacia: Metabolic studies and skeletal histomorphometry, *Bone*, 7, 171, 1986.

59. Driscoll, R.H., Jr. et al., Vitamin D deficiency and bone disease in patients with Crohn's disease, *Gastroenterology*, 83, 1252, 1982.

60. Lo, C.W. et al., Vitamin D absorption in health subjects and in patients with intestinal malabsorption syndromes, *Am. J. Clin. Nutr.*, 42, 644, 1985.

61. Hay, A.W. et al., Essential fatty acid restriction inhibits vitamin D-dependent calcium absorption, *Lipids*, 15, 251, 1980.

62. Rigotti, N.A., Nussbaum, S.R., Herzog, D.B. et al., Osteoporosis in women with anorexia nervosa, *N. Engl. J. Med.*, 311, 1601, 1984.

63. Rigotti, N.A. et al., The clinical course of osteoporosis in anorexia nervosa. A longitudinal study of cortical bone mass, *JAMA*, 265,1133, 1991.

64. Grinspoon, S. et al., Severity of osteopenia in estrogen-deficient women with anorexia nervosa and hypothalamic amenorrhea, *J. Clin. Endocrinol. Metab.*, 84, 2049, 1999.

65. Jacoangeli, F. et al., Osteoporosis and anorexia nervosa: Relative role of endocrine alterations and malnutrition, *Eat. Weight Disord.*, 7, 190, 2002.

66. Ammann, P. et al., Protein undernutrition-induced bone loss is associated with decreased IGF-I levels and estrogen deficiency, *J. Bone Miner. Res.*, 15, 683, 2000.

67. Selby, P.L. et al., Bone loss in celiac disease is related to secondary hyperparathyroidism, *J. Bone Miner. Res.*, 14, 652, 1999.

68. Lichtenstein, G.R., Management of bone loss in inflammatory bowel disease, *Semin. Gastrointest. Dis.*, 12, 275, 2001.

69. Bourrin, S. et al., Dietary protein restriction lowers plasma insulin-like growth factor I (IGF-I), impairs cortical bone formation, and induces osteoblastic resistance to IGF-I in adult female rats, *Endocrinol.*, 141, 3149, 2000.

70. Khan, N. and Jamal, M., Maternal risk factors associated with low birth weight, *J. Coll. Physicians Surg. Pak.*, 13, 25, 2003.

71. Stoch, M.B. and Smythe, P.M., 15-Year developmental study on effects of severe undernutrition during infancy on subsequent physical growth and intellectual functioning, *Arch. Dis. Child*, 51, 327, 1976.

72. Hales, C.N. and Ozanne, S.E., The dangerous road of catch-up growth, *J. Physiol.*, 547, 5, 2003.

73. Stein, Z., *Famine and human development: The Dutch hunger winter of 1944-45*, Oxford University Press, New York, 1975.

74. Wolf, G., Adult type 2 diabetes induced by intrauterine growth retardation, *Nutr. Rev.*, 61,176, 2003.

75. Barker, D.J. et al., Fetal nutrition and cardiovascular disease in adult life, *Lancet*, 341, 938, 1993.

76. Gonzalez-Barranco, J. et al., Effect of malnutrition during the first year of life on adult plasma insulin and glucose tolerance, *Metabolism*, 52, 1005, 2003.

77. van Leth, F.C., Koeleman, J.M., and Manya, A.S., Malnutrition: More than the eye can see, *E. Afr. Med. J.*, 77, 549, 2000.

78. Sathy, N. et al., Growth faltering and developmental delay in children with PEM, *Indian Pediatr.*, 28, 255, 1991.

79. Modan-Moses, D. et al., Stunting of growth as a major feature of anroexia nervosa in male adolescents, *Pediatrics*, 111, 270, 2003.

80. Delemarre-van de Waal, H.A., van Coeverden, S.C., and Engelbregt, M.T., Factors affecting onset of puberty, *Horm. Res.*, 57, 15, 2002.

81. Tomova, A. and Kumanov, P., Sex differences and similarities of hormonal alterations in patients with anorexia nervosa, *Andrologia*, 31, 143, 1999.

82. Ayers, J.W. et al., Osteopenia in hypoestrogenic young women with anorexia nervosa, *Fertil. Steril.*, 41, 224, 1984.

83. Howard, L. and Ashley, C., Nutrition in the perioperative patient, *Annu. Rev. Nutr.*, 23, 263, 2003.

84. Haydock, D.A. and Hill, G.L., Impaired wound healing in surgical patients with varying degrees of malnutrition, *JPEN*, 10, 550, 1986.

85. Haydock, D.A. and Hill, G.L., Improved wound healing response in surgical patients receiving intravenous nutrition, *Br. J. Surg.*, 74, 320, 1987.

86. Schroeder, D. et al., Effects of immediate postoperative enteral nutrition on body composition, muscle function, and wound healing, *JPEN*, 15, 376, 1991.

87. Delany, H.M. et al., Effect of early postoperative nutritional support on skin wound and colon anastomosis healing, *JPEN*, 14, 357, 1990.

88. Ek, A.C., Prediction of pressure sore development, *Scand. J. Caring Sci.*, 1, 77, 1987.

89. Ek, A.C., Prevention, treatment and healing of pressure sores in long-term care patients, *Scand. J. Caring Sci.*, 1, 7, 1987.

90. Myers, S.A. et al., Consistent wound care and nutritional support in treatment, *Decubitus*, 3, 16, 1990.

91. Shukla, V.K. et al., Correlation of immune and nutritional status with wound complications in patients undergoing abdominal surgery, *Am. Surg.*, 51, 442, 1985.

92. Thomas, D.R., Specific nutritional factors in wound healing, *Adv. Wound Care*, 10, 40, 1997.

93. Cariomagno, M.A. et al., T and B lymphocyte function in response to a protein-free diet, *Infect. Immun.*, 38, 195, 1982.
94. Reynolds, J.V. et al., Impairment of macrophage activation and granuloma formation by protein deprivation in mice, *Cell. Immunol.*, 139, 493, 1992.
95. Conzen, S.D. and Janeway, C.A., Defective antigen presentation in chronically protein-deprived mice, *Immunology*, 63, 683, 1988.
96. Chandra, R.K., Chandra, S., and Gupta, S., Antibody affinity and immune complexes after immunization with tetanus toxoid in protein-energy malnutrition, *Am. J. Clin. Nutr.*, 40, 131, 1984.
97. Reddy, V., Raghuramulu, N., and Bhaskaram, C., Secretory IgA in protein-calorie malnutrition, *Arch. Dis. Child*, 51, 87, 1976.
98. Suskind, R. et al., Complement activity in children with protein-calorie malnutrition, *Am. J. Clin. Nutr.*, 29, 1089, 1976.
99. Stiehm, E.R., Humoral immunity in malnutrition, *Fed. Proc.*, 39, 3093, 1980.
100. Kaushik, P.V. et al., Nutritional correlates of acute respiratory infections, *Indian J. Matern. Child Health*, 6, 71, 1995.
101. Bagga, A. et al., Bacteriuria and urinary tract infections in malnourished children, *Pediatr. Nephrol.*,18, 366, 2003.
102. Hagel, I. et al., Defective regulation of the protective IgE response against intestinal helminth Ascaris lumbricoides in malnourished children, *J. Trop. Pediatr.*, 49, 136, 2003.
103. Friedland, I.R., Bacteriaemia in severely malnourished children, *Ann. Trop. Paediatr.*, 12, 433, 1992.
104. Vasquez-Garibay, E. et al., Effect of renutrition on natural and cell-mediated immune response in infants with severe malnutrition, *J. Pediatr. Gastroenterol. Nutr.*, 34, 296, 2002.

6 Nutrition Assessment

Neha Parekh

CONTENTS

Optimal nutritional health is an intricate balance between nutrient intake, absorption, and requirement. In intestinal failure, various physiologic, socioeconomic, and psychological stressors compromise the maintenance of this nutritional equilibrium. Although adequate nutrient intake may be preserved, malabsorption is inherent to the disease and can lead to significant nutrient deficiency over a relatively short period of time. Insufficient funds, lack of family support, generalized weakness, uncontrolled pain, and varying levels of depression are common contributors to noncompliance or poor response to therapy in this population. In addition, nutrient requirements are elevated when faced with active disease states, infection, postsurgical stress, or general need for repletion. Treatment of the patient with intestinal failure should thus involve a thorough evaluation of nutritional status.

Despite the abundance of clinical data surrounding the use of subjective and objective assessment tools to identify malnutrition, no single measure has been proven to be both cost-efficient and effective in all patients. This is in part due to the fact that readily available measures such as anthropometrics and serum proteins are frequently distorted by the parallel influences of malnutrition and disease on body composition and function.[1] Nonnutritional factors interfering with the predictive ability of nutrition assessment techniques include, but are not limited to, errors in measurement, narrowly defined standards for comparison, and alterations in fluid balance in response to illness and injury. The use of more precise assessment methods such as dual energy x-ray absorptiometry or *in vivo* neutron activation analysis is mainly reserved for research purposes due to cost and space constraints.[2] The most appropriate tools and methods of assessment vary with the purposes for conducting the evaluation and the type of patient being evaluated. This chapter will address several components of nutrition assessment that clinicians may find useful in attaining one or more of the following goals:[3]

1. Uncover nutrient deficiencies and evaluate need for repletion.
2. Collect the data necessary for formulation of a nutrition plan of care.
3. Assess adherence to or monitor response to medical and/or nutrition therapy.
4. Evaluate surgical risk and determine need for preoperative nutrition intervention.

COMPONENTS OF NUTRITION ASSESSMENT

A comprehensive nutrition assessment includes four main components: historical background, physical examination, anthropometric studies, and biochemical analysis. Within each category are numerous subcategories of both subjective and objective nutrition assessment techniques. The advantages and drawbacks of each are discussed with a special emphasis on the potential applications of each method in the assessment of the intestinal failure patient.

HISTORICAL BACKGROUND

Information obtained from a detailed history contributes to a more accurate assessment of nutritional status. It prompts the clinician to investigate areas of possible

---

TABLE 6.1
Components of a Nutrition-Focused Historical Assessment [18, 82, 83]

- Clinical History
  - Present and previous illnesses or trauma interfering with nutritional status
  - Diagnostic tests evaluating organ function
  - Chronic diseases and/or surgical procedures affecting the GI tract
  - Length of the remaining small and large intestine and presence of the ileocecal valve
  - Location of any GI tubes, surgical drains, stomas, or fistulas
- History of Present Illness
  - Chewing or swallowing problems
  - Pain, nausea, or vomiting surrounding oral intake
  - Changes in appetite, satiety level, or taste of foods or fluids
  - Changes in urinary or bowel habits
  - Presence of fever, chills, or myalgias
  - Usual level of activity with any remarkable changes
- Diet History
  - Diet restrictions, aversions, or allergies
  - Intake of commercial and/or nonconventional nutritional supplements
  - Enteral, parenteral, oral rehydration, or intravenous fluid and electrolyte regimens
- Medication Usage
  - Vitamin, mineral or herbal supplements
  - Appetite stimulants or suppressants
  - Common to intestinal rehabilitation: antidiarrheals, histamine receptor antagonists, somatostatin analogues, proton pump inhibitors, pancreatic enzymes, bile acid therapy, probiotics, and fiber supplementation
  - Allergies to medications, enteral or parenteral nutrition components, or medical supplies
- Psychosocial Information
  - Altered mental states including depression, anxiety, and confusion
  - Low education and/or income levels
  - Drug or alcohol addiction
  - Absence of social support

---

deficit and forms the basis for a more focused physical examination.[4] The historical portion of nutrition assessment is divided into clinical history, history of present illness, diet history, medication usage, and psychosocial information (Table 6.1).

Clinical History

Gathering data for a clinical history begins with a thorough review of the patient's medical record. However, this information is not always complete or accurate. The patient should be interviewed to provide a more comprehensive picture. Speaking directly with former healthcare providers can help to confirm the data and fill in any missing information. Configuration of the patient's gastrointestinal (GI) tract is often useful in understanding the extent of GI dysfunction. Operative records and directed questions to the surgeon can help to construct an accurate diagram.

History of Present Illness

The onset and duration of the patient's current health problem provides a more recent picture of changes in GI function that may possibly alter nutritional status. An investigation of recent weight changes should start with the weight maintained over the longest period of time in good health. This is considered the usual body weight. Changes from that point are evaluated based on highest or lowest deviation from the usual weight during the onset of present illness. Weight fluctuations are common in bowel disease due to side effects of corticosteroid therapy and dehydration. It is especially important to note any consistently significant increase or decrease in GI losses via stomas, drains, tubes, or fistulae.

Diet History

A record of past and present patterns of nutritional intake can provide valuable information for assessment of nutritional status and formulation of a treatment plan. Nutrient deficiencies are uncovered with relative certainty when an accurate dietary intake record is compared with carefully estimated daily requirements. An evaluation of oral intake against GI losses can assist the clinician in determining whether an adjustment in fluid provisions, antidiarrheals medications, or dietary composition is required. However, the assessment of dietary patterns may be skewed by high intra-individual variability in food intake, frequent withholding of intake for diagnostic testing or surgical procedures, or inaccurate reporting of intake at the patient or caregiver level.[5]

Many different methods of dietary assessment are documented in the literature. In working with the intestinal failure patient both in the clinical and outpatient setting, two techniques seem to stand out as the most useful. The first is a modified Burke-type dietary history in which the patient is asked to verbally report all foods and beverages consumed on a usual day.[6] The clinician then asks probing questions to ascertain the frequency and amounts of consumption of specific foods or food groups. If the patient is made to feel comfortable with the clinician in a nonjudgmental atmosphere, this line of questioning can reveal information regarding compliance with therapy. The second method is a 24- to 72-hour nutrient intake record (NIR). This technique is most often used in the clinical setting to evaluate the adequacy of all food and beverages consumed while transitioning from one feeding modality to another (i.e., from parenteral to oral nutrition). Either the patient or a caregiver can be responsible for recording the data for an NIR; however, instruction must be provided on delineating portion sizes.

An experienced registered dietitian can assess the adequacy of overall energy, protein, fluid, and micronutrient intake based on information obtained from a thorough diet history. Gastrointestinal losses and increased requirements secondary to level of stress should be taken into consideration. An interpretation of findings should be provided with comments on deficiency, estimated requirements, and possible methods for repletion (Table 6.2).

TABLE 6.2
Daily Macronutrient Requirements in Intestinal Failure [84-87]

- Total Calories
  - For the patient of normal weight for height [a]: 25 to 35 kcal/kg actual weight.
  - For the underweight [a] patient: 35 to 45 kcal/kg ideal body weight. [a]
  - For the obese or overweight [a] patient: 15 to 20 kcal/kg actual weight.
  - For the patient with fever or sepsis: Add 5 to 10 kcal/kg actual weight.
  - For the metabolically stressed patient: Begin with 10 to 20 kcal/kg dry weight. Increase as tolerated to goals for stable patient as stress subsides.
- Protein
  - For the normal weight, overweight or obese [a] patient…
    - With average GI losses: 1.0 to 1.5 g/kg actual weight
    - With excessive GI losses: 1.5 to 2.0 g/kg actual weight
    - With metabolic stress: 1.5 to 2.0 g/kg dry weight
  - For the underweight [a] patient…
    - With average GI losses: 1.0 to 1.5 g/kg ideal body weight [a]
    - With excessive GI losses: 1.5 to 2.0 g/kg ideal body weight [a]
    - With metabolic stress: 1.5 to 2.5 g/kg ideal body weight [a]

[a] See Table 6.4 for interpretation of weight for height by body mass index (BMI) and ideal body weight (IBW).
Dry weight = Weight free of fluid retention

Medication Usage

A list of the patient's pertinent prescription and over-the-counter medications is obtained for review. Recent use of corticosteroids, narcotics, immunosuppressants, chemotherapy, antidiarrheals, laxatives, somatostatin analogues, diuretics, and antibiotics should be noted. Each of these medications is capable of exerting significant effects on bowel function, fluid balance, and nutritional status depending on dosage and duration of use.[7]

Psychosocial Information

The maintenance of adequate nutrient intake and compliance with nutrition therapy is often altered in the patient with social, economic, or psychological deficits. This can significantly affect an individual's ability to participate in his or her own nutritional care. For those receiving specialized nutrition therapy, it is important to ensure the patient's ability to obtain and safely administer the therapy as directed. In general, the psychosocial portion of the interview should be used to ascertain areas of need and involve the appropriate ancillary medical staff for assistance with managing these issues.

TABLE 6.3
Physical Signs of Macronutrient and Micronutrient Deficiency[4,18]

- Protein
  - Mental confusion, hyperirritability, apathy
  - Thinning, dull, easily pluckable hair
  - Edema, anasarca
  - Delayed wound healing, decubitus ulcers
  - Hepatomegaly in stress-induced hypoalbuminemia
  - Decreased baseline temperature
- Protein-energy
  - Dry, dull hair
  - Hollowed cheeks
  - Mottled teeth with cavities
  - Loss of balance
  - Muscle weakness and overall wasting
- Essential fatty acids
  - Xerosis (scaly, flaky dermatitis of the extremities)
  - Thrombocytopenia
  - Follicular hyperkeratosis
  - Dry, dull hair
- Thiamine (Vitamin B-1)
  - Wernicke's-Korsakoff encephalopathy
  - Peripheral neuropathy
- Cobalamin (Vitamin B-12)
  - Megaloblastic anemia
  - Pernicious anemia
- Folic Acid
  - Pancytopenia
  - Glossitis
  - Stomatitis
- Ascorbic Acid (Vitamin C)
  - Perifollicular hyperkeratosis
  - Hemorrhage
- Vitamin A
  - Night blindness
  - Bitot's spots
  - Hyperkeratosis of skin
- Vitamin D
  - Osteomalacia
  - Rickets
- Vitamin E
  - Hemolytic anemia
  - Neuropathy
- Vitamin K
  - Bleeding
  - Increased prothrombin time (PT)

(continued)

TABLE 6.3
Physical Signs of Macronutrient and Micronutrient Deficiency[4,18] (Continued)

- Iron
  - Hypochromic microcytic anemia
  - Weakness
  - Cheilosis
- Zinc
  - Apathy
  - Hair loss
  - Reduced wound healing
  - Dysgeusia
- Copper
  - Microcytic hypochromic anemia, leukopenia, neutropenia
  - Menke's syndrome
- Chromium
  - Glucose intolerance
  - Peripheral neuropathy
  - Metabolic encephalopathy
- Selenium
  - Dilated cardiomyopathy
  - Keshan's disease
  - White nails

PHYSICAL ASSESSMENT

A nutrition-focused physical examination is valuable in the detection of nutritional deficiencies or excesses that may not be as apparent with the use of other readily available assessment methods. Physical examination can also provide verification of information uncovered during the medical chart review and patient interview.

Signs of Macro- and Micronutrient Deficiency

Common physical signs of macronutrient and micronutrient deficiencies are listed in Table 6.3. Bodily tissues that are rapidly proliferating (i.e., hair, skin, nails, oral cavity, and eyes) tend to respond more promptly to nutrient deficiencies than other tissues.[8] Thin, dry, easily pluckable hair can signify protein or protein-calorie deficiency, whereas dryness, scaling, or roughened bumps of the skin may indicate essential fatty acid deficiency. Protein deficiency is also observed with excessive bruising, edema, or delayed wound healing.

The most obvious physical markers of chronic protein-calorie deficiency are temporal or skeletal muscle wasting and loss of subcutaneous fat in the face, triceps, thighs, and waist. Body composition studies have shown that profound protein depletion, or greater than 30% loss of total body protein stores, is signaled when the tendons are prominent to palpation.[9] Body mass of patients whose skin can be felt when pinching the triceps and biceps skinfolds between finger and thumb is estimated to be composed of only 10% to 13% fat.[9]

Fluid Balance

Surgical stress or chronic malabsorption can lead to severe hypoalbuminemia and fluid retention presenting as edema, ascites, or anasarca. Dehydration due to substantial fluid loss via gastric suctioning, vomiting, diarrhea, and fistula or wound drainage is physically detected by assessing skin turgor. Physical findings should be integrated with daily weight changes, laboratory values, intake and output records, and appearance of urine and stool to ascertain overall fluid balance.

Gastrointestinal Function

The functional capacity of the patient's GI tract is evaluated using techniques of inspection, auscultation, percussion, and palpation. Bowel sounds, level of abdominal distention, and presence of tenderness is assessed to rule out ileus or bowel obstruction. Data from the physical assessment of bowel function should be combined with radiologic and laboratory tests along with a history of early satiety, postprandial pain, nausea, vomiting, flatus, diarrhea, or constipation to provide a comprehensive evaluation of GI function.

Muscle Function

Deficits in muscle function have been linked to nutritional depletion and higher incidences of postoperative complications among hospitalized patients.[10–12] Muscle function as assessed by ulnar nerve stimulation has been shown to respond more quickly to nutritional repletion than measures of body composition or serum proteins.[10] The deterioration in muscle function assessed by handgrip strength was found by Klidjian et al. to have higher prognostic value for postsurgical complications than anthropometrics or serum albumin levels.[11]

Several methods exist for the assessment of muscle function in the hospital and outpatient setting. One of the more simple functional tests for alert and cooperative patients is grip strength, which is measured with a small, portable handgrip dynamometer. Handgrip dynamometry was able to predict 90% of patients developing postoperative complications among those undergoing major elective abdominal surgery.[13] A grip strength below 85% of standard for age and sex was found by Webb et al. to be the most specific predictor of postoperative risk;, however, research has yet to show the benefits of preoperative nutrition support in the at-risk population.[14] Handgrip strength was also found to be significantly less in chronically energy-deficient and underweight young males as compared to those who were well nourished but underweight or of normal weight status.[15] This implies a potential use of grip strength in the differentiation of patients with similar weights but conflicting nutritional status.

Stimulation of the ulnar nerve with an electrical impulse is used to assess the force of contraction and rate of relaxation of the abductor pollicis muscle as another measure of muscle function. Muscle function measured by ulnar nerve stimulation responds quickly to nutritional repletion. However, studies have shown that the positive response may be more related to restoration of fluid and electrolyte balance rather than body nitrogen repletion.[16,17]

The assessment of pulmonary function provides evidence of possible fluid overload, increased energy requirements, and diminished muscle strength. Labored respirations or respiratory rates exceeding 20 breaths per minute may be indicative of increased energy expenditure.[18] Severe impairment of respiratory muscle strength is present when the patient is unable to move a strip of paper held 10 cm from the lips with a forceful exhalation.[19] An appraisal of muscle function can also be accomplished through a survey of the patient's general activity level, including exercise tolerance, energy capacity, and ability to perform activities of daily living.

Immune Function

The adverse effects of malnutrition on cell-mediated immune function are well documented in the literature.[20,21] Delayed hypersensitivity skin testing (DHST) is a measure of cellular immunity involving the intradermal injection of antigens to elicit induration. The absence of a response is classified as anergy, or significant impairment of immune function. Although nutritional repletion may reverse immunosuppression in the anergic patient, the value of skin testing for use in nutrition assessment remains questionable.[22] In a comparison of skin testing to clinical judgment, the use of skin testing alone was not able to predict increased morbidity or mortality in postoperative gastrointestinal cancer patients.[23] Several common nonnutritional factors, including infection, illness, and medications, can alter the results of DHST, rendering it a nonspecific measure of nutritional status in the hospitalized patient.[24] Skin testing is best applied to nutrition assessment when nonnutritional factors leading to the development of anergy are excluded.[25]

ANTHROPOMETRY AND BODY COMPOSITION ANALYSIS

Indirect Measures

The use of anthropometry to indirectly quantify body composition for nutrition assessment dates back to the nineteenth century.[26] Measures of body height, weight, skinfolds, and circumference are simple anthropometric parameters traditionally used to reflect body composition, classify nutritional status, and predict surgical risk. Several methods are available to interpret body weight for a given height (Table 6.4). Likewise, standards exist to estimate deficits in muscle mass and fat stores from mid-arm circumference (MAC) and triceps skinfold (TSF) measurement.[27] The validity and reproducibility of these interpretations depend on an accurate weight history, calibrated equipment, well-trained observers, applicable standards of reference, and the maintenance of near-normal hydration status.[28]

Despite these limitations, the use of traditional anthropometric parameters for nutrition assessment is supported by the research. A preoperative loss of more than 20% body weight was associated with a significantly higher postoperative mortality rate than a preoperative loss of less than 20% body weight in a 1936 study of elective gastric resection patients.[29] Windsor and Hill in 1987 found that a preoperative loss

TABLE 6.4
Interpretation of Body Weight Data [61,88–90]

- Percentage of Usual Body Weight (UBW)[61, 88]

  - $\% \text{ UBW} = \dfrac{\text{actual weight}}{\text{UBW}} \times 100$

    - Interpretation: 85% to 95% UBW mild malnutrition
      75% to 84% UBW moderate malnutrition
      0% to 74% UBW severe malnutrition
- Percentage of Weight Lost over Time [88]

  - $\% \text{ weight loss} = \dfrac{\text{UBW–actual weight}}{\text{UBW}} \times 100$

  - Interpretation:

Time	Severe Weight Loss
1 week	> 2%
1 month	> 5%
3 months	> 7.5%
6 months	> 10%

- Ideal Body Weight (IBW) [89] and Percentage of IBW[61, 88]
  - IBW for Men = 106 lb for 5 feet in height plus 6 lb for each additional inch of height
  - IBW for Women = 100 lb for 5 feet in height plus 5 lb for each additional inch of height

  - $\% \text{ IBW} = \dfrac{\text{actual weight}}{\text{IBW}} \times 100$

  - Interpretation: 80% to 90% IBW mild malnutrition
    70% to 79% IBW moderate malnutrition
    0% to 69% IBW severe malnutrition
- Body Mass Index (BMI)[90]

  - $\text{BMI} = \dfrac{\text{weight (kg)}}{\text{height}^2 \text{ (m)}}$

  - Interpretation: Underweight   < 18.5
    Normal range   18.5 to 24.9
    Overweight   25.0 to 29.9
    Obese   ≥ 30.0

of greater than 10% body weight in combination with observable functional impairment was able to predict high postoperative risk patients significantly better than weight loss alone.[30]

Studies involving the measurement of MAC in acutely ill patients are inconclusive and conflicting.[31,32] Most practitioners are in agreement that anthropometric measures of muscle mass and body fat are of highest value when used in the ambulatory setting to monitor response to therapy over intervals of one month or more.[33-35] In the hospital setting, skinfold and arm circumference measurements should be reserved for the initial assessment of nutritional status in the nonmorbidly obese patient free of major upper body fluid aberrations.[35]

Direct Measures

More direct and precise methods of assessing body composition have been developed to further partition body weight into components of total body water (TBW), fat-free mass (FFM), and body fat. Bioelectrical impedance analysis (BIA), dual energy x-ray absorptiometry (DXA), total body potassium counting (TBK), and *in vivo* neutron activation analysis (IVNAA) are some of the more common means of direct body composition analysis ranging from least to most expensive and technically difficult.[34] These techniques allow the clinician to uncover malnutrition defined by a low FFM that may be masked by a high adiposity in patients classified as normal or obese based on weight evaluations alone.[36]

Bioelectrical impedance estimates TBW by measuring the opposition of body tissues to the flow of a small electrical current (50 kHz at less than 1mA). Population-specific regression equations are then used to derive estimates of FFM and percent body fat from BIA data.[37] Reliable BIA equations have been developed for use in stable pre- and postoperative liver, lung, and heart transplant patients.[38,39] However, limitations exist in the generalization of these equations to the intestinal transplant candidate. Water and electrolyte disturbances, which are common in intestinal failure, may skew BIA measurements, leading to over- or underestimation of malnutrition in this population.[40] Pichard et al. studied the use of BIA in chronically ill patients and confirmed the need for disease-specific BIA equations.[41] At present, the most valuable application of BIA in intestinal failure and rehabilitation may likely be for assessment of nutritional repletion and response to therapy over time.[42]

Highly precise and reproducible estimates of total body bone mineral content, fat mass, and lean soft tissue are obtainable through the use of DXA, an imaging technique using radiation to detect small changes in body composition.[43] Beams of defined energy are passed through the subject, with attenuation of the beams being proportional to the size and composition of bodily tissues through which they pass.[44] Excellent agreement has been observed between body composition estimates derived from DXA and methods designated as standards of reference.[45] A study of body composition in malnourished patients with Crohn's disease revealed that DXA measurements were more accurate than BIA or TBK in this population.[40] Correlations have been established between measurement obtained from DXA and from simple anthropometry in home parenteral nutrition patients with intestinal failure.[46,47] The use of DXA for monitoring body compositional changes of patients with intestinal failure holds great promise; however, its use in the U.S. is currently limited to research and further study is needed to establish correlation to outcome in hospitalized patients.[34]

BIOCHEMICAL ANALYSIS

Biochemical markers of visceral protein stores, immune function, and micronutrient status are convenient for use in the hospital setting; however, all are susceptible to influence from metabolic derangements of disease, trauma, or surgical stress. Consideration must be given to the patient's clinical state when interpreting laboratory values used in nutrition assessment.[48]

Serum Proteins

Hepatic transport proteins, including albumin, transferrin, prealbumin, and retinol-binding protein, are considered biochemical indicators of visceral or organ, enzymatic, and structural protein stores in the body. Serum levels of these proteins are largely affected by variations in synthesis, degradation, and distribution seen with chronic malnutrition or acute stress. In chronic uncomplicated starvation, serum albumin concentrations are maintained near normal due to decreased catabolism and shifts in distribution from extra- to intravascular spaces.[49] However in acute stress, albumin levels often fall dramatically in response to increased degradation, decreased synthesis with preferential use of amino acids for production of acute phase proteins, and increased vascular permeability with redistribution of albumin to extravascular spaces.[50]

Despite this, serum proteins are strong prognostic indicators of morbidity,[51] mortality,[52] length of hospital stay,[53] and surgical risk[54] among hospitalized patients (Table 6.5). Upon testing the effectiveness of visceral proteins for use in nutrition assessment, prealbumin was found to be more sensitive to changes in nutritional status and response to therapy than albumin or transferrin.[54,55] Retinol-binding protein also reacts quickly to nutrient deprivation and repletion; however, it is not as readily available for clinical use.[56]

TABLE 6.5
Overview of Hepatic Transport Proteins[18,61,91]

Serum Protein	Half-Life	Factors Possibly Increasing Levels	Factors Possibly Decreasing Levels	Clinical Significance
Albumin	2–3 weeks	Dehydration Administration of exogenous albumin Anabolic steroids	Liver disease Acute metabolic stress States of fluid retention	Readily available Prognostic index of clinical outcome Responds slowly to nutritional change
Transferrin	8–10 days	Iron-deficiency anemia Acute hepatitis Chronic blood loss Dehydration	End-stage liver disease Acute metabolic stress States of fluid retention	Highly sensitive to iron status Useful in monitoring response to nutrition therapy over time in stable patients
Prealbumin	2–3 days	Chronic renal failure Dehydration	Liver disease Acute metabolic stress	Good index of short-term changes in nutritional status
Retinol-binding protein	12 hours	Renal dysfunction	Liver disease Acute metabolic stress	Responds quickly to nutritional changes Not readily available

Acute-Phase Reactants

In response to tissue damage and inflammation, cytokines are released to stimulate the preferential production of acute-phase reactant proteins from the circulating amino acid pool.[57] C-reactive protein (CRP) is an acute-phase reactant protein produced during inflammation to help control infection and promote proper tissue repair.[58] Serum levels of CRP rise with the catabolic phase of the stress response (10 to 300 mg/L) and then rapidly fall with anabolism (0.06 to 8 mg/l).[59] Intensive care clinicians have used CRP in conjunction with prealbumin to determine the appropriate time for more aggressive nutrition support.[60]

Nitrogen Balance

Assessment of nitrogen balance is the only biochemical method that reflects both skeletal muscle and visceral protein compartments of the body. Nitrogen balance studies are used to determine protein requirements and evaluate the efficacy of the nutrition support regimen. Twenty-four-hour nitrogen intake (0.0625 g nitrogen per g protein) is subtracted by urinary urea nitrogen (UUN) output over the same period of time to obtain a rough estimate of nitrogen balance. A factor of four is added to account for non-UUN losses such as ammonia via skin, urine, stool, wounds, or the GI tract.[61] Negative nitrogen balance is indicative of net protein catabolism, whereas a positive nitrogen balance reflects net protein synthesis as seen in states of recovery and repletion.[62] The accuracy of nitrogen balance studies relies heavily on accurate intake records and accurate 24-hour urine collections.[63]

Essential Fatty Acid Deficiency

Prolonged malabsorption may lead to clinically significant vitamin, mineral, trace element, or fatty acid deficiency in the patient with intestinal failure. Essential fatty acid deficiency (EFAD) has been reported within one week of receiving lipid-free parenteral nutrition.[64] An essential fatty acid laboratory profile can identify EFAD by displaying a triene-to-tetraene ratio of greater than 0.4 or by an increase in oleic and palmitoleic acids with a decrease in linoleic and arachidonic acids.[65,66]

CLASSIFICATION OF NUTRITIONAL STATUS

PROTEIN-CALORIE MALNUTRITION

From evidence obtained through a complete nutrition assessment, patients identified as malnourished may be classified by type and intensity of malnutrition. Protein-energy or protein-calorie malnutrition (PEM or PCM) is a general term for inadequate macro-nutrient intake, absorption, or utilization in relation to macronutrient requirement. PCM encompasses a broad spectrum of illnesses ranging from marasmus, or chronic nutrient deprivation, to kwashiorkor, a reaction to acute protein loss and increased nutrient requirement associated with major trauma or sepsis (Table 6.6).

TABLE 6.6
Types of Protein-Calorie Malnutrition (PCM)[19,61]

	Semi-Starvation	Stress-Induced Hypoalbuminemia	Mixed
Clinical and Diet History	Prolonged deficit in intake and/or utilization of food Possible chronic illness	Recent exposure to stress of major surgery, trauma, or serious sepsis leaving the individual unable to currently eat or utilize food Previously normal intake pattern	Prolonged or acute deficit in intake and/or utilization of food Exposure to stress of trauma, surgery, acute illness or sepsis
Weight History	Significant weight loss over time	Weight intact or increased	Significant weight loss acutely or over time
Physical Assessment	Evident loss of fat and muscle stores Relatively intact immune function	Normal or near normal fat and muscle stores Generalized edema Depressed immune function	Evident loss of fat and muscle stores Possible lower extremity edema Depressed immune function
Laboratory Findings	Normal serum proteins	Low serum proteins	Low serum proteins

PROGNOSTIC INDICES

Upon assimilating research data on the numerous tools readily available for nutrition assessment, the conclusion may be made that no single parameter is of consistent value in all types of patients. Several indexes and techniques have been developed by assembling the predictive power of single assessment tools to more accurately pinpoint nutritional risk.

Prognostic Nutritional Index (PNI)

PNI is calculated from a mathematical equations using serum albumin, serum transferrin, delayed hypersensitivity skin tests, and triceps skinfold measurements. Mullen and colleagues developed and validated the PNI to identify patients who may benefit from preoperative nutrition repletion.[67,68] Smith and Hartemink tested this application in a randomized, prospective, controlled trial of patients undergoing upper GI surgery.[69] All patients admitted to the trial were deemed at some level of surgical risk by PNI. A trend toward decreased morbidity and mortality was observed in the patients receiving at least 10 days of preoperative intravenous nutrition versus those undergoing surgery at the next convenient time.

Nutritional Risk Index (NRI)

The NRI is a simple and clinically validated measure of nutritional status defined on the basis of serum albumin and percentage weight loss.[70] Severe malnutrition as classified by NRI was strongly linked to higher postoperative mortality among patients with gastric cancer.[71] The Veterans Affairs Cooperative Study revealed that preoperative patients undergoing major abdominal or thoracic surgery and classified as severely malnourished by NRI could benefit from receiving parenteral nutrition preoperatively.[72]

Subjective Global Assessment (SGA)

Baker et al.[73] and Detsky et al.[74] developed the technique of Subjective Global Assessment (SGA) based on the principle that findings from a routine clinical examination can correlate with objective measurements and predict clinical outcomes with greater accuracy than objective measurements in a wide range of patient populations.[75,76] (See Table 6.7.) The method has been tested for interrater reproducibility among nurses and medical residents with 91% agreement,[77] and among medical residents and specialists in clinical nutrition with 79% agreement.[78]

A recent comparison of SGA to BIA measurements of FFM found that FFM was significantly lower in patients classified as severely malnourished by SGA than in those classified as well nourished by SGA.[79] SGA classification did not correlate with BIA measurements of FFM in a study of 47 intestinal failure patients receiving home parenteral nutrition.[80] However, the authors concluded that SGA in combination with a weight history is sufficient for the assessment of PCM in this population. Preoperative nutrition assessment by SGA was able to predict outcome of liver transplantation in a 2001 study by Stephenson et al.[81] Significantly more complications were observed in the severely malnourished versus moderate and mildly malnourished patients as classified by SGA.

TABLE 6.7
Features of Subjective Global Assessment (SGA)[77,92]

- History
  - Change in weight over time
  - Change in dietary intake patterns over time
  - Presence of gastrointestinal symptoms persisting for > 2 weeks
  - Change in functional capacity over time
  - Primary diagnosis and level of metabolic demand
- Physical
  - Degree of loss of subcutaneous fat
  - Degree of muscle wasting
  - Degree of edema
  - Degree of ascites
  - Presence of mucosal, cutaneous, or hair abnormalities

CONCLUSION

A thorough assessment of nutritional status provides a strong foundation for the development of the most effective plan of nutrition care for the intestinal failure patient. Estimation of nutrient requirements, determination of route of feeding, and selection of dietary components all depend on an accurate collection and interpretation of data gathered during nutrition assessment. Unfortunately, a definitive tool for the determination of when to initiate aggressive nutrition support or when to adjust nutrient content for maximal benefit does not yet exist. Clinical judgment based on a careful history and physical examination, anthropometry, laboratory data, and measures of functional capacity is currently the most effective means of evaluating nutritional status in the intestinal failure population.

REFERENCES

1. Klein, S., Kinney, J., and Jeejeebhoy, K., Nutrition support in clinical practice: Review of published data and recommendations for future research directions, *JPEN*, 21, 133, 1997.
2. Charney, P., Nutrition assessment in the 1990's: Where are we now? *Nutr. Clin. Pract.*, 10, 131, 1995.
3. ASPEN Board of Directors and the Clinical Guidelines Task Force, Guidelines for the use of parenteral and enteral nutrition in adult and pediatric patients, *JPEN*, 26, 9SA, 2002.
4. Hammond, K., History and physical examination, in *Contemporary Nutrition Support Practice*, 2nd ed., Matarese, L.E. and Gottschlich, M.M., Eds., WB Saunders, Philadelphia, 2003, chap. 2.
5. Dwyer, J., Dietary assessment, in *Modern Nutrition in Health and Disease*, 9th ed., Shils, M.E., Olson, J.A., Shike, M. et al., Eds., Lippincott, Williams and Wilkins, Baltimore, 1999, chap. 58.
6. Burke, B.S., The dietary history as a tool in research, *J. Am. Diet. Assoc.*, 23, 1041, 1947.
7. Weseman, R.A., Adult small bowel transplantation, in *Comprehensive Guide to Transplant Nutrition*, Hasse, J.M. and Blue, J.S., Eds., ADA, 2002, 106–22.
8. Morrisson, S.G., Clinical nutrition physical examination, *Support Line*, 19, 16, 1997.
9. Hill, G.L., Body composition research: Implications for the practice of clinical nutrition, *JPEN*, 16, 197, 1992.
10. Russell, D.McR. et al., Skeletal muscle function during hypocaloric diets and fasting: A comparison with standard nutritional assessment parameters, *Am. J. Clin. Nutr.*, 37, 133, 1983.
11. Klidjian, A.M. et al., Relation of anthropometric and dynamometric variables to serious postoperative complications, *BMJ*, 281, 899, 1980.
12. Hunt, D.R., Rowlands, B.J., and Johnston, D., Handgrip strength — A simple prognostic indicator in surgical patients, *JPEN*, 9, 701, 1985.
13. Klidjian, A.M. et al., Detection of dangerous malnutrition, *JPEN*, 6, 119, 1982.
14. Webb, A.R. et al., Handgrip dynamometry as a predictor of postoperative complications: Reappraisal using age standardized grip strengths, *JPEN*, 13, 30, 1989.
15. Vaz, M. et al., Maximal voluntary contraction as a functional indicator of adult chronic undernutrition, *Brit. J. Nutr.*, 76, 9, 1996.

16. Brooks, S.D. and Kearns, P.J., Muscle function analysis: an alternative nutrition assessment technique, *Support Line,* 19, 12, 1997.
17. Russell, D. et al., A comparison between muscle function and body composition in anorexia nervosa: The effect of refeeding, *Am. J. Clin. Nutr.,* 38, 229, 1983.
18. Shronts, E.P., Fish, J.A., and Hammond, K.P., Nutrition assessment, in *The ASPEN Nutrition Support Practice Manual,* Souba Jr., W.W., Ed., ASPEN, 1998, chap. 1.
19. Hill, G.L., The clinical assessment of adult patients with protein energy malnutrition, *Nutr Clin Pract* 10:129–130, 1995.
20. Dominioni, L. and Dionigi, R., Immunological function and nutritional assessment, *JPEN,* 11, 70S, 1987.
21. Langkamp-Henken, B. and Wood, S.M., Evaluating immunocompetence, in *Contemporary Nutrition Support Practice, 2nd Ed.,* Matarese, L.M. and Gottschlich, M.M., Eds., WB Saunders, Philadelphia, 2003, chap. 5.
22. Meakins, J.L. et al., Delayed hypersensitivity: Indicator of acquired failure of host defenses in sepsis and trauma, *Ann. Surg.,* 186, 241, 1977.
23. Ottow, R.T., Bruining, H.A., and Jeekel, J.I., Clinical judgment versus delayed hypersensitivity skin testing for the prediction of postoperative sepsis and mortality, *Surg. Gynecol. Obstet.* 159, 475, 1984.
24. Twomey, P., Ziegler, D., and Rombeau, J., Utility of skin testing in nutritional assessment: A critical review, *JPEN,* 6, 50–58, 1982.
25. Ing, A.F., Meakins, J.L., McLean, A.P. et al., Determinants of susceptibility to sepsis and mortality: malnutrition vs. anergy, *J. Surg. Res.,* 32, 249, 1982.
26. Shiveley, L.R. and Thuluvath, P.J., Assessment of nutritional status via anthropometry, *Nutrition,* 13, 714, 1997.
27. Frisancho, A.R., New norms of upper limb fat and muscle areas for assessment of nutritional status, *Am. J. Clin. Nutr.,* 34, 2540, 1981.
28. Hark, L., Bowman, M., and Bellini, L., Nutrition assessment in medical practice, in *Medical Nutrition and Disease,* 2nd ed., Morrison, G., Hark, L., Eds., Blackwell Science, Malden, 1999, 3.
29. Studley, H.O., Percentage of weight loss. A basic indicator of surgical risk in patients with chronic peptic ulcer, *JAMA,* 106, 458, 1936.
30. Windsor, J.A. and Hill, G.L., Weight loss with physiological impairment. A basic indicator of surgical risk, *Ann. Surg.,* 207, 290, 1988.
31. Green, C.J. et al., Energy and nitrogen balance and changes in mid-upper arm circumference with multiple organ failure, *Nutrition* 11, 739, 1995.
32. Ravasco, P. et al., A critical approach to nutritional assessment in critically ill patients, *Clin. Nutr.,* 21, 73, 2002.
33. Hillhouse, J., Reliability of commonly used anthropometrics in adult hospitalized patients, *Support Line,* 18, 9, 1996.
34. Howell, W.H., Anthropometry and body composition analysis, in *Contemporary Nutrition Support Practice,* 2nd ed., Matarese, L.E. and Gottschlich, M.M., Eds., WB Saunders, Philadelphia, 2003, chap. 3.
35. Heymsfield, S.B., Baumgartner, R.N., and Pan, S.F., Nutritional assessment of malnutrition by anthropometric methods, in *Modern Nutrition in Health and Disease,* 9th ed., Shils, M.E., Olson, J.A., Shike, M. et al., Eds., Lippincott, Williams and Wilkins, Baltimore, 1999, 903.
36. Kyle, U.G. et al., Body composition in 995 acutely ill or chronically ill patients at hospital admission: a controlled population study, *J. Am. Diet. Assoc.,* 102, 944, 2002.
37. Janssen, I. et al., Estimation of skeletal muscle mass by bioelectrical impedance analysis, *J. Appl. Physiol.,* 89, 465, 2000.

38. Kyle, U.G. et al., Reliable bioelectrical impedance analysis estimate of fat-free mass in liver, lung and heart transplant patients, *JPEN,* 25, 45, 2001.

39. Ellis, K.J. et al., Bioelectrical impedance methods in clinical research: A follow-up to the NIH technology assessment conference, *Nutrition,* 15, 874, 1999.

40. Royall, D. et al., Critical assessment of body composition measurements in malnourished subjects with Crohn's disease: The role of bioelectric impedance analysis, *Am. J. Clin. Nutr.,* 59, 325, 1994.

41. Pichard, C., Kyle, U.G., and Slosman, D.O., Fat-free mass in chronic illness: Comparison of bioelectrical impedance and dual-energy x-ray absorptiometry in 480 chronically ill and healthy subjects, *Nutrition,* 15, 668, 1999.

42. NIH Technology Assessment Panel, Bioelectrical impedance analysis in body composition measurement, *Nutrition,* 12, 749, 1996.

43. Going, S.B. et al., Detection of small changes in body composition by dual-energy X-ray absorptiometry, *Am. J. Clin. Nutr.,* 57, 845, 1993.

44. Lang, P. et al., Osteoporosis. Current techniques and recent developments in quantitative bone densitometry, *Radiol. Clin. N. Am.,* 29, 49, 1991.

45. Fuller, N.J. et al., Four-component model for the assessment of body composition in humans: Comparison with alternative methods, and evaluation of the density and hydration of fat-free mass, *Clin. Sci.,* 82, 687, 1992.

46. Matarese, L.E. et al., Body composition changes in cachectic patients receiving home parenteral nutrition, *JPEN,* 26, 366, 2002.

47. Tjellesen, L., Staun, M., and Nielsen, P.K., Body composition changes measured by dual energy x-ray absorptiometry in patients receiving home parenteral nutrition, *Scand. J. Gastroenterol.,* 32, 686, 1997.

48. Mattox, T.W., Biochemical markers of nutritional status, *Support Line,* 13, 1, 1991.

49. Smith, G., Weidel, S.E., and Fleck, A., Albumin catabolic rate and protein energy depletion, *Nutrition,* 10, 335, 1994.

50. Vanek, V., The use of serum albumin as a prognostic or nutritional marker and the pros and cons of IV albumin therapy, *Nutr. Clin. Pract.,* 13, 110, 1998.

51. Anderson, C.F. and Wochos, D.N., The utility of serum albumin values in the nutritional assessment of hospitalized patients, *Mayo Clin. Proc.,* 57, 181, 1982.

52. Apelgren, K.N. et al., Comparison of nutritional indices and outcome in critically ill patients, *Crit. Care. Med.,* 10, 305, 1982.

53. dos Santos Junqueira, J.C. et al., Nutritional risk factors for postoperative complications in Brazilian elderly patients undergoing major elective surgery, *Nutrition,* 19, 321, 2003.

54. Mears, E., Outcomes of continuous process improvement of a nutritional care program incorporating serum prealbumin measurements, *Nutrition,* 12, 479, 1996.

55. Church, J.M. and Hill, G.L., Assessing the efficacy of intravenous nutrition in general surgical patients: Dynamic nutritional assessment with plasma proteins, *JPEN,* 11, 135, 1987.

56. Winkler, M.F. et al., Use of retinol-binding protein and prealbumin as indicators of the response to nutrition therapy, *J. Am. Diet. Assoc.,* 89, 684, 1989.

57. Gabay, C. and Kushner, I., Acute-phase proteins and other systemic responses to inflammation, *New Eng. J. Med.,* 340, 448, 1999.

58. Liepa, G.U. and Basu, H., C-reactive proteins and chronic disease: What role does nutrition play? *Nutr. Clin. Pract.,* 18, 227, 2003.

59. Russell, M., Laboratory monitoring, in *Contemporary Nutrition Support Practice,* 2nd ed., Matarese, L.E. and Gottschlich, M.M., Eds., WB Saunders, Philadelphia, 2003, chap. 4.

60. Boosalis, M.G. et al., Relationship of visceral proteins to nutritional status in chronic and acute stress, *Crit. Care Med.,* 17, 741, 1989.
61. Shopbell, J., Hopkins, B., and Shronts, E., Nutrition screening and assessment, in *The Science and Practice of Nutrition Support. A Case-Based Core Curriculum,* Gottschlich, M.M., Ed., Kendall/Hunt Publishing, Dubuque, 2001, chap. 6.
62. Konstantinides, F.N., Nitrogen balance studies in clinical nutrition, *Nutr. Clin. Pract.* 7, 231, 1992.
63. Kopple, J.D., Uses and limitations of the balance technique, *JPEN,* 11, 79S, 1987.
64. McCarthy, M.C. et al., Topical corn oil in the management of essential fatty acid deficiency, *Crit. Care Med.,* 11, 373, 1983.
65. Holman, R.T., The ratio of trienoic:tetraenoic acids in tissue lipids as a measure of essential fatty acid requirement, *J. Nutr.,* 70, 405, 1960.
66. McCarthy, M.C., Nutritional support in the critically ill surgical patient, *Surg. Clin. North Am.,* 71, 831, 1991.
67. Mullen, J.L. et al., Prediction of operative morbidity and mortality by preoperative nutritional assessment, *Surg. Forum,* 30, 80, 1979.
68. Buzby, G.P. et al., Prognostic nutritional index in gastrointestinal surgery, *Am. J. Surg.,* 139, 160, 1980.
69. Smith, R.C. and Hartemink, R., Improvement of nutritional measures during preoperative parenteral nutrition in patients selected by the prognostic nutritional index: A randomized controlled trial, *JPEN,* 12, 587, 1988.
70. Prendergast, J.M. et al., Clinical validation of a nutrition risk index, *J. Commun. Health,* 14, 125, 1989.
71. Rey-Ferro, M. et al., Nutritional and immunologic evaluation of patients with gastric cancer before and after surgery, *Nutrition,* 13, 878, 1997.
72. The Veterans Affairs Total Parenteral Nutrition Cooperative Study Group, Perioperative total parenteral nutrition in surgical patients, *N. Engl. J. Med.,* 325, 525, 1991.
73. Baker, J.P. et al., Nutritional assessment. A comparison of clinical judgment and objective measurements, *N. Engl. J. Med.,* 306, 969, 1982.
74. Detsky, A.S. et al., Evaluating the accuracy of nutritional assessment techniques applied to hospitalized patients: Methodology and comparisons, *JPEN,* 8, 153, 1984.
75. Jeejeebhoy, K.N. et al., Critical evaluation of the role of clinical assessment and body composition studies in patients with malnutrition and after total parenteral nutrition, *Am. J. Clin. Nutr.,* 35, 1117, 1982.
76. Detsky, A.S. et al., Predicting nutrition-associated complications for patients undergoing gastrointestinal surgery, *JPEN,* 11, 440, 1987.
77. Detsky, A.S. et al., What is subjective global assessment of nutritional status? *JPEN,* 11, 8, 1987.
78. Hirsch, S. et al., Subjective global assessment of nutritional status: further validation, *Nutrition,* 7, 35, 1991.
79. Kyle, U.G. et al., Nutrition status in patients younger and older than 60 years at hospital admission: A controlled population study in 995 subjects, *Nutrition,* 18, 463, 2002.
80. Egger, N.G., Carlson, G.L., and Shaffer, J.L., Nutritional status and assessment of patients on home parenteral nutrition: Anthropometry, bioelectrical impedance, or clinical judgment? *Nutrition,* 15, 1, 1999.
81. Stephenson, G.R., Moretti, E.W., and El-Moalem, H., Malnutrition in liver transplant patients: Preoperative subjective global assessment is predictive of outcome after liver transplantation, *Transplantation,* 72, 666, 2001.

82. ASPEN Board of Directors and the Clinical Guidelines Task Force, Standards for specialized nutrition support: adult hospitalized patients, *Nutr. Clin. Pract.,* 17, 384, 2002.

83. Newton, J.M., Halsted, C.H., Clinical and functional assessment of adults, in *Modern Nutrition in Health and Disease,* 9th ed., Shils, M.E., Olson, J.A., Shike, M. et al., Eds., Lippincott, Williams and Wilkins, Baltimore, 1999, 895.

84. Griffiths, A.M., Inflammatory bowel disease, in *Modern Nutrition in Health and Disease,* 9th ed., Shils, M.E., Olson, J.A., Shike, M. et al., Eds., Lippincott, Williams and Wilkins, Baltimore, 1999, 141.

85. Schneeweiss, B. et al., Energy and substrate metabolism in patients with active Crohn's disease, *J. Nutr.* 129, 844, 1999.

86. Beyer, P.L., Nutrient considerations in inflammatory bowel disease and short bowel syndrome, in *Nutrition in the Prevention and Treatment of Disease,* Coulston, A.M. et al., Eds., Academic Press, San Diego, 2001, 577.

87. Lennon, E.A. and Speerhas, R., Estimating nutritional requirements, in *Nutrition Support Handbook,* Parekh, N.R. and DeChicco, R., Eds., Cleveland Clinic Foundation, Cleveland, 2004, chap. 4.

88. Blackburn, G.L. et al., Nutritional and metabolic assessment of the hospitalized patient, *JPEN,* 1, 11, 1977.

89. Hamwi, G.J., Changing dietary concepts, in *Diabetes Mellitus: Diagnosis and Treatment,* Danowski, T.S., Ed., American Diabetes Association, New York, 1964, 73.

90. National Institutes of Health: Clinical guidelines on the identification and treatment of overweight and obesity in adults — The evidence report, *Obes. Res.,* 6, 51S, 1998.

91. Cresci, G., Nutrition assessment and monitoring, in *Nutritional Considerations in the Intensive Care Unit,* Shikora, S.A., Martindale, R.G., and Schwaitzberg, S.D., Eds., ASPEN Kendall/Hunt, Iowa, 2002, chap. 3.

92. Jeejeebhoy, K.N., Assessment of fluid and nutritional status, in Intestinal Failure, Nightingale, J., ed., Greenwich Medical Media, London, 2001, 263.

7 Malnutrition: Vitamin and Trace Mineral Deficiencies

James S. Scolapio and Andrew Ukleja

CONTENTS

Deficiency of micronutrients, including vitamins and trace elements, can occur in patients with intestinal failure either from short bowel syndrome or extensive mucosal disease, such as radiation enteritis. Because water-soluble vitamins are absorbed from the proximal jejunum, it is unusual for these deficiencies to occur. It is possible, however, that these deficiencies do occur but are not clinically recognized. In contrast, vitamin B_{12} and fat-soluble vitamins require adequate distal small bowel function for adequate absorption. Therefore, vitamin B_{12} and fat-soluble vitamin deficiencies are more common in patients with intestinal failure. This chapter will focus on vitamin and trace mineral deficiency in patients with short bowel syndrome.

VITAMINS

Because water-soluble vitamins are absorbed in the proximal jejunum, it is unusual for deficiency to develop in short bowel syndrome.[1] Table 7.1 lists the dietary sources and signs and symptoms of specific vitamin deficiencies. Since thiamine, B_{12}, and fat-soluble vitamin deficiencies are the most common to occur in short bowel syndrome, they will be discussed here. Regarding the administration of vitamins and trace elements to parenteral nutrition (PN) solutions we refer the reader to the article "Safe practices for parenteral nutrition formulations."[2] Refer to Table 7.2 and Table 7.3 for PN requirements. The multivitamin preparations should be added to the PN directly prior to the infusion given the unstable nature of these products.[2]

0-8493-1803-3/05/$0.00+$1.50
© 2005 by CRC Press LLC

TABLE 7.1
Vitamins

Vitamin	Dietary Source	Deficiency
Thiamine (B_1)	Cereals, grains, pork, legumes, wheat grain	Wernicke's-Korsakoff encephalopathy, high-output congestive heart failure, lactic acidosis, peripheral neuropathy, nystagmus
Cobalamin (B_{12})	Meat, eggs, dairy	Megaloblastic anemia, subacute combined degeneration of spinal cord, pernicious anemia, progressive neuropathy
Folic acid	Yeast, liver, vegetables, fruits	Pancytopenia, megaloblastic anemia, glossitis, stomatitis
Ascorbic acid	Citrus fruit, tomatoes, green vegetables	Perifollicular hyperkeratosis (scurvy), hemorrhage
Biotin	Milk products, eggs, liver	Scaly dermatitis, alopecia, lethargy, hypotonia, lactic acidosis
Vitamin A	Fish oils, liver, egg yolk, milk, carotenoids, green leaf vegetables	Night blindness, xerosis, Bitot's spots, hyperkeratosis of skin
Vitamin D	Fortified milk, breads	Osteomalcia, rickets, reduced serum calcium
Vitamin E	Whole wheat, vegetable oils	Hemolytic anemia, spinocerebellar degeneration, neuropathy, opthalmoplegia
Vitamin K	Green leafy vegetables	Bleeding, increased prothrombin time (PT)

TABLE 7.2
Daily Vitamin Requirements for Adult PN Solutions[a]

Vitamin	Intake Amount
Thiamin (B_1)	6.0 mg
Riboflavin (B_2)	3.6 mg
Niacin (B_3)	40 mg
Folic acid	600 µg
Pantothenic acid	15 mg
Pyridoxine (B_6)	4 mg
Cyanocobalmin (B_{12})	5 µg
Biotin	60 µg
Ascorbic acid (C)	200 mg
Vitamin A	5000 IU
Vitamin D	400 IU
Vitamin E	30 IU
Vitamin K	150 µg

[a] Federal Register, 2000

TABLE 7.3
Daily Trace Element
Requirements for Adult PN
Solutions (2)

Trace Element	Intake Amount
Chromium	10–15 μg
Copper	0.3–0.5 mg
Manganese	60–100 μg
Zinc	2.5–5 mg
Selenium	60–100 μg

Deficiency of thiamine (Vitamin B-1) presenting as Wernicke's encephalopathy has been reported in PN-dependent short bowel patients during a recent vitamin shortage in which thiamine was not added to the PN.[3,4] Replacement of thiamine resulted in the resolution of symptoms. Active thiamine absorption is greatest in the jejunum and ileum, and primary excretion is through the urine. Thiamine is not stored in large amounts in the body; therefore, daily intake is important. Dietary sources of thiamine included yeast, cereals, grains, lean pork, legumes, and wheat grain. Alcohol can reduce thiamine absorption, making alcoholics predisposed to deficiency. Thiamine in the form of thiamine triphosphate (TTP) serves biochemically as the coenzyme for alpha keto acid decarboxylation and transketolation. Thiamine is important in neurotransmission and nerve conduction. Deficiency of thiamine can result in Wernicke's-Korsakoff syndrome, which is marked by nystagmus followed by ophthalmoplegia, ataxia, and altered mental status.[5] Confusion, coma, and death can result if thiamine is not replaced. "Dry beriberi" clinical features also include symmetric peripheral neuropathy affecting sensory and motor reflex functions. "Wet beriberi" refers to high-output left-ventricular heart failure associated with thiamine deficiency. Lactic acidosis has also been reported in overt thiamine deficiency. The most reliable means of the diagnosis of thiamine deficiency is an increase in serum erythrocyte transketolase activity (ETKA) when thiamine pyrophosphate is added to an *in vitro* assay.[6] Standard multivitamin supplements in PN contain 3.0 mg of thiamine. If deficiency is suspected, 100 mg of thiamine given intravenously for at least 3 consecutive days is recommended.

Vitamin B_{12} (cobalamin) is the other water-soluble vitamin that may become deficient in patients with intestinal failure. Meat, fish, and eggs are the predominate dietary source of vitamin B_{12}. Vitamin B_{12} is not present in plants and, therefore, is not found in vegetables and fruits. Given the large store of vitamin B_{12} in the human body, which is primarily stored in the liver, it takes years of insufficient dietary intake for signs and symptoms of clinical deficiency to occur. Ingested vitamin B_{12} is released from food in the stomach by gastric acid. The free B_{12} then binds to intrinsic factor (IF), which is synthesized from the parietal cells of the stomach, forming a complex that binds to high-infinity receptors of the terminal ileum for absorption.[7] Therefore, when the distal 60 cm of the ileum is diseased or resected, absorption of vitamin B_{12}

can be impaired.[8] Low serum cobalamin levels are a marker of deficiency. However, serum methylmalonic acid (MMA) and homocysteine levels are often elevated earlier than reduced serum cobalamin levels, and they appear to be earlier markers of B_{12} deficiency. Vitamin B_{12} is a coenzyme for both MMA and homocysteine. The best available test for evaluating B_{12} absorption is the Schilling test. In this test, a 24-hour urine collection is performed after the administration of radiolabeled B_{12}.[7] If the test is abnormal after giving IF, the test may be repeated after patients are treated with either antibiotics for possible bacterial overgrowth or with pancreatic enzymes in patients suspected of having pancreatic insufficiency. Gastrointestinal disorders that reduce the absorption of B_{12} include inadequate IF production as a result of antibodies produced against IF (pernicious anemia) or after total gastrectomy. Pancreatic exocrine insufficiency and bacterial overgrowth of the small intestine can also result in malabsorption of vitamin B_{12}. The diphyllobothrium latum fish tapeworm (found in Scandinavian countries) can also result in B_{12} deficiency. Ileal disorders, including Crohn's disease, radiation enteritis, and ileal resections of greater than 60 cm, can also result in vitamin B_{12} malabsorption.[8] Megaloblastic anemia and myelopathy presenting as subacute combined degeneration resulting in upper motor neuron paralysis are some of the signs and symptoms of vitamin B_{12} deficiency. These complications are seen primarily in patients with pernicious anemia. Patients with suspected vitamin B_{12} deficiency should receive monthly replacement usually given as an intramuscular injection. Patients requiring PN receive 5 µg per day of B_{12} as part of the multivitamin preparation added to the PN.

The absorption of the fat-soluble vitamins (A, D, E, and K) requires micellar solubilization by bile salt micelles. Diseases that reduce small bowel surface area or reduce the bile salt pool, such as terminal ileal resections, are more likely to result in fat-soluble vitamin deficiencies. The use of the medication cholestryramine may also result in binding of bile acids and subsequent fat-soluble vitamin deficiency.

Dietary sources of vitamin A include liver, yellow green leafy vegetables, eggs, and whole milk products. Absorption is completed by reesterification to retinyl esters, incorporation into chylomicrons, and delivery into the lymphatics.[9] The primary storage site for vitamin A is the liver. Therefore, in patients with short bowel syndrome, if sufficient amounts of bile salts are lost, reduced micellar solubilization occurs resulting in subsequent vitamin A malabsorption. Vitamin A is important in cell differentiation and proliferation. The primary clinical effects of vitamin A are related to the role of retinal as a precursor of the visual pigment, rhodopsin. Vitamin A of the 11-cis retinal forms is vital for night vision.[10] Deficiency of vitamin A may result in night blindness. Xerosis of the eyes may occur with vitamin A deficiency, resulting in the clinical finding of Bitot's spots and irreversible blindness. Unlike water-soluble vitamins, excess vitamin A intake may be harmful. However, this is unlikely to occur in short bowel syndrome. Excess intake of supplemental or dietary vitamin A may result in liver damage and signs and symptoms of increased intracranial pressure. Caution should be noted since plasma levels of vitamin A may not correlate with hepatic concentrations.[11] Patients with short bowel syndrome requiring TPN can have vitamin A added to the PN formula. The standard dose of vitamin A in PN is 5000 IU (international units). Oral vitamin A preparations may be given to select short bowel patients that are not PN dependent.

Dietary sources of vitamin D include fortified milk and bread. In the intestine vitamin D is absorbed by passive diffusion. Vitamin D is also produced from the skin during sunlight exposure. Vitamin D is hydroxylated to 25-hydroxy D in the liver and then hydroxylated to its active form 1, 25-dihydroxy D in the kidney. The 1, 25 form of vitamin D regulates calcium absorption from the intestine.[7] A deficiency of vitamin D results in low serum calcium and phosphorus levels. Bone mineralization is reduced in vitamin D–deficient individuals, resulting in osteopenia in adults and rickets in children. In patients with short bowel syndrome, serum levels of 1, 25 vitamin D should be evaluated and vitamin D should be replaced if deficient. Other biochemical evidence for vitamin D deficiency include a 24-hour urinary calcium level less than 100 mg/day, elevated parathyroid hormone, and elevated alkaline phosphatase and urinary hydroxyproline.[7] Excess intake of vitamin D can result in marked hypercalcemia and hyperphosphatemia with associated symptoms, which include anorexia, nausea, and vomiting. The standard dose of vitamin D in PN is 400 IU.

Vitamin E is a potent peroxyl radical scavenger and protects polyunsaturated fatty acid (PUFA) within phospholipids of biological membranes and in plasma lipoproteins.[12] Micellar solubilization by bile salts is also needed for the absorption of vitamin E. Dietary sources of vitamin E include vegetable, soybean, and corn oils and unprocessed cereal grains and nuts. The primary storage site for vitamin E is adipose tissue. Vitamin E is an antioxidant protecting against the action of superoxide.[12] Vitamin E deficiency increases lipid peroxidation. Hemolytic anemia, ataxia and peripheral neuropathy have also been reported with vitamin E deficiency.[13–14] Vitamin E deficiency can result in degeneration of large caliber axons in the sensory neurons. Ophthalmoplegia, pigmented retinopathy has also been reported with vitamin E deficiency. Prior to the addition of selenium in PN, patients required more than five times the RDA of vitamin E.[15] It is thought that the addition of polyunsaturated fatty acids (PUFA) in the lipid emulsion of PN increases the need for vitamin E.[7] Serum levels of vitamin E should be calculated by using the ratio of serum vitamin E to total lipids. The standard dose of vitamin E in PN is 30 IU. Unlike vitamin A, serum levels of vitamin E appear to correlate with hepatic concentrations.[16]

The predominant dietary sources of vitamin K are green leafy vegetables. Also the colonic flora produces vitamin K. Therefore, vitamin K deficiency is uncommon in patients with intact colons. Healthy individuals on a vitamin K–deficient diet will not develop vitamin K deficiency unless the colonic flora is disrupted. Vitamin K is required for the synthesis of clotting factors in the liver, which include factors II, VII, IX, and X. Vitamin K is required for gamma-carboxylation of glutamic acid, which results in the synthesis of these factors by the liver.[5] The small intestine normally absorbs 30%–70% of daily-ingested vitamin K, which is sufficient to meet daily needs. Since little of vitamin K is stored, dietary supplementation is important. Besides vitamin K deficiency occurring in situations of fat malabsorption such as short bowel syndrome, the use of broad-spectrum antibiotics may reduce the bacteria flora of the gastrointestinal tract, also resulting in vitamin K deficiency. The primary symptom of vitamin K deficiency is bleeding. The prothrombin time (PT) becomes prolonged. Vitamin K has only recently been routinely added to PN at a dose of 150 µg.

TRACE ELEMENTS

The following essential trace elements are thought to be necessary for normal health and function in humans: iron, zinc, copper, chromium, selenium, iodine, and cobalt. Refer to Table 7.4 for dietary sources and deficiency of specific trace elements. A deficiency of one of these trace elements may result in altered cellular function and the associated clinical signs and symptoms.[17,18] Trace elements are absorbed throughout the gastrointestinal tract and circulate as protein-bound complexes. The tissue stores of these trace elements may not be sufficient during periods of insufficient oral intake, increased metabolic stress, or intestinal malabsorption. The gastrointestinal tract is also the primary route of excretion of these trace elements. It was not until 1979 that a trace element package containing zinc, copper, chromium, and manganese was available that could be added to PN.[17] A few years later, case studies of selenium deficiency were reported in patients with intestinal failure, which resulted in selenium also becoming part of the trace element package.

Iron is essential for normal hemoglobin and myoglobin function. Red meats are the primary dietary source of iron. Iron stores are regulated by the absorption of iron from the gastrointestinal tract. Iron is absorbed predominantly in the duodenum and jejunum, and there is very little excretion of iron from the gastrointestinal tract. Iron is best absorbed in the ferrous (Fe^{+2}) state. Acid in the stomach reduces Fe^{+3} to Fe^{+2}, thus enhancing absorption. Therefore, gastrointestinal causes of decreased iron absorption include diseases that affect the proximal small intestine, such as the postgastrectomy state associated with achlorhydria. Gastric acid is also required to release protein-bound iron from food, for example, red meats. Vitamin C and other organic acids promote the absorption of iron from the gastrointestinal tract. Iron deficiency results in a hypochromic, microcytic anemia. Although the best means of accessing tissue store for deficiency is stainable iron on bone marrow biopsy, this is an invasive test that should not be routinely done.[19] In the absence of active

TABLE 7.4
Trace Elements

Trace Element	Dietary Source	Deficiency
Iron	Red meat, fish, oysters, dried beans	Hypochromic microcytic anemia, cheilosis, weakness
Zinc	Shellfish, meat, eggs	Acrodermatitis enteropathica, diarrhea, apathy, growth retardation, hair loss, skin rash, dysgeusia, reduce wound healing
Copper	Liver, legumes, shellfish, nuts	Microcytic, hypochromic anemia, leukopenia, neutropenia, osteoporosis, Menke's syndrome
Chromium	Brewer's yeast, vegetable oils, liver, cereals	Glucose intolerance, peripheral neuropathy, metabolic encephalopathy
Selenium	Meat, poultry, fish, cereal, grains, seafood	Dilated cardiomyopathy, myositis, weakness, white nails, Keshans's disease

inflammation, reduced plasma ferritin levels and transferrin saturation are a marker of deficiency. Provided there is no chronic gastrointestinal blood loss, oral iron replacement is usually sufficient to replete iron stores. The usual adult dose of iron is one tablet (325 mg) of ferrous sulfate three times a day.[20] In patients with short bowel syndrome oral iron alone may not be sufficient to correct the deficiency and intravenous replacement is required. Because of the risk of anaphylaxis, iron is not routinely placed in PN.[20] After a test dose of intravenous iron, iron dextran can be given alone or added to the crystalloid PN solution. Iron should not be added to the all-in-one fat containing solutions.[5]

Zinc is found in many foods, including shellfish and meats. Zinc is an important co-factor in over 100 metalloenzymes and is very important in protein and amino acid metabolism, including nucleic acid metabolism.[21] Zinc is important for cell proliferation, night vision, taste, wound healing, and immune function. A deficiency of zinc can result in growth retardation, reduced wound healing, dysgeusia, night blindness, alopecia, and a skin rash.[22] There is a condition of zinc deficiency known as *acrodermatitis enteropathica*. This is a rare autosomal recessive disease of zinc metabolism and impaired intestinal uptake.[5] Symptoms of this syndrome include diarrhea, growth retardation, alopecia, and eczematous skin rash. Adult PN patients have also been reported to have mental depression, diarrhea, bullous dermatitis, alopecia, and stomatitis within 4 weeks of not having zinc placed in the PN.[22] Although zinc is absorbed throughout the gastrointestinal tract, greater absorption occurs from the jejunum with zinc binding to a surface receptor before being absorbed. The process is saturable; therefore, absorption decreases with high zinc intake.[23] In plasma, zinc is loosely bound to albumin and transferred to peripheral tissues for use. Diarrhea and fistula losses are the primary reasons for zinc deficiency to occur. Zinc supplementation should be given to persons at risk of developing deficiency or those with documented low serum levels of zinc. Oral zinc sulfate (220–440 mg) given twice daily is suggested.[1] Many patients do not tolerate this oral dose because of gastrointestinal upset. Standard multiple trace element solutions (MTE) that are added to the PN contain 2.5–5.0 mg of zinc. Depending on stool losses, more zinc may be required.[25] Plasma zinc levels should be measured periodically to assess requirements. Reduced serum alkaline phosphatase can also be found in zinc deficiency.

Copper is part of the enzymes of cytochrome C oxidase, superoxide dismutase, and lysyl oxidase. Copper is important for normal function of the central nervous system, skeletal collagen, and elastin formation as well as normal red and white blood cell maturation.[26-27] Liver, legumes, shellfish, nuts, and poultry are excellent dietary sources of copper. Copper is primarily absorbed from the stomach and proximal small intestine. Infants with short bowel syndrome treated with PN without copper have been reported to have anemia, hypoplastic bone marrow, and osteoporosis.[28–29] Scurvy-like bone disease responsive to copper has been described in infants nourished solely with milk.[29] Menke's syndrome is a genetic defect in copper absorption.[5] Ninety percent of circulating copper is in the form of ceruloplasmin.[30] Copper is also important for iron transfer throughout the body. The primary storage site for copper is the liver and brain. Copper is excreted via the bile. In patients with cholestatic liver disease, copper may accumulate in the liver, resulting in hepatic injury. Zinc, iron, and other divalent minerals inhibit copper absorption.[31] Although copper deficiency is rare in otherwise healthy adults, deficiency has been reported in short bowel patients receiving PN without copper.[32] Copper deficiency may present clinically as microcytic, hypochromic anemia, leukopenia, and neutropenia. The standard MTE in PN contains 0.30–0.50 mg of copper. In those patients with cholestatic liver disease, the amount of copper in PN should be reduced.[32]

Chromium deficiency in animals has been reported to cause glucose intolerance. Its deficiency has also been reported in patients after extensive intestinal resection.[33–36] Chromium is important in promoting insulin action in peripheral tissue. In vitro chromium increases insulin stimulation of glucose oxidation and lipogenesis in adipose tissue. Dietary sources of chromium include brewer's yeast, vegetable oils, whole grain, cereals, and liver. A decline of body chromium stores caused by age may contribute to glucose intolerance of the elderly.[37] Peripheral neuropathy has also been reported with chromium deficiency.[35] Chromium is excreted in the urine. Plasma chromium levels are reduced in deficiency but may also be reduced by acute illness. Therefore, it is an unreliable means of accessing body stores.[38] Disappearance of glucose intolerance after chromium replacement is a good diagnostic test for deficiency. A total of 10–15 µg of chromium is included in the standard MTE of a PN formula.

Selenium is an antioxidant important in the function of glutathione peroxidase, an enzyme made up of four subunits each containing selenocysteine.[39] This enzyme protects against tissue damage from peroxides. Selenium is incorporated into tissue protein as selenocysteine.[40] Selenium is present in high concentrations in seafood. In blood, selenium is present in both plasma and red cells. Selenium is efficiently absorbed from the duodenum, and its main route of excretion is urine. Selenium deficiency has been reported in patients with short bowel syndrome to cause dilated cardiomyopathy, myositis, white fingernail beds, and weakness.[41–44] In China, where soil content of selenium is low, children can present with dilated congestive cardiomyopathy and cardiac arrhythmia known as Keshan's disease. Sixty micrograms of selenium are in certain MTE solutions of PN.

Other trace elements include cobalt, iodine, fluoride, molybdenum, manganese, cadmium, lead, boron, aluminum, arsenic, mercury, vanadium, nickel, tin, and silicon. Deficiency of iodine, fluoride, and molybdenum has been reported in short bowel syndrome. Iodine is important for normal thyroid function. Seafood and table salt are rich sources of iodine. Iodine deficiency is now rare in the U.S. Fluoride is needed for normal growth and reproduction. Major sources of fluoride include drinking water, tea, and sardines. Low intake is associated with dental caries and increased risk of osteoporosis. Molybdenum is important for the metabolism of purines and sulfur-containing compounds. Dietary sources include beef, cereals, and legumes. There is one reported case of molybdenum deficiency in a patient treated with PN who developed tachypnea, headache, nausea, and vomiting.[45] Toxicity of molybdenum may cause gout-like syndrome. Manganese is also part of the MTE in standard PN. Excess of manganese can result in toxicity manifesting as neuropsychiatric and Parkinson-like symptoms.[46–47] On T-1 weighted magnetic resonance imaging (MRI) increased deposits of manganese can be found in the globus pallidus. Manganese, like copper, is excreted via the bile and, therefore, its amount given in

PN should be reduced in cholestatic liver disease. The standard MTE of PN contains 60–100 μg of manganese.

SUMMARY

In summary, deficiency of vitamin and trace elements results from inadequate intestinal absorption. This is usually the consequence of short bowel syndrome. Except for vitamin B_{12}, which is absorbed from the terminal ileum, deficiency of other water-soluble vitamins is less common. In contrast deficiency of fat-soluble vitamins (A, D, E, K) is more common than water-soluble vitamin in patients with short bowel syndrome since bile salts are necessary for micellar solubilization and subsequent intestinal absorption. Dietary sources of vitamins and deficiency state are reported in Table 7.1.

Trace elements are necessary for normal health and cellular function. Besides deficiency states excess of manganese and copper in PN can result in adverse clinical effects. Both manganese and copper are hepatically excreted and therefore should be reduced or eliminated in the PN of patients with cholestatic liver disease. Deficient states of trace elements are reported in Table 7.4.

REFERENCES

1. Buchman, A.L., Scolapio, J., and Fryer, J., AGA technical review on short bowel syndrome and intestinal transplantation, *Gastroenterology,* 124, 1111–1134, 2003.
2. Safe Practices for Parenteral Nutrition Formulation, *JPEN,* 22, 49–66, 1998.
3. Hahn, J.S., Berquist, W., Alcorn, D.M. et al., Wernicke encephalopathy and beriberi during TPN attributable to multivitamin shortage, *Pediatrics,* 101E, 10, 1998.
4. Alloju, M., and Ehrinpreis, M.N., Shortage of intravenous multivitamin solution in the US, *NEJM,* 337, 54–55, 1998.
5. Heizer, W.D. and Holcombe, B.J., Approach to the patient requiring nutritional supplementation, In *Textbook of Gastroenterology,* 2nd ed., Yamada, T., Alpers, D.H., Owyang, C., Eds., J.B. Lippincott Co., 1995, 1044–1090.
6. Tanphaichitr, V., Thiamin. In *Modern Nutrition in Health and Science,* 9th ed., Shils, M.E., Olson, J.A., Shike, M., Eds., Philadelphia: Williams and Wilkins Co., 1999, 381–389.
7. Jeejeebhoy, K.N., Nutrient requirements and nutrient deficiencies in gastrointestinal diseases. In *Gastrointestinal Disease,* 5th ed., Sleisenger, M.H. and Fordtran, J.S., W. B. Saunders, 1993, 2017–2047.
8. Behrend, C., Jeppesen, P.B., and Mortensen, P.B., Vitamin B-12 absorption after ileorectal anastomosis for Crohn's disease: Effect of ileal resection and time span after surgery, *Eur J Gastro Hepat.,* 7, 397–400, 1995.
9. Norum, K.R. and Blomnoff, R. Vitamin A absorption, transport, cellular uptake and storage, *Am J Clin Nutr.,* 56, 735–44, 1992.
10. Wald, G., The molecular basis of visual excitation, *Nature,* 219, 800, 1968.
11. Ukleja, A., and Scolapio, J.S., Nutritional assessment of serum and hepatic stores of vitamin A in patients with cirrhosis, *JPEN,* 26, 184–188, 2002.
12. Sitren, H.S., Vitamin E. In *Clinical Guide to Parenteral Micro Nutrition,* 2nd ed., Baumgartner, T.G., Ed., Lyhomed, 1991, 389.

13. Howard, L. et al., Reversible neurological symptoms caused by vitamin E deficiency in a patients with short bowel syndrome, *Am J. Clin Nutr.,* 36, 1243–1249, 1982.

14. Sokol, R.J., Vitamin E deficiency and neurological disease, *Annu Rev Nutr.,* 8, 351–373, 1988.

15. Thurlow, P.M., and Grant, J.P., Vitamin E and TPN, *Annals NY Acad. Sci.,* 393, 121–132, 1982.

16. Ukleja, A. et al., Serum and hepatic vitamin E assessment in cirrhotics before liver transplantation, *JPEN,* 27, 71–73, 2003.

17. Shils, M.E., Historical aspects of minerals and vitamins in parenteral nutrition, *Federation Proceedings,* 3, 263–267, 1979.

18. McClain, C.J., Trace metal abnormalities in adults during hyperalimentation, *JPEN,* 5, 424–429, 1981.

19. Morgon, E.H. and Walters, M.N.I., Iron storage in human disease. Fractionation of hepatic and splenic iron into ferritin and hemosiderin with histochemical correlations, *J Clin. Pathol.,* 16, 101, 1963.

20. Bolinger, A.M. and Korman, N.R., Anemia. In *Applied Therapeutics: The Clinical Use of Drugs,* 4th ed., Young, L.L., Koda-Kimble, M.A., Eds., Vancouver, WA: Applied Therapeutics, 1983, 1051.

21. Shenkin, A., Micronutrients. In *Enteral and Tube Feeding,* 3rd ed., Rombeau, J.L. and Rolandelli, R.H., Eds., Philadelphia: W.B. Saunders, 1997:96–111.

22. Kay, R.G. et al., A syndrome of acute zinc deficiency during total parenteral alimentation in man, *Ann Surg.,* 183, 331–340, 1976.

23. Davies, N.T., Studies on the absorption of zinc by rat intestine, *Br. J. Nutr.,* 43, 189–203, 1980.

24. Jeejeebhoy, K.N., Zinc and chromium in parenteral nutrition, *Bull. NY Acad. Med.,* 60, 118–124, 1984.

25. Wolman, S.L. et al., Zinc in total parenteral nutrition. Requirements and metabolic effects, *Gastroenterology,* 76, 458–467, 1979.

26. Shike, M., Copper in parenteral nutrition, *Bul. NY Acad. Med.,* 60, 132–143, 1984.

27. Shike, M., et al., Copper metabolism and requirements in total parenteral nutrition, *Gastroenterology,* 81, 290–297, 1981.

28. Karpel, J.T. and Peden, V.H., Copper deficiency in long-term parenteral nutrition, *J. Pediatr.,* 80, 32–36, 1972.

29. Goyens, D., Brasseur, D., and Cadranel, S., Copper deficiency in infants with active celiac disease, *J. Pediatr. Gastroenterol. Nutr.,* 4, 677–680, 1985.

30. Cartwright, G.E. and Wintrobe, M.M., Copper metabolism in normal subjects, *Am. J. Clin. Nutr.,* 14, 224, 1964.

31. Hall, A.C., Young, B.W., and Bremmer, I., Intestinal metallothionein and the mature antagonism between copper and zinc in the rat, *J. Inorg. Biochem.,* 11, 57–66, 1979.

32. Fleming, C.R., Trace element metabolism in adult patients requiring total parenteral nutrition, *Am. J. Clin. Nutr.,* 49, 573–579, 1989.

33. Freund, H., Atamian, S., and Fischer, J.E., Chromium deficiency during total pareneteral nutrition, *JAMA,* 241, 496–498, 1979.

34. Brown, R.O. et al., Chromium deficiency after long-term parenteral nutrition, *Dig. Dis. Sci.* 31, 661–664, 1986.

35. Jeejeebhoy, K.N. et al., Chromium deficiency, glucose intolerance, and neuropathy reversed by chromium supplementation, in a patient receiving long-term total parenteral nutrition, *Am. J. Clin. Nutr.,* 30, 531–538, 1977.

36. Rudman, D. and Williams, P., Nutrient deficiencies during TPN, *Nutrition Reviews,* 43, 1–12, 1985.

37. Schroeder, H.A., The role of chromium in mammalian nutrition, *Am. J. Clin. Nutr.,* 21, 230–244, 1968.
38. Pekarek, R.S. et al., Relationship between serum chromium concentrations and glucose utilization in normal and infected subjects, *Diabetes,* 24, 350–3, 1975.
39. Rotruck, J.T. et al., Selenium: Biochemical role as a component of glutathione peroxidase, *Science,* 179, 588–590, 1973.
40. Dickson, R.C. and Tomlinson, R.N., Selenium in blood and human tissue, *Clinica Chimica Acta,* 16, 311–321, 1967.
41. Fleming, C.R. el al., Selenium deficiency and fatal cardiomyopathy in a patients on home parenteral nutrition, *Gastroenterology,* 83, 689–693, 1982.
42. Johnson, R.A. et al., An accidental case of cardiomyopathy and selenium deficiency, *NEJM,* 304, 1210–1212, 1981.
43. Brown, M.R. et al., Proximal muscle weakness and selenium deficiency associated with long-term parenteral nutrition, *Am. J. Clin. Nutr.,* 43, 549–554, 1986.
44. Kien, C.L. and Ganther, H.E., Manifestations of chronic selenium deficiency, *Am. J. Clin. Nutr.,* 37, 319–28, 1983.
45. Abumrad, N.N., Schneider, S.D, and Rogers, L.S., Molybdenum — is it an essential trace metal? *Am. J. Clin. Nutr.,* 34, 2551–2559, 1981.
46. Mehta, R. and Reilly, J.J., Manganese levels in a jaundiced long term TPN patient: Potential for hepatobiliary toxicity? Case report and literature review, *JPEN,* 14, 428–430, 1990.
47. Fitzgerald K. et al., Hypermanganesemia in patients receiving TPN, *JPEN,* 23, 333–336, 1999.

8 Physiologic and Laboratory Testing for Malabsorption and Short Bowel Syndrome

Charlene W. Compher and David C. Metz

CONTENTS

One of the most difficult aspects of providing clinical advice and nutritional care for patients with intestinal failure (IF) is that the anatomy alone does not necessarily predict the actual function of the remaining bowel. This is most evident when there is a superimposed gastrointestinal disorder that aggravates digestion and absorption, such as Crohn's disease or radiation enteritis or a mucosal disease that may be symptomatically silent, such as celiac disease. Finally, even with no increase in bowel length, patients with short bowel syndrome (SBS) may experience improvement in bowel function as adaptation occurs. Thus, a familiarity with measures of intestinal absorptive function is needed to optimally manage these patients, even though the methods used may require adjustment for patients with severe bowel disease.

0-8493-1803-3/05/$0.00+$1.50

This chapter describes the various tests of malabsorption in patients with severe diarrhea, paying special attention to causes of diarrhea in patients with IF receiving parenteral nutrition (PN) (Table 8.1). It should also be noted that chronic malabsorption itself leaves patients susceptible to deficiencies of key nutrients that can further complicate their clinical picture. Therefore, biochemical tests used to evaluate metabolic bone disease, inflammation, and malabsorption of minerals are also described (Table 8.1). Testing for vitamin status evaluation is described in Chapter 7.

TABLE 8.1
Tests of Malabsorption in Patients with Short Bowel Syndrome

Transit time
    Lactulose breath hydrogen testing
    Marker studies
Fat malabsorption (Steatorrhea)
    Sudan stain
    72-hr fecal fat collection
Measurement of the stool osmotic gap
D-Xylose absorption
Bile salt malabsorption
    Empiric administration of a bile salt binding resin (e.g., Cholestyramine)
    ^{75}Se-homotaurocholate testing
Lactose tolerance testing
    Lactose breath hydrogen testing
    Endoscopic biopsy
Bacterial overgrowth
    Quantitative small bowel bacterial culture
    Breath hydrogen testing
Tests for coexisting disease states
    Celiac disease antibodies
    Protein-losing enteropathy
    Others (e.g., thyroid disease, diabetes, neuroendocrine syndromes)
Tests of systemic effects of malabsorptive states
    Tests of inflammation
    Calprotein
Nutrient balance studies
Divalent cation and metabolic bone disease studies
    Calcium and magnesium excretion
    Osteoblastic activity
    Osteoclastic activity

TRANSIT TIME

An important factor in patients with IF is the small intestinal transit time, since the period that food components remain accessible within the intestinal lumen may have a profound influence on nutrient absorption. Transit time testing can be measured radiographically, by breath hydrogen testing (BHT), and by the time to appearance of an ingested marker dye.

Breath hydrogen testing depends on gut flora (especially lactobacilli) that are able to metabolize lactulose, glucose, or lactose to hydrogen and methane. Since lactobacilli do not normally inhabit the small intestine, the appearance of hydrogen in breath samples signifies the arrival of the ingested sugar into the cecum (Figure 8.1), and the time to breath hydrogen generation above baseline levels is an indirect measurement of oro-cecal transit time. Normal breath hydrogen concentrations are less than 10 ppm,[1] though cigarette smoking can cause an elevated baseline breath hydrogen concentration. A rise of 10 ppm greater than baseline concentrations signifies the arrival of lactulose into the large bowel, or greater than 12 ppm if glucose and greater than 20 ppm if lactose sugars are used. If baseline breath hydrogen concentration is greater than 10 ppm, in the absence of cigarette smoking, a presumptive diagnosis of small bowel bacterial overgrowth (SBBO) is suggested.[2] Approximately 10% of individuals may be labeled as nonresponders, since their gut flora do not generate hydrogen. Small bowel bacterial overgrowth will preclude the use of BHT because the baseline hydrogen concentration is so high that a threshold increase may not be discernible. Since antibiotic use eliminates the GI flora, patients

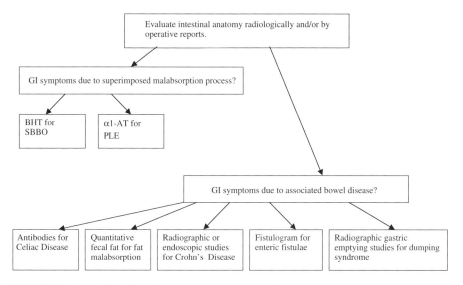

FIGURE 8.1 Algorithm for physiological evaluation of patients with intestinal failure.

with current or recent antibiotic use will gain limited information from the test. Patients who have end ostomy anatomy will not be good candidates for BHT because they have no ileocecal valve as well as direct exposure of the small intestine to the outside world, predisposing to bacterial overgrowth.

The standard protocol used for BHT in other subjects requires modification for patients with SBS. Lactulose has the propensity to produce diarrhea even in patients with normal anatomy, and this effect may be more pronounced in patients with SBS. Thus, a smaller dose than the customary 20 g should be used in patients with SBS. In addition, the transit time in patients with SBS is so much shorter than other patients, that the peak in breath hydrogen generation may be missed if the typical timing of sample collection (baseline, 15, 30, 60, 90, 120, 150, 180 minutes)[3] is used. Thus, the following protocol has been adjusted for the patient with SBS in terms of lactulose dose and timing of breath sample collection.

Patients should fast from midnight prior to the BHT for transit time. At time 0, 10 g lactulose syrup is given orally. Forty ml samples of expired alveolar air are collected in breath testing bags at times –20, –10, 5, 10, 15, 20, 25, 30 minutes relative to the lactulose ingestion and every 15 minutes thereafter for 2 hours. The air samples are injected into the breath hydrogen analyzer.[4] A sustained increase of 10 ppm hydrogen above the baseline reading is considered the oro-cecal transit time. The mean transit time for lactulose BHT in subjects with normal anatomy is 70–75 minutes;[4] thus, shorter times are expected with SBS.

For patients who do not have a colon in circuit or who have had recent antibiotic exposure or SBBO, an alternative method of transit time testing is needed. Early trials reporting on the use of colored marker appearance in stool samples used dyes that are not available for human use in the U.S. currently. The rapid transit time in patients with SBS makes monitoring of the appearance of a blue color marker in fecal samples fairly easy to do in a hospital or research center setting. The protocol listed here has been modified for patients with rapid intestinal transit.

After a 10-hour fast, patients will ingest 12 drops of blue food color (McCormick) mixed in 30 ml water, followed by 240 cc water. From that time point, all fecal and ostomy output will be monitored for the first evidence of blue color. Patients with ostomies will empty them every 10 minutes or with sensation of fecal passage. The transit time will be noted as the time required for the first appearance of color. Total transit time is expected to be within minutes to a few hours.

Published data on transit time in patients with IF or chronic diarrhea are summarized here. Total transit time, by colored marker passage, was < 3 hours in 8 ostomates[5] and < 10 hours in 43 patients with IF.[6] By scintigraphy, mouth to ostomy transit was < 5 minutes for liquids (normal 18 minutes) and 60 minutes for solids (normal 103 minutes) in patients with IF.[7] Mouth to cecum transit time by BHT in 45 patients with chronic diarrhea (including 2 with SBS) was 29 minutes compared to a normal control value of 75 minutes.[4]

FECAL FAT TEST

Some authorities prefer a Sudan stain for fat on a stool smear,[8,9] a qualitative measure of fat malabsorption. However, since stool fat output depends on the oral fat intake, a positive Sudan stain should be confirmed with a formal 72-hour stool collection on an appropriate diet. Conversely, Sudan staining may be false negative in patients who have ingested insufficient oral fat to render the test positive. The 72-hour fecal fat test is used to confirm steatorrhea, if collected under appropriate conditions. Steatorrhea, defined as an excess amount of fat in the stool, may be due to pancreatic lipase deficiency (e.g., chronic pancreatitis), deficiency of bile salts (e.g., severe terminal ileal disease or resection), or from luminal disease states preventing absorption of fat (e.g., mucosal disease or even bacterial overgrowth).[8,9]

Many patients find it very difficult to collect complete and continuous stool specimens for a 72-hour fecal fat test at home. Dietary fat intake must be around 100 g daily, a challenge for the patient who has symptoms of fat malabsorption. In fact, many patients automatically limit their fat intake because they know it causes diarrhea. In hospitalized patients, the 100 g fat diet must be ordered, and this level of fat intake cannot be attained with clear liquid diets. It may be difficult to interpret the results if the collection is incomplete or the dietary fat intake was less than 100 g.[8,9]

MEASUREMENT OF THE STOOL OSMOTIC GAP

Measurement of the stool osmotic gap is useful to distinguish secretory diarrhea from osmotic diarrhea. The former results from endogenous (e.g., neurohumoral) or exogenous (e.g., toxins) substances that stimulate enterocytes to secrete fluid and electrolytes, whereas the latter is due to an increase in nonabsorbed osmotically active agents that draw fluid into the intestinal lumen overwhelming the absorptive capacity of the gut. Since most osmotically active luminal factors are ingested, osmotic diarrhea tends to decrease in the face of fasting, whereas secretory diarrhea continues unabated, providing the patient remains adequately hydrated. Patients taking magnesium salts need to discontinue these osmotically active compounds prior to stool osmatic gap measurement. Stool osmotic gap is assessed by calculating the difference between estimated stool osmolarity (twice measured stool sodium plus potassium concentration) from the measured stool osmolarity. However, stool osmolarity should equal serum osmolarity, so that many investigators assume a "normal" stool osmolarity of approximately 290 mOsm. Normal stool osmotic gap is < 50 mOsm. Values > 100 mOsm are indicative of osmotic diarrhea (e.g., lactose intolerance), whereas values in the normal range reflect secretory diarrhea (e.g., a VIPoma, hyperthyroidism, hypergastrinoma). Very high or low stool osmolarity measurements are suggestive of factitious diarrhea in which the stool has been diluted with urine or water, respectively.[9]

D-XYLOSE ABSORPTION

The d-xylose absorption test was widely used in earlier times, and is fairly easy to perform. D-xylose is a naturally occurring sugar that is normally incompletely absorbed in the proximal small bowel, 35% metabolized in the liver, and 25% excreted in urine.[9] Following an orally administered 25 g dose of d-xylose, failure to collect more than 4 g in urine is indicative of malabsorption. Test results, though, are nonspecific since many GI conditions increase intestinal permeability to d-xylose.[8,9] Thus a positive d-xylose absorption test only confirms the presence of a malabsorptive state. It provides no information on the underlying cause of the malabsorption. Furthermore, false-positive test results occur in patients with renal insufficiency, delayed gastric emptying, and ascites.

BILE SALT MALABSORPTION

Since bile salt malabsorption is a common cause of diarrhea in Crohn's disease, SBS, after cholecystectomy and idiopathically,[8] a useful subjective test includes evaluation of symptoms before and after initiation of a bile salt binding resin. A more precise test, however, requires ingestion of ^{75}Se-homotaurocholate, a synthetic bile acid, followed by whole body counting at 7 days, when less than 15% retention of the initial dose indicates malabsorption.[8]

LACTOSE MALABSORPTION

Secondary lactose intolerance is a common clinical finding in patients with Crohn's or Celiac disease or SBS. Primary or congenital lactose intolerance also occurs in certain ethnic groups (especially among Africans, Chinese, and Jews) due to lactase deficiency. It is a common genetic deficiency inherited as an autosomal dominant condition with high penetrance.[9] This may be present from a young age or it can develop well into adulthood, making it appear as if a new problem has been acquired. In subjects with normal intestinal function, lactose is absorbed and does not reach the colon intact for bacterial fermentation. Subjects with lactose intolerance, however, absorb only a small amount of lactose and most of it passes to the colon, where it is metabolized by colonic flora and hydrogen is released. The BHT response to a 25–50 g oral lactose challenge diagnoses lactose malabsorption.[8] Figure 8.2 illustrates results of a lactose tolerance BHT in a patient with lactose intolerance. Lactase deficiency specifically can be diagnosed by assessing lactose enzyme activity in biopsy specimens obtained endoscopically, although this test is generally not required in adults.

SMALL BOWEL BACTERIAL OVERGROWTH

To detect small bowel bacterial overgrowth (SBBO), a quantitative culture of small bowel aspirate can be obtained and is viewed as positive if $> 10^6$ organisms/ml are counted.[2] Since such a bacterial count is sometimes found with healthy individuals, a functional test may be more helpful. BHT (as outlined earlier) using glucose or lactulose provides a functional test of SBBO, when the initial reading is high and does not increase markedly.[8] A double-bump pattern is most diagnostic in patients with intact colons, the first peak due to the generation of lactic acid by lactobacilli abnormally located in the small bowel and the second peak due to action of normally resident lactobacilli in the colon indicative of oro-cecal transit time. This

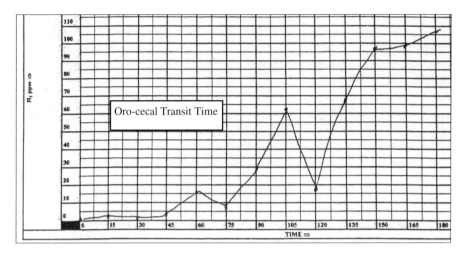

FIGURE 8.2 Example of an oro-cecal transit test using lactulose-breath hydrogen testing.

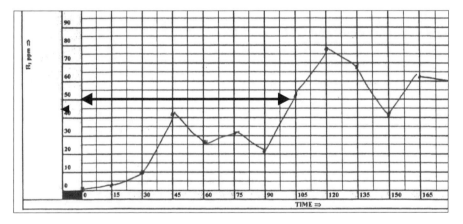

FIGURE 8.3 Example of a positive test for bacterial overgrowth with lactulose. The bold arrow marks the oro-cecal transit time.

double-bump pattern has been criticized for limited sensitivity compared to culture of small intestinal bacterial aspirates.[2] Figure 8.3 demonstrates an abnormal lactulose hydrogen breath test in a patient with SBBO.

OTHER CAUSES OF DIARRHEA THAT MAY COEXIST WITH ENTERIC FAILURE

Diarrhea in patients with SBS may sometimes be due to superimposed conditions, including bacterial overgrowth (discussed earlier), enteric infections, or even the subsequent appearance of additional disease states. The latter group of conditions includes common disease states such as diabetes mellitus (in which the diarrhea is due in part to motility disturbances as a consequence of autonomic neuropathy) or other endocrinopathies (such as thyrotoxicosis in which the diarrhea is due to the action of excessive thyroid hormone) as well as rare conditions such as neuroendocrine tumor syndromes (such as the VIPoma Syndrome or the Carcinoid Syndrome). Specific testing for these conditions is beyond the scope of this chapter (although stool osmolarity and electrolyte testing to identify secretory versus osmotic diarrhea was described earlier). However, celiac disease (also called celiac sprue or gluten sensitive enteropathy) is a relatively common disorder that warrants special mention because it has now become clear that silent or latent forms of the disease exist, such that the condition may become apparent only after an additional insult (such as bowel resection) that further reduces absorptive capacity.

Celiac disease, an immune-mediated enteropathy triggered by reaction to wheat, barley, or rye, affects approximately 1:130–300 of the population in Western Europe and likely similar numbers in the U.S.[10, 11] The prevalence is increased to 1:22 in first-degree relatives of celiac disease patients[10] and to 8% in those with Type I diabetes mellitus.[14] Celiac disease also has specific predilection for specific HLA subtypes. This magnitude of disease prevalence has been increased in part due to the advent of new serologic tests for antigliadin antibodies (AGA), anti-endomysial antibodies (EMA) and tissue transglutaminase (tTG), which have become preferred diagnostic methods.[15] Serum IgA and IgG AGA are assayed by ELISA,[11,12] IgA EMA by immunofluorescence, and tTG IgA by ELISA.[0] In a recent trial from France and Italy, the EMA and tTG test results were concordant in 94% of patients, while AGA assays had lower sensitivity and specificity.[13] These authors suggest screening with the anti-tTG assay, and following with IgA for EMA when tTG is positive. In fact, they would not require intestinal biopsy if both blood tests are positive,[13] though others support the use of a biopsy any time there is clinical suspicion of celiac disease,[14] a philosophy with which we concur.

Protein-losing enteropathy (PLE) is a rare cause of hypoalbuminemia. The condition is characterized by the presence of low serum protein levels and peripheral edema in the absence of other obvious causes for protein loss (i.e., without cirrhosis or the nephrotic syndrome) as a consequence of leakage of serum proteins into the GI lumen at a rate that exceeds synthetic capability. By itself, PLE rarely leads to frank diarrhea or steatorrhea, but this may supervene in the presence of superimposed SBS or if the underlying mucosal (e.g., Crohn's or celiac disease, ulcerative jejunitis or graft versus host disease) or submucosal disease (e.g., lymphangiectasia or constrictive pericarditis) is severe. Low serum levels of smaller proteins such as albumin, gamma globulin, or ferritin with normal levels of the larger serum proteins such as fibrinogen or alpha-2-macroglobulin are an important clue to the presence of PLE.[15] The diagnosis can be confirmed by measurement of radioactive chromium clearance after an IV chromium dose, a demanding procedure with a 6–10 day hospital admission, or by identifying the clearance of unusual proteins within stool especially α-1-antitrypsin (α-1-AT). The α-1-AT clearance is calculated as stool volume fecal chromium concentration/serum chromium. Normal α-1-AT clearance is 13 ± 3, and excretion is 40 ± 3ml/d. Tecnetium-labeled albumin clearance also can be obtained. Lymphopenia is characteristic of conditions that obstruct lymph flow (e.g., lymphangiectasia or constrictive pericarditis).[9]

INFLAMMATION

In the diagnostic evaluation of patients with diarrhea, inflammatory markers such as C-reactive protein (CRP) and erythrocyte sedimentation rate (ESR) are used to distinguish organic from functional disorders. Rarely will these tests, which have the advantage of being clinically available, together with a complete blood count and biochemistry profile, be normal in organic conditions.[8]

For patients with Crohn's disease, systemic inflammatory markers have been evaluated for their ability to predict disease relapse. CRP is an acute phase reactant from the α-globulin family that reacts with the C-polysaccharide of pneumococci. CRP is synthesized by the liver in response to mediators such as IL-6 and IL-1β.[16] In Crohn's patients in remission for 12 months, a persistently elevated CRP predicted a higher relapse rate in the second year than those with normal CRP concentration. CRP may have greater prognostic value in children than adults. Elevated IL-6 concentration was also associated with, but not predictive of, frequent disease relapse, with 73% sensitivity and 96% specificity.[16] Soluble IL-2 receptor concentration had a sensitivity of 88% and specificity of 65% for predicting relapse of Crohn's disease within 1 year.[16] Clinical assays for IL-6, IL-1β, and soluble IL-2 receptors are not yet available. ESR has been reported as elevated with greater frequency in colonic than ileal Crohn's disease flares.[9] Mild elevations in WBC and low albumin concentration are also seen with active inflammatory disorders, though specific biochemical tests to diagnose flares are not yet available.[9]

Calprotectin, a calcium-binding protein comprising up to 60% of the cytosolic protein content of neutrophils, is stable during intestinal transit but increases during intestinal inflammation. A single stool assay by ELISA gave a 90% sensitivity and 83% specificity of Crohn's disease relapse in a group of 43 patients, with a tenfold relative risk of relapse (95% CI, 2.5-45.8) if the calprotectin concentration was > 50 mg/L.[16] In this trial, ESR and CRP were not predictive, in contrast to fecal calprotectin.

NUTRIENT BALANCE STUDIES

Quantitative measurements of nutrient malabsorption are most readily obtained in a clinical research center. Complete collection of fecal output and dietary intake over an extended time period is distasteful and difficult for patients to do at home. One small advantage that patients with rapid transit have is that they do not require a 4-day period of adaptation to a special diet, as is standard for nutrient balance testing in normal volunteers. In fact, many patients with SBS will clear the contents of their entire intestinal tract in < 24 hours. If transit time is tested at baseline, it may be possible to customize a time of NPO prior to the admission to the research center for nutrient balance testing. In a group of 45 intestinal failure patients, mean total transit time was < 10 hours,[6] suggesting that a 10-hour fast should be adequate to eliminate any impact of the previous day's food intake from balance studies on the following day. The protocol outlined here was designed for patients with SBS.

Patients are admitted to the clinical research center in the morning after a 10-hour fast. Patients' usual PN infusion schedules need not be modified in any way prior to their participation in the nutrient balance tests. Patients are permitted to select a diet that resembles their usual food patterns for each admission, since there is little to be gained from study of a short-term change in dietary pattern. From the time of admission until discharge 48 hours later, all food and fluid intake are measured and recorded. For research purposes, it is helpful also to collect, blend, and freeze a duplicate sample of all food and fluid intake, and a separate collection of any food left over by the patient, for assay of nutrient content. The nutrient intake would be that in the duplicate diet sample minus that in the food left over sample.[18] Otherwise, the nutrient content can be estimated from comparison with nutrient databases. Such a 48-hour balance period was adequate to evaluate nutrient balance in SBS patients.[6] Complete collections of all fecal output are measured, refrigerated during the collection period, pooled, blended, and frozen at $-80°C$. Patients with ostomies empty them every 2 hours during the admission.

Frozen samples (both food aliquot and fecal output) can be assayed in commercial laboratories for nitrogen (by Kjehldahl method[18]) and fat content (by chloroform-methanol extraction[18]). The energy content of freeze-dried fecal samples can be combusted by bomb calorimetry.[6] Total carbohydrate content can be assayed by anthrone detection.[19] Alternatively, carbohydrate can be estimated by subtraction of fat and nitrogen (9.35 and 5.65 and kcal/g respectively) from the measured kcal of the fecal collection, using a factor of 4.20 kcal/g for carbohydrate.[18] Patients with SBS secrete variable amounts of gastric acid and intestinal fluids in response to oral foodstuffs. Thus, the accepted measure of fluid absorption is a comparison of the total weight of food plus fluid intake with the stool output.[6] Calcium and magnesium can be assayed by atomic absorption spectroscopy.[21] Nutrient balance is calculated as the nutrient intake minus the fecal output of the particular nutrient. Clinically available metabolic laboratories in the U.S. will assay stool samples for nitrogen, fat, calcium, sodium, and potassium content.

In long-term PN patients with SBS, dietary fat absorption is generally less efficient than that of protein and carbohydrates. Carbohydrate is absorbed at 61%–79%, protein at 61%–81% but fat at only 52%–54% of that ingested.[22] Unless patients are able to absorb > 84% of basal energy requirements and > 1.4 liters of fluid daily, which may actually require intake of up to 400% of energy needs and 7 liters of fluid daily, as a rule they do not become independent of PN support.[6]

DIVALENT CATION BALANCE AND METABOLIC BONE DISEASE

Calcium status can be difficult to evaluate, since the body's homeostatic mechanisms will often produce normal serum calcium, and changes in hydration may artificially impact calcium concentration. To evaluate adequacy of body calcium content, particularly in a patient who complains of muscle cramping during the PN run, ionized calcium concentration may be helpful, though these measures will be insensitive to early signs of negative calcium balance. To evaluate calcium status for a metabolic bone disease evaluation, concurrent serum concentrations of calcium, phosphorus, magnesium, alkaline phosphatase, parathyroid hormone, and vitamin D (25-hydroxy and 1-, 25-dihydroxy) are recommended, along with annual dual x-ray absorptiometry scans.

To evaluate excess calcium excretion or limited magnesium excretion as a component of metabolic bone disease, urine collections are used. Urine samples may be measured in 30 ml (spot) samples excluding the first daily void in patients with malabsorption syndromes, if the results are normalized to creatinine concentration. In patients with PN, a complete 24-hour urine collection is needed to reflect calcium or magnesium[24] excretion with accuracy. Urine samples are assayed by atomic absorption spectroscopy for total calcium and/or magnesium content.[21,24]

Useful biochemical tests of bone activity can be grouped by measurement of osteoblast (bone specific alkaline phosphatase, procollagen 1 carboxy terminal peptide, and osteocalcin) and osteoclast activity (urine deoxypyridinoline and N-telopeptide of type-I collagen). For serum alkaline phosphatase, the bone specific isozyme is most informative, assayed by ELISA, and has normal concentrations of 8–24 U/l.[25] Procollagen 1 carboxy terminal peptide is assayed by RIA,[26] and serum total osteocalcin, also called bone gla-protein, by ELISA[26] or immunoradiometric (IRMA) assay.[27] Urine samples for osteoclast activity can be measured in 30 ml (spot) samples excluding the first daily void in patients with malabsorption syndromes, but patients with PN require a complete 24-hour urine collection. Deoxypyridinoline is measured by HPLC,[25,26,28] with a normal range of 1.5–6.1 mM/mM creatinine.[25] N-telopeptide type 1 collagen protein is measured using RIA[26] or ELISA[25,27,29] with normal range of 5–60 mM/mM creatinine.[25,29]

CONCLUSION

While a clinical presentation that includes diarrhea may be challenging to decipher, the availability of clinical tests for transit time, nutrient malabsorption, and serologic markers can provide insight. Noninvasive measures of inflammation may assist in the management of Crohn's disease. The chronic comorbid conditions associated with malabsorption syndromes, including metabolic bone disease, are further clarified by the measurement of osteoclastic and osteoblastic activity, as well as calcium and magnesium excretion. In patients with severe diarrhea, including SBS, many of these standard test procedures will require modification to obtain best results and to avoid exacerbating the patient's GI symptoms.

REFERENCES

1. Miller, M.A. et al., Comparison of scintigraphy and lactulose BHT for assessment of orocecal transit (lactulose accelerates small bowel transit), *Dig. Dis. Sci.* 42:10–18, 1997.
2. Riordan, S.M. et al., The lactulose BHT and small intestinal bacterial overgrowth, *Am. J. Gastroent.* 91:1795–1803, 1996.
3. Hamilton, L.H., *Breath Tests and Gastroenterology,* 2nd ed. Quintron, Milwaukee, WI, 1998.

4. Lin, H.C., Van Citters, G.W., Heimer F., and Bonorris G., Slowing of gastrointestinal transit by oleic acid, *Dig. Dis. Sci.,* 46, 223, 2001.

5. Woolf G.M. et al., Diet for patients with a SBS: Evaluation of fluid, calorie, and divalent cation requirements, *Dig. Dis. Sci.,* 32, 8, 1983.

6. Jeppesen, P.B. and Mortensen, P.B., Intestinal failure defined by measurements of intestinal energy and wet weight absorption, *Gut,* 46, 701, 2000.

7. Nightingale, J.M.D. et al., Disturbed gastric emptying in the SBS. Evidence for a 'colonic brake', *Gut,* 34, 1181, 1993.

8. Forbes, A., Investigation of diarrhoea in adults, *Clin. Med.,* 2, 410, 2002.

9. Yamada, T. et al., *Textbook of Gastroenterology,* 3rd ed. Lippincott & Co., Philadelphia, 890, 1999.

10. Fasano, A. et al., Prevalence of celiac disease in at-risk and not-at-risk groups in the United States, *Arch. Int. Med.,* 63, 286, 2003.

11. Abdulkarim, A.S. and Murray J.A., Review article: the diagnosis of coeliac disease, *Aliment. Pharmacol.Ther.,* 17, 987, 2003.

12. Kumar, V. et al., Celiac disease and immunoglobulin A deficiency: How effective are the serological methods of diagnosis?, *Clin. Diag. Laboratory Immunol.,* 9, 1295, 2002.

13. Tonutti, E. et al. The role of antitissue transglutaminase assay for the diagnosis and monitoring of celiac disease: a French-Italian multicentre study, *J. Clin. Pathol.;* 56, 389, 2003.

14. Cronin, C., Exploring the iceberg—the spectrum of celiac disease, *Am. J. Gastro.,* 98, 518, 2003.

15. Florent, C. et al., Intestinal clearance of alpha1-antitrypsin, a sensitive method for the detection of protein-losing enteropathy, *Gastroenterology* 82:777–780, 1982.

16. Arnott, I.D.R., Watts, D., and Ghosh, S., Review article: is clinical remission the optimum therapeutic goal in the treatment of Crohn's disease, *Aliment. Pharmacol. Ther.* 16, 857, 2002.

17. Seguy, D. et al., Low-dose growth hormone in adult home parenteral nutrition-dependent SBS patients: A positive study, *Gastroenterology,* 124, 293, 2003.

18. Williams, D., Ed., *Official Methods of Analysis of the Association of Official Analytical Chemists,* American Organization of Analytical Chemists, Arlington, VA, 1984.

19. Ameen, V.Z. and Powell G.K., A simple spectrophotometric method for quantitative fecal carbohydrate measurement, *Clin. Chim. Acta.,* 152, 3, 1985.

20. Ameen, V.Z., Powell, G.K., and Jones, L.A., Quantitation of fecal carbohydrate excretion in patients with SBS, *Gastroenterology,* 92, 493, 1987.

21. Haderslev, K.V., Jeppesen, P.B., Mortensen, P.B., and Staun, M., Absorption of calcium and magnesium in patients with intestinal resections treated with medium chain fatty acids, *Gut,* 46, 819, 2000.

22. Woolf, G.M., Miller, C., Kurian, R., and Jeejeebhoy, K.N., Nutritional absorption in SBS, *Dig. Dis.Sci.,* 32, 8, 1987.

23. Messing, B. et al., Intestinal absorption of free oral hyperalimentation in the very SBS, *Gastroenterology,* 100, 1502, 1991.

24. Fleming, C.R. et al., The importance of urinary magnesium values in patients with gut failure, *Mayo Clinic Proc.,* 71:21–24, 1996.

25. Schulte, C. et al., Bone loss in patients with inflammatory bowel disease is less than expected: A follow-up study, *Scand. J. Gastroenterol.,* 34, 696, 1999.

26. Bjarnason, I. et al., Reduced bone density in patients with inflammatory bowel disease, *Gut,* 40, 228, 1997.

27. Dresner-Pollak, R. et al., Increased urinary N-telopeptide cross-linked type 1 collagen predicts bone loss in patients with inflammatory bowel disease, *Am. J. Gastro.*, 95, 699, 2000.

28. Haderslev, K.V. et al., Short-term administration of glucagons-like peptide-2. Effects on bone mineral density and markers of bone turnover in short-bowel patients with no colon, *Scand. J. Gastroenterol.*, 37, 392, 2002.

29. Schulte, C.M.S. et al., Genetic factors determine extent of bone loss in inflammatory bowel disease, *Gastroenterology*, 119, 909, 2000.

9 The Role of Diet and Specific Nutrients

Theresa A. Byrne, Suzanne Cox,
Maria N. Karimbakas, and
Rebecca A. Weseman

CONTENTS

Few clinical scenarios present a more challenging long-term nutritional problem than that which confronts the patient with intestinal failure, specifically those with short bowel syndrome (SBS). The prolonged and severe diarrhea and malabsorption that characterize this syndrome results in dehydration, metabolic disturbances, micronutrient deficiencies, and progressive malnutrition. Over the past 3 decades enormous resources have been devoted to advancing the provision of parenteral nutrition (PN) to these patients, resulting not only in the significant improvement in patient survival but also allowing many of these individuals to resume full and productive lives. Despite these advances, this mode of nutrition support is not aimed at improving the function of the remnant and/or diseased bowel. In contrast, despite encouraging results demonstrating that luminal nutrients play an important role in bowel adaptation in several animal models of SBS, there has been relatively little focus on the role that specific nutrients or oral or enteral diets might play in facilitating adaptation in patients with SBS. There is also limited consensus on the role that oral diets play in the compensation of the residual bowel, and thereby the management of these patients. This review will attempt to define the potential role that specific nutrients and/or diets may play in bowel adaptation and in the rehabilitation of patients with SBS.

INTESTINAL ADAPTATION IN ANIMALS

In animals subjected to massive small bowel resection, the residual intestine undergoes a patterned adaptive response, which is characterized by structural (increases in intestinal crypt depth and villus height) and functional (increased absorptive capacity per centimeter remaining bowel) changes.[1,2] This process of intestinal adaptation is achieved by the interaction of numerous factors of which oral or enteral nutrients are thought to play a critical role.[2,3]

THE ROLE OF LUMINAL NUTRIENTS

Following intestinal resection, adaptive mucosal hyperplasia of the remnant small bowel occurs only if nutrients are present in the intestinal lumen.[4] The absence of luminal nutrients inhibits intestinal hyperplasia even when adequate calories are provided intravenously.[5] Luminal nutrients may stimulate bowel adaptation by several interrelated mechanisms, including (1) the direct contact and uptake by the mucosal surface, (2) by provoking the release of pancreatico-biliary secretions and (3) by triggering the release and circulation of specific hormones.[2,3]

SPECIFIC NUTRIENTS

In an attempt to determine the effect of a single nutrient on the adaptive response, specific nutrients have been infused into the gastrointestinal tract of experimental animals otherwise nourished via PN. Long-chain triglycerides given intragastrically to rats after resection promote intestinal adaptation to a greater extent than proteins and polysaccharides.[6] This same effect was not observed with medium-chain triglycerides.[7] Free fatty acids have been shown to be a more potent stimulator of small bowel adaptation than long-chain triglycerides,[8] particularly specific polyunsaturated long-chain fatty acids.[9,10]

The effect of specific sugars on small bowel adaptation has also been studied in experimental animals. Infusions of the disaccharides sucrose, maltose, and lactose resulted in significantly greater mucosal growth than with equal concentrations of the monosaccharides glucose, fructose, and galactose.[11] Similarly, some studies have suggested that whole proteins such as casein are more potent than hydrolysates in inducing mucosal hyperplasia in rats undergoing intestinal resection.[12] Others have also found that polymeric diets (containing protein, polysaccharide, and fat) can contribute to better intestinal mucosal regeneration than a monomeric diet (containing amino acid, glucose, disaccharide, and triglyceride) in rats following intestinal resection.[13]

It has been suggested that the nonessential amino acid glutamine, which serves as a major fuel source for both the enterocytes and the colonocytes, may also play a role in bowel adaptation. In animals, glutamine supplementation has been shown to accelerate postresection hyperplasia following extensive intestinal resection.[14,15] In addition to structural or morphological effects, others have questioned the potential functional effects glutamine might have on absorption. Gardemann et al.[16] demonstrated that the administration of luminal, but not vascular, glutamine enhances glucose absorption in the rat. Others have described the ability of enteral glutamine to enhance sodium and chloride absorption in various animal models.[17,18]

Non-nutritive components of foods such as dietary fibers have also been implicated as agents, which may influence bowel adaptation. In an animal model of massive small bowel resection, the addition of the water-soluble fiber pectin to an elemental diet enhanced small bowel mucosal adaptation, as indicated by mucosal weight, DNA content, mucosal thickness, and disaccharidase activity.[19] Others have demonstrated that pectin increases stool solidity and improves colonic water absorption in the rat following extensive small bowel resection.[20] The fermentation of specific soluble fibers and carbohydrates results in the production of short chain fatty acids (SCFA),[21] and the administration of these agents has also been shown to reduce mucosal atrophy associated with the PN following extensive bowel resection[22] and exert trophic effects both on the small bowel and in the colon in animal models.[23]

In addition to evaluating the stimulatory effect of the exogenous administration of a given nutrient or the non-nutritive components of foods, others have evaluated the effect of a specific nutrient deficiency on bowel adaptation following resection in experimental animals. Deficiencies of zinc,[24] Vitamin A,[25] and essential fatty acids[26] have been shown to impair mucosal adaptation.

BOWEL ADAPTATION/COMPENSATION IN HUMANS

Clinically, the patient with SBS progresses from a phase of massive diarrhea and the related severe fluid and electrolyte disturbances to a period associated with a decrease in diarrhea, an apparent improvement in nutrient absorption, and a corresponding decrease in the need for parenteral support. However, the mechanisms underlying this process in humans have not been elucidated. A recent study by Ziegler et al.[27] found no evidence that adaptation to the extensive loss of intestinal surface area in humans involves hyperplasia of either the small bowel or colonic mucosa. Rather, these authors observed up-regulation of the peptide transporter PepT1 in the colon of patients with SBS, suggesting that the colon can increase the luminal transport of di- and tripeptides derived from the diet or other sources. This study, along with a small body of evidence[28–30], raises the critical question of whether the vast body of animal data evaluating bowel adaptation is relevant to humans with SBS.

In addition, it may be more appropriate to refer to the observed changes in some of the human studies as bowel compensation, rather than adaptation, for the functional improvement (e.g., improved absorption, decreased diarrhea) to a given intervention (e.g., administration of an appropriate diet) often disappears if the intervention is stopped. Thus, the positive response is a result of the intervention that allows the bowel to compensate, but does not necessarily induce the lasting changes that have been associated with the defined process of bowel adaptation.

THE ROLE OF LUMINAL NUTRIENTS

The limited size of the SBS patient population, the complexity and invasive techniques involved with examination of the small bowel, and ethical concerns related to the randomization of patients to a treatment arm that may impair the normal adaptive response are all factors that have contributed to the limited number of studies evaluating changes in bowel morphology and/or nutrient absorption in patients with SBS. For instance, there are no prospective, randomized trials comparing the effects of luminal vs. no luminal nutrition on bowel adaptation during the early postoperative phases. Often the potential clinical implications of a given nutrient or diet have been derived from other patient populations or from descriptive reports of unique findings in patients with SBS.

For example, case reports have been published encouraging the use of early enteral feedings in patients following extensive resection.[31,32] In a larger report by Levy et al.[33] of 62 patients who had recently undergone extensive resection resulting in remnant small bowel lengths of 30 to 150 cm, the authors describe their experience with the use of continuous enteral feedings during the early adaptive stages. Despite their aggressive utilization of enteral feedings in this challenging group of patients, they described a marked reduction in stool volumes. In addition, PN was discontinued in all patients at a mean of 36 days from the initiation of the enteral feedings. Although there was no comparative group or evaluation of bowel morphology, the authors concluded that the early use of enteral feedings stimulates adaptive changes in the residual small intestine, allowing oral alimentation to be resumed after a relatively short period of time. These authors also described that despite the theoretical advantage of providing a readily absorbable elemental diet, their clinical experience revealed that these solutions, which have a high osmolality, offer no advantage over polymeric formulas.

THE ROLE OF SPECIFIC NUTRIENTS

Limited clinical data are available on the role that specific nutrients play at enhancing bowel adaptation or compensation; thus, implications are often based on related human data. The parenteral administration of the amino acid glutamine has been shown to prevent bowel atrophy and the deterioration in gut permeability in patients receiving PN.[34] In a preliminary study[35] of 8 patients with ileostomies, the ingestion of 50 g of glutamine resulted in an increase in nitrogen absorption and nitrogen balance; however, these changes were expected given that the subjects increased their consumption of protein during the experimental period. Water and electrolyte losses were unaffected. Other studies in patients with SBS have utilized glutamine, in combination with growth hormone, with[36-39] or without[40] a modified diet. Some of these reports describe positive changes in nutrient absorption and PN dependency;[36,37,39] others[38] describe no change in bowel morphology, a delay in gastric emptying, and limited improvement in selected markers of nutrient absorption; and others[40] describe no change in nutrient absorption. However, it was not the intent of any of these studies to differentiate the effect of glutamine from the other interventions (growth hormone and/or a modified diet), making it impossible to define the potential effects of glutamine alone from these studies.

In an attempt to further clarify the specific role of glutamine in patients with SBS, Scolapio et al.[41] conducted a randomized, double-blind, placebo-controlled crossover study in 8 patients with short bowel syndrome. All patients consumed a high-carbohydrate, low-fat diet during the outpatient active and placebo treatment periods, which were each 8 weeks in duration with no washout period. Active treatment was oral glutamine 0.45g kg^{-1}day^{-1}. For 3 days, on two separate occasions, 8 weeks apart, the patients were admitted to a hospital where studies of nutrient absorption, bowel morphology, and gastrointestinal transit were conducted. During the two evaluation periods, the patients received a diet that apparently differed in composition from that which they consumed during the outpatient placebo and treatment periods. Further, the diets utilized during the two evaluation periods did not appear to be constant. The authors describe no changes in small bowel morphology, as might be expected based on the recent finding by Ziegler et al.[27] described earlier. They also found no change in gastrointestinal transit, d-xylose absorption, or stool losses; however, the lack of clarity regarding the diet used during the evaluation periods makes it difficult to interpret these results.

Because of some of the positive morphological and functional effects of specific fibers in animal models of SBS, it has been suggested that the addition of dietary fibers might facilitate bowel adaptation or compensation and thereby assist in the management of patients with SBS. Overall, when discussing the role of fiber in humans it is useful to divide fiber into soluble and insoluble types. In general, the insoluble fibers tend to increase stool bulk and decrease transit time, whereas specific soluble fibers do not increase fecal weight and have been shown to delay gastric emptying, slow total intestinal transit time, and have a mild antidiarrheal effect in adults subjects.[42-44]

Fermentable, soluble fibers such as pectin (as well as unabsorbed or resistant starches) may assist in bowel adaptation and/or the in the management of the patient with short bowel, particularly those with intact colon. The anaerobic bacterial metabolism of these fibers and carbohydrates that either resist digestion or escape absorption in the upper intestinal tract result in the production of short-chain fatty acids (SCFA), hydrogen gas, carbon dioxide, methane, and water in the colon.[21,45] The SCFA, the major by-product of bacterial fermentation, is readily absorbed by the colonic mucosa and utilized for energy in animals as well as in man.[46] The energy derived from this process can be considerable in patients with short bowel syndrome.[47] In addition, a case report of a child with short bowel indicated that the use of a diet supplemented with the soluble fiber pectin resulted in a slight improvement in nitrogen absorption and slowing of stomach to anus transit time.[48]

Although such effects have positive clinical implications for patients with SBS, others report on the potential negative effects associated with the use of specific soluble fibers. Fuse et al.[49] describe a decrease in fatty acid and glucose absorption with increasing concentrations of pectin in healthy subjects. Others describe an inverse relationship between fat absorption and soluble fiber intake in patients with SBS.[36]

Medium-chain triglycerides (MCT), which do not require digestion by pancreatic lipase or co-lipase, are often used clinically in an attempt to reduce steatorrhea in patients with SBS; however, few studies have clearly defined their role. In a relatively recent report, Jeppesen and Mortensen[50] compared 2 high fat (50% of total calories) diets in 19 patients who had undergone an intestinal resection, 9 *without colon* (mean residual small bowel length, 203 cm; range, 125–300) and 10 *with colon* (mean residual small bowel length, 143 cm, range 50–250 cm). The patients were randomized in a crossover design to a diet that consisted of either long-chain triglycerides or long-chain triglycerides plus MCT. The diet enriched with MCT resulted in an improvement in fat absorption (from 23% to 58%) and overall energy absorption (from 46% to 58%) for patients with colon. For patients without colon, the diet enriched with MCT resulted in an increase in fat absorption (from 37% to 46%), but did not improve overall energy absorption because malabsorption of carbohydrate and protein increased. The authors suggest that the colon serves as a digestive organ for MCT, which are probably absorbed as medium-chain fatty acids. Like SCFA, the medium-chain fatty acids are water-soluble. Despite the long-standing assumption that MCT may be beneficial to patients with SBS because they are more readily absorbed by the small bowel, these authors conclude that only patients with colon seem to benefit from the use of MCT.

More recently,[51] the use of an emulsion containing the specific fatty acid, oleic acid, has been shown to slow gastrointestinal transit and reduce stool frequency and stool volume in patients with chronic diarrhea of diverse etiologies, including SBS. The consumption of the oleic acid-containing emulsion prior to a meal apparently activated nutrient-triggered inhibitory feedback mechanisms, slowing transit and reducing stool output.

MANAGEMENT OF SBS: THE ROLE OF SPECIFIC DIETS

A very limited number of studies have attempted to determine if a given diet or diet prescription (rather than a specific nutrient) can assist in the management of patients with SBS by either enhancing nutrient absorption, decreasing stool or ostomy output, and/or reducing PN requirements. Although early reports[52–54] concluded that no significant therapeutic benefit can be achieved via the manipulation of the diet, these studies were conducted in a very small number of patients, predominately those without colon.

A later study by Nordgaard et al.[55] recognized that patients with colon differ in their response to dietary manipulation than those without colon. These authors compared the effect of a high-carbohydrate diet (60:20:20%, carbohydrate:fat:protein) to a high-fat diet (20:60:20% carbohydrate:fat:protein) in 14 patients with short bowel, 8 with colon, and 6 without. For those patients with colon, the high-carbohydrate diet significantly reduced the fecal loss of calories in comparison to the high-fat diet, and the absorption of energy increased from 49% to 69%. The authors concluded that the presence of colon allowed carbohydrate calories that would otherwise be lost due to upper-intestinal malabsorption to be fermented by the colonic bacteria to SCFA, absorbed, and utilized for energy. For patients without colon, the high carbohydrate diet increased ostomy output by more than 700 cc per day compared to outputs on the high-fat diet; however, these differences were not statistically significant.

The importance of diet was further emphasized in a preliminary report describing the findings of a prospective, randomized, placebo-controlled trial in 41 PN dependent patients (the majority with colon) with SBS.[56] In this study, the control group was treated with an optimized oral diet, which was also supplemented with glutamine. These patients experienced a significant reduction in PN requirements over their baseline PN needs. However, the extent of the reduction was greatest in those patients who, in addition to the optimized diet supplemented with glutamine, also received growth hormone.

In addition to this study, the positive effects of diet intervention in 10 PN dependent SBS patients with colon are shown in Table 9.1 and Table 9.2. Table 9.1 compares 3 days of calorie and fluid intake, stool output, and "fluid" absorption (fluid intake–liquid stool output) while consuming an ad lib diet to 3 days while consuming an optimized diet. The optimized diet was designed utilizing the guidelines presented in Table 9.3. Patients recorded food intake and stool output and worked with dietitians who manipulated the diet based on the measured responses to arrive at an optimized diet plan. They continued on this plan for an average of 13 months (range 6–36 months). During that time, PN was gradually reduced, as tolerated. Table 9.2 compares PN requirements, weight, and serum albumin levels prior to diet intervention to PN requirements, weight and serum albumin levels on average 13 months after the initiation of diet intervention.

Overall, the reduction in PN was well tolerated. One patient experienced a >5% reduction in weight; however, this weight loss was gradual and desired, for the patient was 157% above her ideal body weight prior to diet intervention, and she continued to remain above her ideal body weight at the time of the follow-up evaluation. One patient experienced a fall in serum albumin below the lower limits of normal. In addition to weight and albumin, the hydration and micronutrient status of the patients were closely monitored. Objective parameters (data not shown), such as BUN:Cr, urine volumes, serum electrolytes, and vitamin and trace element and essential fatty acid profiles, revealed that the patients were able to maintain hydration and micronutrient status, despite the marked reduction in PN. Like the study by Nordgaard et al.,[55] these data demonstrate that patients with colon respond favorably to diet intervention, and with the appropriate follow-up and monitoring, these responses can result in clinically significant changes in PN requirements with maintenance of nutrition and hydration status in most patients.

For patients without colon, there is less consensus on the potential role that diet intervention might play in the management of these individuals. Some authors feel that these individuals do not benefit from diet intervention.[57] Because the proportion

TABLE 9.1
Ad Lib vs. Optimized Oral Diet in Patients with Colon

Pt. #	Jejunum/Ileum (cm)	Colon (%)	Ad Lib Diet				Optimized Diet			
			Calorie Intake (kcal)	Fluid Intake (cc)	Stool Output (cc)	Enteral Balance (cc)	Calorie Intake (kcal)	Fluid Intake (cc)	Stool Output (cc)	Enteral Balance (cc)
1	45	100	1,929	2390	1412	+978	2,466	3620	1250	+2370
2	62	50	1,445	1380	663	+727	2,403	1635	725	+910
3	40	100	2,011	1320	683	+637	2,446	2300	617	+1683
4	150	75	1,479	1780	308	+1472	2,410	2310	833	+1477
5	100	66	2,922	1665	1850	−185	3,526	2445	1590	+855
6	135	33	2,925	2165	1452	+713	2,545	3443	2158	+1285
7	30	66	1,734	1553	1560	−6	1,784	2160	1217	+943
8	10	75	3,465	3560	4167	−607	3,604	4207	3700	+507
9	120	66	2,900	2660	2550	+110	3,722	4680	1600	+3080
10	56	100	1,221	1540	958	+582	1,769	2400	1150	+1250
Median	59	70	1,970	1723	1432	+609	2,456	2423	1234	+1268

TABLE 9.2
Comparison of PN Requirements, Weight, and Serum Albumin Before and After Diet Treatment

Patient #	Baseline			Follow-up		
	PN Days	Weight (kg)	Albumin	PN Days	Weight (kg)	Albumin
1	7	69.2	3.6	0	71.0	4.4
2	7	54.6	3.3	0	48.2	4.7
3	7	89.6	3.8	0	71.8	4.3
4	7	59.1	4.8	0	56.1	4.4
5	7	70.0	4.0	0	71.6	4.3
6	6	70.5	4.3	0	68.0	3.7
7	7	72.7	3.3	3.5	72.0	3.1
8	7	57.6	3.6	0	63.6	3.9
9	4	65.5	3.5	2	64.1	2.8
10	7	58.2	3.5	0	58.2	4.1
Median	7.0	67.4	3.6	0.0	66.1	4.2

TABLE 9.3
Diet Prescription

	Colon	No Colon
Carbohydrate	50%–60% of total calories (limit simple sugars)	40%–50% of total calories (restrict simple sugars)
Protein	20%–30% of total calories	20%–30% of total calories
Fat	20%–30% of total calories primarily as essential fats)	30%–40% of total calories primarily as essential fats)
Fluid	Isotonic or hypo-osmolar fluids	Isotonic, high-sodium oral rehydration solutions
Soluble Fiber	5–10 grams/day (if stool output is > 3 L/day)	5–10 grams/day (if stool output is > 3 L/day)
Oxalates	Limit intake	
Meals/Snacks	5–6 meals per day	4–6 meals per day

From Byrne, T.A., *Nutrition in Clinical Practice*, 15, 306, 2000. With permission.

of fat absorbed in these individuals is constant,[52,54] others argue that an increased intake can lead to a greater absorption of energy.[58] Also, because the jejunum differs than the ileum and colon in the handling of water and sodium, others stress the importance of the composition of fluid intake in these patients whose primary challenge often revolve around issues related to fluid management rather than calorie absorption.[58,59]

Our own experience has shown that some, but not all, patients without colon respond favorable to dietary manipulation. Table 9.4 compares the calorie and fluid intake, stool output, and enteral balance while consuming an ad lib intake versus an optimized diet in a small group of patients without colon. The optimized diet was designed utilizing the prescription guidelines in Table 9.3. On average, these patients experienced a reduction in stool output of approximately 500 cc and improvement in fluid absorption of nearly one liter. Though these results may not be as consistent as what can be achieved in patients with intact colon, clinically they are important to the patient. In our experience, patients with less than 50 cm of small bowel and no functional colon rarely demonstrate significant clinical benefit from diet manipulation.

PRACTICAL CONSIDERATIONS

The initial step in designing diets is establishing the prescription. Recommendations for diet prescriptions for patients with and without colon are shown in Table 9.3. These recommendations are derived from our experience of testing the effects of different diets on stool or ostomy output in approximately 400 patients with SBS, and then monitoring their long-term nutritional and hydration status.

CALORIES

During the early postoperative period, total daily calorie intake is initially restricted (to approximately 500 calories/per day) to avoid further exacerbation of diarrhea. As tolerance to oral intake improves, caloric intake can be gradually increased. (If oral foods are not tolerated, a polymeric enteral formula should be initiated.) Though energy absorption is variable in patients who have stabilized following resection, many patients absorb about two-thirds as much energy as normal and thus need to increase their dietary intake by a half to maintain weight.[60,61] While some absorb more and others less, this is a reasonable starting point in establishing a daily calorie goal in a stable patient, if the intent is to sustain the patient without PN. Though many patients are hyper-phagic and have no difficulty consuming this number of calories, others find it more challenging. If absorption of fluid is adequate and not adversely affected by increased intake, a nocturnal tube feeding can be trialed in these patients. In some patients, particularly those with no colon, the increased intake of calories can actually aggravate fluid losses, making it necessary to reduce the established goal. Careful monitoring of weight, stool, and ostomy output and other parameters of nutritional and hydration status can help to determine if the oral calorie goal needs to be adjusted and/or if PN is required.

CARBOHYDRATE

In an effort to reduce osmotic load, complex carbohydrates such as those found in pasta, potatoes, rice, bread, are favored over simple sugars (sucrose, fructose, lactose). Patients with colon appear to derive the most benefit from a high carbohydrates diet due to the energy derived from the fermentation of malabsorbed carbohydrates

TABLE 9.4
Ad Lib vs. Optimized Oral Diet in Patients without Colon

Patient #	Jejunum/ Ileum (cm)	Colon %	Ad Lib Diet				Optimized Diet			
			Calorie Intake (kcal)	Fluid Intake (cc)	Stool Output (cc)	Enteral Balance (cc)	Calorie Intake (kcal)	Fluid Intake (cc)	Stool Output (cc)	Enteral Balance (cc)
1	115	0	2,641	3330	3100	+230	3,224	3662	2685	+977
2	107	0	1,934	2240	1768	+472	1,760	2453	1250	+1200
3	62	0	992	1797	2558	−762	1,376	2540	2000	+540
Median	107	0	1934	2240	2558	230	1,760	2540	2000	+977

by the colonic flora. Though lactose-containing diets have been shown to be relatively well tolerated in patients with SBS,[62] lactose (particularly milk) restriction may reduce stool or ostomy output in some patients, particularly in those with a preexisting intolerance.

PROTEIN

Most patients with SBS tend to tolerate protein. High biological value proteins (such as those found in chicken, turkey, fish, beef, pork) are encouraged.

FAT

In patients with no colon, the proportion of fat absorbed from the diet appears to be constant;[54] thus, an increased intake can result in greater absorption of calories. In our experience, intakes of greater than 40% of total calories are typically not well tolerated long-term. In contrast, fat restriction (to approximately 20%–30% of total calories) is often helpful for patients with small bowel in continuity with colon. The restriction can reduce steatorrhea and diarrhea, decrease in losses of magnesium and calcium, and decreased oxalate absorption.[58] As described earlier, the use of diets containing MCT appear to be helpful for patients with colon (but not those without)[50]; however, in our experience they are often not well accepted long-term. In addition, the use of fats/oils which contain the appropriate proportion of essential fats (e.g., safflower oil, soybean oil) can help prevent essential fatty acid deficiency, which can be common in this population.[63]

FLUID

Like calories, oral fluid intake should be limited (to approximately 500 cc/day) during the very early postoperative period. As the patient stabilizes, the intake of fluid can gradually progress. Patients with jejunostomies require an isotonic, high sodium (90 mmol/L or greater), glucose–containing solutions, sipped throughout the day. Examples of such solutions include Oral Rehydration Salts (Jianas Brothers Packaging Co.; Kansas City, MO) and Cera-Lyte (Cera Products, LLC; Jessup, MD). In a stable patient, often 3–3.5 liters are required per day; however, if ostomy output exceeds intake despite the appropriate diet and fluid modifications, supplemental intravenous fluids are required. Both hypo- and hyper-osmolar beverages should be avoided. Because the colon avidly absorbs sodium against steep electrochemical gradients,[58] the composition of the oral fluid is not as critical in patients with colon. However, care should be taken to assure that the diet is adequate in sodium. In the stable patient, fluid intakes between 2.5 and 3.5 liters per day are often well tolerated and adequate to replace losses. Intake of hyper-osmolar beverages (e.g., regular soda, fruit juices) are often not well tolerated, particularly in large volumes, and should be restricted.

FIBER

Though fermentable fibers have a theoretical benefit for the patient with colon, the same benefits can be derived from a high-carbohydrate diet. In our experience, supplemental fiber contributed to increased gas and bloating in some patients. We also observed an inverse relationship between fat absorption and soluble fiber intake.[36] We reserve the use of soluble fiber for those patients with large stool or ostomy outputs (> 3 liters/day). The intent of using these fibers in these patients is to gelatinize the stool and help control fluid losses, an effect that has been observed in some, but not all patients.

OXALATES

Patients with colon are at increased risk of oxalate nephropathy. A low-oxalate diet reduces oxalate absorption, and thus urinary excretion. Foods high in oxalates include spinach, rhubarb, parsley, beets, cocoa, and tea. Patients with jejunostomies do not need an oxalate restriction.

MEALS AND SNACKS

Meals and snacks should be distributed throughout the day. Each meal should contain the protein, fat, and carbohydrate, with the intent to avoid the overconsumption of a given food item or calories source at any one time. It is possible for patients to be compliant to the prescribed diet but to select an inappropriate diet. An example of this is provided in Table 9.5. Both the "appropriate diet" and the "less appropriate" diet provide 2,400 calories, 50% carbohydrate, 20% protein, and 30% fat; however, the foods have a marked difference on output. Figure 9.1 compares the effect of two "appropriate" diet prescriptions on stool output and fluid absorption in the same patient (45 cm small bowel, 100% colon). Both Diet 1 and Diet 2 provided the recommended percentage of carbohydrate, protein, and fat for a patient with colon; however, Diet 1 contained less appropriate food choices whereas Diet 2 consisted of more appropriate foods. Stool output decreased by more than 50% and fluid absorption improved by nearly 2 liters while consuming Diet 2.

VITAMIN AND MINERAL SUPPLEMENTS

Nutrient abnormalities and deficiencies are common in patients with SBS, even those infusing PN.[64,65] In addition to the debility that can result from these deficiencies, nutrient deficiencies can impair bowel adaptation in animals. Routine (semiannual) assessments are recommended. For patients receiving no or reduced quantities of PN, oral vitamin and mineral supplements need to be provided. All patients who have lost their terminal ileum need regular injections of vitamin B12. Adequate calcium and vitamin D are required to avoid bone-related abnormalities.

TABLE 9.5
"Appropriate" and "Less-Appropriate" Meal Patterns

2400 calories, 50% carbohydrate, 20% protein, 30% fat

Diet # 1- "Appropriate"	Diet # 2- "Less Appropriate"
Breakfast:	**Breakfast:**
1 cup of Oatmeal	8 ounces of orange juice
2 ounces of lactose-free milk	1 cheese and fruit-filled danish
1 egg	
2 slices of toast or 1 English Muffin	
2 teaspoons of margarine	
1 teaspoon of diet jelly	
4 ounces of coffee	
Morning Meal:	**Morning Meal:**
1 bagel	Nothing
$^{1}/_{2}$ ounce of cheese	
1 teaspoon of margarine	
1 small banana	
4 ounces of water	
Lunch:	**Lunch:**
3 ounces of baked ham	1 slice cheese pizza
$^{1}/_{2}$ cup of rice	12 ounces of regular soda
$^{1}/_{2}$ cup of carrots	
2 small dinner rolls	
2 teaspoons of margarine	
4 ounces of water or diet soda	
Dinner:	**Dinner:**
4 ounces of roasted chicken	12 ounces of T-bone steak
1 large baked potato	1 large baked potato
2 dinner rolls	1 cup of spinach
2 teaspoons of margarine	12 ounces of beer
4 ounces of water or diet soda	
Evening Snack:	**Evening Snack:**
1 roast beef sandwich prepared with:	3-4 cups of popcorn
2 slices of bread	1 cup of raspberry sorbet
1 ounce of roast beef	12 ounces of diet soda
1 teaspoon of mayonnaise	
1 teaspoon mustard	
1 ounce of pretzels	
4 oz water or diet soda	
Additional Fluid:	**Additional Fluid:**
1.5 to 2.0 liters of oral rehydration solution	1.5 to 2.0 liters of water

From Byrne, T.A., *Nutrition in Clinical Practice,* 15, 306, 2000. With permission.

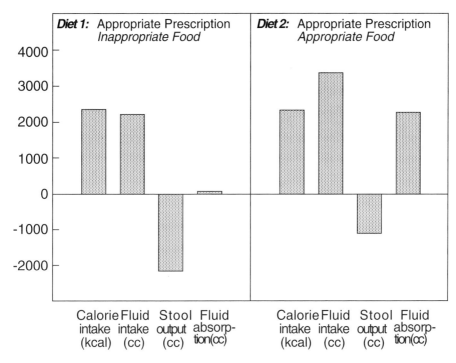

FIGURE 9.1 The effect of two appropriate diet prescriptions on stool output and fluid absorption in a patient with SBS (45 cm small bowel, 100% colon). Though the composition of both diets are the same (2,400 calories, 50% carbohydrate, 20% protein, and 30% fat), Diet 1 contained inappropriate food choices, whereas Diet 2 contained appropriate foods which resulted in a reduction in stool output and improvement in fluid absorption. (Adapted from Byrne, T. A., *Nutrition in Clinical Practice*, 15, 306, 2000.)

MONITORING AND EDUCATION

The most efficient and accurate way to arrive at an optimized diet is to obtain daily food intake and stool/ostomy output records. In comparison to metabolic balance studies, we have found that such data provides a relatively inexpensive way to objectively monitor progress to various diet manipulations and allows clinicians to identify specific foods, which may not be well tolerated. Though this process may seem overly cumbersome, most patients are receptive to providing this information. To assure that the information is accurate, patients require training on how to record and collect the requested data. In addition, once the optimal diet plan is identified, compliance to the diet is best achieved and maintained if the patient receives adequate education and long-term monitoring. The optimal diet prescription needs to be translated into food and meal patterns that meet the individual preferences and lifestyle requirements of the patient. Overall, due to the complexities involved with managing these patients, consideration should be given to referring these individuals to specialized centers who are experienced in caring for large numbers of these patients.

CONCLUSION

Although specific nutrients have been shown to accelerate bowel adaptation in animal models, much less is known about their role in enhancing morphological changes or improving nutrient absorption in patients with SBS. Clinically, the early provision of luminal nutrients during the postoperative period appears to facilitate the eventual reduction in PN and transition to oral or enteral nutrition. The use of specific nutrients or non-nutritive components of foods may assist the management of select patients. However, perhaps more important than a given nutrient is the composition of the entire oral diet. Long-term, the use of appropriate oral diets, coupled with adequate patient education and monitoring, allow most patients with SBS to achieve an improved clinical outcome.

REFERENCES

1. O'Brien, D.P. et al., Intestinal adaptation: structure, function and regulation, *Semin. Pediatr. Surg.,* 10, 56, 2001.
2. Weser, E., Nutritional aspects of malabsorption: Short gut adaptation, *Clin. Gastroenterol.,* 12, 443, 1983.
3. Lentze, M.J., Intestinal adaptation in short-bowel syndrome, *Eur. J. Pediatr.,* 148, 294, 1989.
4. Levine, G.M., Deren, J.J., and Yezdimir, E., Small bowel resection. Oral intake is the stimulus for hyperplasia, *American Journal of Digestive Diseases,* 21, 542, 1976.
5. Feldman, E.J. et al., Effects of oral versus intravenous nutrition on intestinal adaptation after small bowel resection in the dog, *Gastroenterology,* 70, 712, 1976.
6. Morin, C.L., Grey, V.L., and Garofalo, C., Influence of lipids on intestinal adaptation after resection, in *Mechanisms in Intestinal Adaptation*, Robinson J.W.L., Dowling R.H., Riecken E.O., Eds, MTP Press, Lancaster, 1982, 175.
7. Vanderhoof, J.A. et al., Effect of high percentage medium chain triglyceride diet on mucosal adaptation following massive bowel resection in the rat, *J. Parenter. Enter. Nutr.,* 8, 685, 1984.
8. Grey, V.L. et al., The adaptation of the small intestine after resection in response to free fatty acids, *Am. J. Clin. Nutr.* 40, 1235, 1984.
9. Kollman, K.A., Lien, E.L., and Vanderhoof, J.A., Dietary lipids influence adaptation after massive bowel resection, *J. Pediatr. Gastroenterol. Nutr.,* 28, 41, 1999.
10. Vanderhoof, J.A. et al., Effects of dietary menhaden oil on mucosal adaptation after small bowel resection in rats, *Gastroenterology,* 106, 95, 1994.
11. Weser, E., Babbitt, J., and Hoban, M., Intestinal adaptation: Different growth responses to disaccharides compared to monosaccharides in rat small bowel, *Gastroenterology,* 91, 1521, 1986.
12. Vanderhoof, J.A. et al., Effect of casein versus casein hydrolysate on mucosal adaptation following massive bowel resection in infant rats, *J. Pediatr. Gastroenterol. Nutr.,* 3, 262, 1984.
13. Lai, H.S. et al., Effects of monomeric and polymeric diets on small intestine following massive resection, *J. Formosan Med. Assoc.,* 88, 982, 1989.
14. Gouttebel, M.C. et al., Influence of N-Acetylglutamine or glutamine infusion on plasma amino acid concentrations during the early phase of small-bowel adaptation in the dog, *J. Parenter. Enter. Nutr.,* 16, 117, 1992.

15. Tamada, H. et al., Alanyl glutamine-enriched total parenteral nutrition restores intestinal adaptation after either proximal or distal massive resection in rats, *J. Parenter. Enter. Nutr.,* 17, 236, 1993.
16. Gardemann, A. et al., Increases in intestinal glucose absorption and hepatic glucose uptake elicited by luminal but not vascular glutamine in the jointly perfused small intestine and liver of the rat, *Biochem. J.*, 283, 759, 1992.
17. Rhoads, J.M. et al., L-glutamine stimulates jejunal sodium and chloride absorption in pig rotavirus enteritis, *Gastroenterology*, 100, 683, 1991.
18. Rhoads, J.M. et al., L-glutamine with d-glucose stimulates oxidative metabolism and NaCl absorption in the piglet jejunum, *Am. J. Physiol.*, 263, G960, 1992.
19. Koruda, M.J. et al., The effect of a pectin supplemented elemental diet on intestinal adaptation to massive small bowel resection, *J. Parenter. Enter. Nutr.*, 10, 343, 1986.
20. Roth, J.A. et al., Pectin improves colonic function in rat short bowel syndrome, *J. Surgical Research*, 58, 240, 1995.
21. Rombeau, J.L. and Kripke, S.A., Metabolic and intestinal effects of short-chain fatty acids, *J. Parenter. Enter. Nutr.*, 14, 181S, 1990.
22. Koruda, M.J. et al., Effect of parenteral nutrition supplemented with short-chain fatty acids on adaptation to massive small bowel resection, *Gastroenterology*, 95, 715, 1988.
23. Kripke, S.A. et al., Stimulation of intestinal mucosal growth with intracolonic infusion of short-chain fatty acids, *J. Parenter. Enter. Nutr.*, 13, 109, 1989.
24. Tamada, H. et al., Zinc-deficient diet impairs adaptive changes in the remaining intestine after massive small bowel resection in the rat, *Br. J. Surg.*, 79, 959, 1992.
25. Swartz-Basile, D.A., Rubin, D.C., and Levin, M.S., Vitamin A status modulates intestinal adaptation after partial small bowel resection, *J. Parenter. Enter. Nutr.* 24, 81, 2000.
26. Hart, M.H. et al., Essential fatty acid deficiency and postresection mucosal adaptation in the rat, *Gastroenterology*, 94, 682, 1988.
27. Ziegler, T.R. et al., Distribution of the H+/peptide transporter PepT1 in human intestine: up-regulated expression in the colonic mucosa of patients with short bowel syndrome, *Am. J. Clin. Nutr.*, 75, 922, 2002.
28. Porrus, R.L., Epithelial hyperplasia following massive resection in man, *Gastroenterology*, 48, 753, 1965.
29. DeFrancesco, A. et al., Histological findings regarding jejunal mucosa in short bowel, *Transplantation Proceedings*, 26, 1455, 1994.
30. O'Keefe, S.J.D. et al., Long-acting somatostatin anologue therapy and protein metabolism in patients with jejunostomies, *Gastroenterology*, 107, 379, 1994.
31. Votik, A.J. et al., Use of elemental diet during the adaptive stage of short gut syndrome, *Gastroenterology*, 65, 419, 1973.
32. Rodriguez, D.J. and Clevenger, F.W., Successful enteral refeeding after massive small bowel resection, *West. J. Med.,* 159, 192, 1993.
33. Levy, E. et al., Continuous enteral nutrition during the early adaptive stage of the short bowel syndrome, *Br. J. Surg.,* 75, 549, 1988.
34. Van Der Hulst, R.R.W.J. et al., Glutamine and the preservation of gut integrity, *Lancet*, 341, 1363, 1993.
35. Bouteloup, C. et al., Effect of oral glutamine on absorptive function of ileostomised patients, *Clin. Nutr.*. 13, 61S (abstr.), 1994.
36. Byrne, T.A. et al., Growth hormone, glutamine and a modified diet enhance nutrient absorption in patients with severe short bowel syndrome, *J. Parenter. Enter. Nutr.*, 19, 296, 1995.

37. Byrne, T.A. et al., A new treatment for patients with short bowel syndrome, *Ann. Surg.* 222, 243, 1995.

38. Scolapio, J.S. et al., Effect of growth hormone, glutamine and diet on adaptation in short-bowel syndrome: a randomized, controlled trial, *Gastroenterology* 113, 1074, 1997.

39. Zhu, W. et al., Rehabilitation therapy for short bowel syndrome, *Chin. Med. J.*, 115, 776, 2002.

40. Szkudlarek, J., Jeppesen, P.B., and Mortensen, P.B., Effect of high dose growth hormone with glutamine and no change in diet on intestinal absorption in short bowel patients: a randomized, double-blind, crossover placebo controlled study, *Gut*, 47, 199, 2000.

41. Scolapio, J.S. et al., Effect of glutamine in short-bowel syndrome, *Clin Nutr,* 20, 319, 2001.

42. Jenkins, D.J.A. et al., Fiber and starchy foods: Gut function and implications in disease, *Am. J. Gastroenterol.*, 81, 920, 1986.

43. Spiller, G.A. et al., Effect of purified cellulose, pectin, and a low-residue diet on fecal volatile fatty acids, transit time, and fecal weight in humans, *Am. J. Clin. Nutr.*, 33, 754, 1980.

44. Schwartz, S.E. et al., Sustained pectin ingestion delays gastric emptying, *Gastroenterology*, 83, 812, 1982.

45. Ahmed, R., Segal, I., and Hassan H., Fermentation of dietary starch in humans, *Am. J. Gastroenterol.*, 95, 1017, 2000.

46. McNiel, N.I., The contribution of the large intestine to energy supplies in man, *Am. J. Clin. Nutr.*, 39, 338, 1984.

47. Nordgaard, I., Hansen, B.S., and Mortensen, P.B., Importance of colonic support for energy absorption as small-bowel failure proceeds, *Am. J. Clin. Nutr.*, 64, 222, 1996.

48. Finkel, Y. et al., The effects of a pectin-supplemented elemental diet in a boy with short gut syndrome. *Acta. Paediatr. Scand.,* 79, 983, 1990.

49. Fuse, K., Bamba, T., and Hosoda, S., Effects of pectin on fatty acid and glucose absorption and on the thickness of the unstirred water layer in rat and human intestine, *Digestive Diseases and Sciences*, 34, 1109, 1989.

50. Jeppesen, P.B. and Mortensen, P.B., The influence of a preserved colon on the absorption of medium chain fat in patients with small bowel resection, *Gut*, 43, 478, 1998.

51. Lin, H.C. et al., Slowing of gastrointestinal transit by oleic acid. A preliminary report of a novel, nutrient-based treatment in humans, *Digestive Diseases and Sciences*, 46, 223, 2001.

52. McIntyre, P.B. Fitchew, M., and Lennard-Jones, J.E., Patients with a high jejunostomy do not need a special diet, *Gastroenterology*, 91, 25, 1986.

53. Ovesen, L., Chu, R., and Howard, L., The influence of dietary fat on jejunostomy output in patients with severe short bowel syndrome, *Am. J. Clin. Nutr.*, 38, 270, 1983.

54. Woolf, G.M. et al., Diet for patients with a short bowel: high fat or high carbohydrate? *Gastroenterology*, 84, 823, 1983.

55. Nordgaard, I., Hansen B.S., and Mortensen, P.B., Colon as a digestive organ in patients with short bowel, *Lancet*, 343, 373, 1994.

56. Byrne, T.A. et al., Recombinant human growth hormone reduces parenteral nutrition (PN) requirements in patients with the short bowel syndrome: a prospective, randomized, double-blind, placebo-controlled study, *J. Parenter. Enter. Nutr.*, 27, S17 (abstract #034), 2003.

57. Scolapio, J.S., Short bowel syndrome, *J. Parenter. Enter. Nutr.*, 26, S11, 2002.

58. Lennard-Jones, J.E., Review article: practical management of the short bowel, *Aliment. Pharmacol. Ther.*, 8, 563, 1994.
59. Lennard-Jones, J.E., Oral rehydration solutions in short bowel syndrome, *Clinical Therapeutics*, 12, Suppl. A., 129, 1990
60. Rodigues, C.A., Lennard-Jones, J.E., and Thompson, D.G., Energy absorption as a measure of intestinal failure in the short bowel, *Gut,* 30, 176, 1989.
61. Messing, B., Pigot, F., and Rongier, M., Intestinal absorption of free oral hyperalimentation in the very short bowel syndrome, *Gastroenterology*, 100, 1502, 1991.
62. Marteau, P. et al., Do short bowel patients need a lactose-free diet? *Nutrition,* 13, 13, 1997.
63. Jeppesen, P.B., Hoy, C.E., and Mortensen, P.B., Deficiencies of essential fatty acids, vitamin A and E and changes in plasma lipoproteins in patients with reduced fat absorption or intestinal failure, *Eur. J. Clin. Nutr.*, 54, 632, 2000.
64. Cox, S., Karimbakas, M., and Byrne, T., The incidence of nutrient abnormalities in patients dependent upon long-term PN, *Nutrition in Clinical Practice*, 17, 61 (abstr. #N40), 2002.
65. Burnes, J.U. et al., Home parenteral nutrition — a 3-year analysis of clinical and laboratory monitoring, *J. Parenter. Enter. Nutr.*, 16, 327, 1992.

10 Medications: Antidiarrheals, H$_2$ Blockers, Proton Pump Inhibitors, and Antisecretory Therapy

Hossam M. Kandil and Stephen J.D. O'Keefe

CONTENTS

Patients with short bowel syndrome, particularly those with end-jejunostomies, have high gastric and pancreatic secretory rates, which, when coupled with the fact that the proximal gut mucosa is "leaky" and passively loses fluid when food is eaten, means that fluid and electrolyte losses are the predominant management problems. Consequently, the first lines of management have to be directed toward suppressing secretory losses and reducing osmotic forces. Medications can also improve nutrient absorption by slowing the rate of transit of nutrients through the remaining gut, and therefore allowing more time for digestion and absorption. Consequently, medical management is based on therapies that a) reduce secretory loses, and b) decrease gut motility. Newer lines of therapy are based on trophic hormones that enhance mucosal function.

0-8493-1803-3/05/$0.00+$1.50
© 2005 by CRC Press LLC

ANTIDIARRHEALS

Increased gastrointestinal motility and faster gastric emptying contribute to the increased diarrhea and stomal output in patients with short bowel syndrome, particularly in patients with loss of the ileal brake and colon. This may be secondary to low plasma peptide YY (PYY) levels, as PYY is chiefly synthesized and released from the distal bowel.[1] Increased motor activity has been measured in short bowel syndrome patients in the fasting state, although the response to feeding may not be different from healthy subjects.[2]

In order to counteract these changes, opiates and their derivatives form an integral part of long-term management of patient with short bowel syndrome. Loperamide is one of the most commonly used drugs because of its lack of extraintestinal effects. Loperamide does not appear to affect the frequency of contractions during fasting. In addition, it may stimulate eating in some patients.[2] Although some case reports show positive effects for loperamide on water and salt balance,[3] this has not been a constant finding.[4] High doses of up to 16 mg 3 times a day an hour prior to meals may be needed,[5] as absorption may be low, and the safety index is high. More potent opiates, such as codeine phosphate, are more effective in slowing transit but have more unwanted central side effects.

Octreotide decreases intestinal motility, gastric emptying, and gallbladder contraction while increasing intestinal electrolyte and water absorption.[6,7] However, it is expensive and has to be given subcutaneously. There is concern that octreotide might cause growth retardation in children due to its effects on growth hormone secretion. Long-term administration (i.e., greater than 1 month) of octreotide has been associated with the formation of cholesterol gallstones. There is also concern that it may inhibit intestinal adaptation postresection. Its use should be limited to patients with the highest stomal outputs.

ANTISECRETORY AGENTS

HISTAMINE RECEPTOR ANTAGONISTS AND PROTON PUMP INHIBITORS

Gastric hypersecretion and gastrin hyperactivity occur immediately after intestinal resection.[8–10] This may be related to decreased intestinal inhibitory hormones after bowel resection, such as cholecystokinin and somatostatin.[10] The effect may be transient and may improve with the resumption of oral intake, but can result in peptic ulcer disease and severe erosive esophagitis.[11] Increased intra-duodenal acidity may reduce fat digestion and absorption through the inhibition of pancreatic enzyme activity and precipitation of bile salts.[12–14] Treatment with intravenous proton pump inhibitors is routine in the immediate postoperative period and can be changed to oral treatment with resumption of oral intake.

The effects of H-2 receptor antagonists and proton pump inhibitors on nutrient absorption remain unclear. A decrease in stool wet weight has been shown in response to proton pump inhibitors and intravenous cimetidine, particularly in patients with large stool output.[15] On the other hand, the effects on fat, nitrogen, energy, sodium, and potassium absorption are inconsistent, with most studies showing no beneficial

TABLE 10.1
Effect of Intravenous Ranitidine and Omprazole Twice Daily on Fecal Excretion. Crossover Double-Blind Control Study in 13 Patients with Short Bowel (Median of 150 cm) and > 1500 g Stool/Day

Fecal Excretion	Control Period	Ranitidine (150 mg BID)	Omeprazole (40 mg BID)
Weight (kg/d)	2.9 (2.3–4.4)	2.5 (2.2–3.3)[a]	2.4 (2.1–2.6)[a]
Sodium (mmol/d)	248 (228–335)	230 (208–335)[a]	228 (200–257)[a]
Potassium (mmol/d)	49 (34–67)	43 (28–50)	36 (29–49)
Calcium (mmol/d)	37 (29–46)	33 (28–45)	33 (28–47)
Magnesium (mmol/d)	14 (8–20)	20 (13–21)	14 (13–20)
Energy (MJ/d)	5.1 (4.7–6.2)	4.8 (4.7–5.3)	5.3 (4.8–6.4)
Nitrogen (g/d)	9.1 (8–10)	8.7 (7.6–9.6)	9.7 (7.8–12.1)

Data are Median (25%–75%).

[a] Significant from control period.

Modified from Jeppesen, P.B., *Gut* 1998; 43:763–769.

effects.[9,15–18] (See Table 10.1.) The importance of gastric acid secretion on absorption of divalent cations is controversial. Although some studies suggest that calcium absorption from insoluble salts such as carbonates may be inhibited in achlorhydric patients, particularly in the fasting states,[19] other studies demonstrate that gastric acidity has no significant effects on calcium absorption irrespective of its source.[15,20,21]

Bacterial growth in the normal small intestine is suppressed by multiple mechanisms, including gastric acid secretion, pancreatic enzyme activity, normal antegrade peristaltic activity, normal enterocyte turnover, and the presence of ileocecal valve. One or more of these barriers are broken in patients with short bowel syndrome, and bacterial overgrowth is common. Bacteria in the small intestine can interfere with fat absorption by deconjugating bile acids. For this reason it is important to reassess the need for acid suppression, bearing in mind that gastric hypersecretion decreases with time. Overgrowth proven by endoscopic aspiration should be treated with cyclical courses of broad-spectrum antibiotics.[22]

SOMATOSTATIN AND ITS ANALOGUES

Somatostatin is an inhibitory hormone produced by neuroendocrine cells throughout the gastrointestinal tract and pancreas. Its chief effect is the tonic control of gastrointestinal function, mainly on the suppressive side. Clinical studies have shown that it is very effective in controlling hypersecretory states and severe diarrhea.[23] It is a potent suppressor of gastric and pancreatic secretion.[24] The half-life of the native compound is short (minutes), which has led to the development of long-acting analogues, such as octreotide, with a half-life of several hours so that it can be given

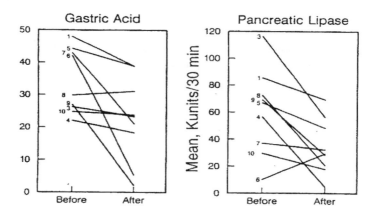

FIGURE 10.1 The effect of octreotide 100 µg sc tid for 7 days on gastric and pancreatic secretion stimulated by pentagastrin and CCK-8 in 10 patients with adapted end-jejunostomies (After O'Keefe, S.J.D., Peterson, M.E., and Fleming, C.R., Octreotide as an adjunct to home parenteral nutrition in the management of permanent end-jejunostomy syndrome, *J. Parenter. Enteral Nutrition* 1994; 18:26–34.), showing significant ($p < 0.05$) suppression of secretion.

as a subcutaneous injection thrice a day. More recently, lantreotide has been developed that has a half-life of several days.[25]

Octreotide can be particularly helpful in patients with high output stomas, that is, more than 4 liters/day, resulting in decreased diarrhea and improved quality of life.[26] In our study of patients with high-output end-jejunostomies,[23] octreotide reduced stomal outputs from 12 to 9 L/d, and sodium losses from 369 to 245 mEq/d (Table 10.2). It appears to do this by reducing gastric and pancreatic exocrine secretion, and may improve fluid and electrolyte reabsorption by reducing motility and increasing mucosal contact time (Figure 10.1). In one patient, the reduction in fluid loss was so great that she gained 4 Kg after the first injection overnight, and developed mild heart failure. On average, however, the gain in fluid balance was modest, resulting in a diminution of TPN fluid requirements of 0.5 L/d. The downside of the hormone is its negative effects on virtually all GI peptides, including insulin, CCK, gastrin, epidermal growth factor (EGF), and GH.[27] It can therefore precipitate diabetes and pancreatic exocrine insufficiency. More important, perhaps, in patients with short bowel is the antiadaptation effects. Mucosal turnover and blood flow is suppressed, mucosal transport is inhibited, and stasis can exacerbate bacterial overgrowth and gallstone formation.[28] Moreover, octreotide may inhibit small bowel adaptation, which may be mediated through decreased secretion of trophic factors such as EGF, and decrease gut hormones such as growth hormone and mucosal protein synthesis.[29,30]

BILE SALT-BINDING RESINS

One function that is irreversibly lost in ileal resections is the active transport mechanisms for bile salt reabsorption. Unabsorbed bile salts enter the colon and stimulate water and salt secretion.[31,32] In addition, bile salt deficiency may result in malabsorption

---

TABLE 10.2
The Effect of Octreotide 100 μg
sc tid for 7 days on 72h Stomal
Outputs in 10 Patients with
Adapted End-Jejunostomies

Daily Stomal Output Rates Effect of Octreotide		
	Before	After
Volume (L)	12.3(8.7)	5.8(2.1)[a]
Fat (g)	67(39)	64(48)
Nitrogen (g)	23(8)	15(7)[a]
Sodium (meq)	605(301)	316(109)[a]
Potassium (mEq)	148(92)	92(28)[a]
Chloride (mEq)	614(273)	363(109)[a]

[a] p <0.05 vs. pre-treatment
After O'Keefe, S.J.D., Peterson, M.E., and
Fleming, C.R., Octreotide as an adjunct to
home parenteral nutrition in the management
of permanent end-jejunostomy syndrome, *J.
Parenter. Enteral Nutrition* 1994; 18:26–34.

---

of fat and fat-soluble vitamins. Undigested fat in the colon binds calcium, which usually combines with dietary oxalate, preventing its absorption. With steatorrhea, the free oxalate is reabsorbed and excreted in the urine, where it can produce renal stones. Should this occur, it may be necessary to prescribe a low-fat diet and bile salt-binding resins, such as cholestyramine. However, these resins may further worsen bile salt deficiency, with exacerbation of the malabsorption of calcium and fat-soluble vitamins. It is therefore important to provide additional calcium and fat-soluble vitamin supplements given 2–3 hours apart from resin.

An often overlooked problem is chronic bile salt deficiency, due to the break in enterohepatic circulation in short bowel patients. Hofmann's group has lead the research into the clinical significance of the deficiency, demonstrating significant improvement of fat absorption with supplementation of the diet with synthetic secondary bile salts that are resistant to bacterial decongugation. For example, cholysarcosine reduced stool fat loss from 65 g/day to 35 g/day in a short bowel patient.[33]

HORMONAL MEDICATIONS

GROWTH HORMONE

Growth hormone is involved in the regulation of bowel growth.[34] Many of the anabolic effects of growth hormone are mediated via the generation of insulin-like growth hormone (IGF-1). In animal models, treatment with growth hormone has been shown in some studies to stimulate intestinal hypertrophy in adult animals,[35,36] although these effects were not seen in growing animals.[37]

The use and efficacy of GH in the treatment of patients with short bowel has produced variable and somewhat controversial effects. Early studies were uncontrolled and complicated by co-treatment with dietary modification and supplementation, and so it was difficult to ascribe specific benefits to GH. Wilmore's group in Boston were enthusiastic for the use of GH in rehabilitating patients with intestinal failure following the analysis of their first study in 47 patients with short bowel syndrome who were treated with growth hormone in addition to glutamine and dietary modification (high-carbohydrate, low-fat diet). After 3 weeks of treatment, they observed significant improvements in nutrient absorption and decreased stool losses. The net effect was a reduction of parenteral nutrition (PN) requirements.[38] In a subsequent study of patients who had been treated with total parenteral nutrition for a mean of 4.3 years, treatment with glutamine and growth hormone along with modified diet resulted in decreased dependence on parenteral nutrition.[39] However, it is common experience to be able to reduce PN requirements by dietary modification alone, and clearly there was a need for a controlled trial. As a next step, Mortensen's group examined the efficacy of GH and glutamine without dietary modification in a controlled blind crossover study of 8 patients with short bowel syndrome dependent on PN for 3–11 years. They found no improvement in the absorption of water, nitrogen, carbohydrates, sodium, potassium, magnesium, and calcium. Their enthusiasm was further dampened by the observation that all subjects in the treatment arm developed side effects.[40] Just when the pendulum had swung against GH, Messing's group from Paris published their results on the use of low-dose GH in 12 HPN-dependent SBS patients with a residual intestinal length 0–120 cm.[41] Nine out of 12 had some colon remaining in continuity. The trial took the form of a randomized double-blind, placebo-controlled, crossover trial of GH 0.05 mg/kg/d for 3 weeks. The results showed an increase in energy absorption of 15% ($p = 0.0002$), nitrogen of 14% ($p = 0.04$), carbohydrates of 10% ($p = 0.04$), and fat of 12% (ns). In addition, d-xylose absorption increased, and the net result was increased body weight and lean body mass. The end result was that there was an increase in absorption of 427 Kcal/day, which could be translated into a reduction of 37% of PN needs.

GLUCAGON-LIKE PEPTIDE 2 (GLP-2)

GLP-2 is one of the intestinal proglucagon-derived peptides, secreted by intestinal mucosa after food ingestion. In animal studies, GLP-2 administration has been shown to induce enterocyte proliferation,[42] and improve absorptive capacity after massive small bowel resection.[43] The interesting thing about the peptide from the SBS point of view is that it is predominantly synthesized by the distal gut and may therefore become deficient in patients with massive resection, raising the intriguing possibility of supplementation in SBS patients.

Glucagon-like immunoreactivity (GLI), also known as enteroglucagon and pro-glucagon derived peptides (PGDPs), were detected by radioimmunoassay in pancreatic extracts and the small and large intestine. Several patients with glucagonomas were reported to exhibit small bowel villus hyperplasia that receded following tumor resection, suggesting trophic effects for PGDPs on the intestine.[44] Intestinal resection was consistently associated with increased circulating levels of the PGDPs and up-regulation of intestinal proglucagon mRNA transcripts in the intestinal remnant.[45,46] Subsequent studies in mice demonstrate that GLP-2 is the PGDP with the greatest intestinotrophic effect.[42] GLP-2-secreting enteroendocrine L cells are most abundant in the ileum and colon. The presence of nutrients in the gastrointestinal tract constitutes the primary stimulus for GLP-2 secretion with its levels low in the fasted state and increase rapidly following nutrient ingestion.[47,48] The kidney plays an important role in the degradation of both GLP-1 and GLP-2 so that circulating levels of total GLP-2 immunoreactivity are increased in patients with renal failure.[47] An intact colon is an important determinant of the levels of circulating GLP-2. Short bowel patients with a jejunostomy lacking a colon exhibited normal basal levels but markedly impaired meal stimulated levels of GLP-2.[49] Exogenous GLP-2 administration increased wet weights in the rodent jejunum and ileum, in association with enhanced crypt cell proliferation, reduced apoptosis in the enterocyte and crypt compartments, and increased thickness of the epithelial mucosa. These effects are not associated with increased food consumption over a 10-day period in mice.[50] GLP-2 administration is associated with both structural and functional changes in the gut mucosal epithelium. Small bowel epithelial cells from mice treated with h[Gly^2]-GLP-2 for 10 days appear significantly narrower and longer, and the length of enterocyte microvilli are significantly increased. The GLP-2-treated epithelium exhibited reduced paracellular permeability.[51] Coinfusion of GLP-2 and parenteral nutrition prevented mucosal atrophy, and significantly attenuated loss of protein and DNA content in the small bowel but not in the colon of parenterally fed rats. Furthermore, GLP-2-treated rats exhibited significantly increased villus height and total mucosal thickness in the duodenum, jejunum, and ileum.[52] In rat models, circulating levels of GLP-2 are increased following 75%–80% intestinal resection. However, exogenous administration of h[Gly^2]-GLP-2 produced significant increases in segmental and mucosal wet weights following 6 and 21 days of peptide administration. Furthermore, crypt-villus height and mucosal sucrase activity were significantly increased in the jejunum along with increased intestinal absorptive capacity. In addition, an inhibitory effect on gastric motility was demonstrated. These results established that administration of GLP-2 in rats significantly augments the endogenous adaptive response to intestinal resection.[53-55]

Consequently, the trophic potential of GLP-2 in enhancing intestinal adaptation to surgical resection is of considerable interest. In an initial clinical trial, GLP-2 was administered to eight patients with short bowel syndrome in the form of two injections of human GLP-2, 400 μg subcutaneously for 35 days. Four of the patients were dependent on parenteral nutrition (mean remnant bowel length 83 cm) and four were not (mean remnant length 106 cm). At the end of the treatment period,

GLP-2-treated patients exhibited a modest increase in energy and nitrogen absorption, increased body weight and lean body mass, decreased fat mass, and increased crypt height and villus depth. Although the relative magnitude of changes in these parameters was small, the positive results suggest that further examination of the potential therapeutic role of GLP-2, or more potent degradation resistant GLP-2 analogues, in patients with intestinal failure is warranted.[56] An international multi-center controlled trial of one such analogue is planned for 2004.

CONCLUSION

The combined use of dietary modification, antimotility drugs, antisecretory agents, and intestinal trophic factors can significantly reduce fluid and electrolyte losses in the stools of stomas of patients with severe short bowel syndrome, thus reducing diarrhea and dependence on IV fluids. Their effect on nutrient absorption is, however, more modest and unlikely, with present therapy, to make patients with severe malabsorption PN-free.

REFERENCES

1. Nightingale, J.M.D., Kamm, M.A., Van Der Sijp, J.R.M., Morris, G.P., Walker, E.R., Mather, S.J., Britton, K.E., and Lennard-Jones, J.E., Disturbed gastric emptying in the short bowel syndrome. Evidence for a 'colonic break,' *Gut* 1993; 34:1171–1176.
2. Remington, M., Malagelada, J.R., Zinsmeister, A., and Fleming C.R., Abnormalities in gastrointestinal motor activity in patients with short bowels: effect of a synthetic opiate, *Gastroenterology.* 1983; 85:629–636.
3. Nightingale, J.M.D., Lennard-Jones, J.E., and Walker, E.R., A patient with jejunostomy liberated from home intravenous therapy after 14 years; Contribution of balance studies, *Clin. Nutr.* 1992; 11:101–105.
4. Rodrigues, C.A., Lennard-Jones, J.E., Thompson, D.G., and Farthing, M.J., The effects of octreotide, soy polysaccharide, codeine and loperamide on nutrient, fluid and electrolyte absorption in the short-bowel syndrome, *Aliment Pharmacol. Therap.* 1989; 3:159–169.
5. Camilleri, M., Prather, C.M., Evans, M.A., and Andresen-Reid, M.L., Balance studies and polymeric glucose solution to optimize therapy after massive intestinal resection, *Mayo Clinic Proceedings* 1992; 67:755–760.
6. Katz, M.D. and Erstad, B.L., Octreotide, a new somatostatin analogue, *Clin. Pharm.* 1989; 8:255–273.
7. Nightingale, J.M., Lennard-Jones, J.E., Walker, E.R., and Farthing, M.J., Jejunal efflux in short bowel syndrome, *Lancet* 1990; 336:765–768.
8. Tang, S.J., Nieto, J, Jensen, D.M., Ohning, G.V., and Pisegna, J.R., The novel use of an intravenous proton pump inhibitor in a patient with short bowel syndrome, *J. Clin. Gastroenterol.* 2002; 34:62–63.
9. Jeppesen, P.B., Staun, M., Tjellesen, L., and Mortensen, P.B., Effect of intravenous ranitidine and omeprazole on intestinal absorption of water, sodium, and macronutrients in patients with intestinal resection, *Gut* 1998; 43:763–769.

10. Aly, A., Barany, F., Kollberg, B., Monsen, U., Wisen, O., and Johansson, C., Effect of an H2-receptor blocking agent on diarrhoeas after extensive small bowel resection in Crohn's disease, *Acta. Med. Scand.* 1980; 207:119–122.

11. Fielding, J.F., Cooke, W.T., and Williams, J.A., Gastric acid secretion in Crohn's disease in relation to disease activity and bowel resection, *Lancet* 1971; 1:1106–1107.

12. Buxton, B., Small bowel resection and gastric hypersecretion, *Gut* 1974; 15:229–238.

13. Go, V.L., Poley, J.R., Hofmann, A.F., and Sunnerskil, W.H., Disturbances in fat digestion induced by acidic jejunal pH due to gastric hypersecretion in man, *Gastroenterology* 1970; 58:638–646.

14. Williams, N.S., Evans, P., and King, R.F., Gastric acid secretion and gastrin production in the short bowel syndrome, *Gut* 1985; 26:914–919.

15. Malagelada, J.R., Pathophysiological responses to meals in the Zollinger-Ellison syndrome: 2. Gastric emptying and its effect on duodenal function, *Gut* 1980; 21:98–104.

16. Cortot, A., Flemming, C.R., and Malagelada, J.R., Improved nutrient absorption after cimetidine in short-bowel syndrome with gastric hypersecretion, *N. Engl. J. Med.* 1979; 300:79–80.

17. Murphy, J.P. Jr., King, D.R., and Dubois, A., Treatment of gastric hypersecretion with cimetidine in the short-bowel syndrome, *N. Engl. J. Med.* 1979; 300:80–81.

18. Nightingale, J.M., Walker, E.R., Farthing, M.J., and Lennard-Jones, J.E., Effect of omeprazole on intestinal output in the short bowel syndrome, *Aliment Pharmacol. Ther.* 1991; 5:405–412.

19. Jacobsen, O., Ladefoged, K., Stage, J.G., and Jarnum, S., Effects of cimetidine on jejunostomy effluents in patients with severe short-bowel syndrome, *Scand. J. Gastroenterol.* 1986; 21:824–828.

20. Recker, R.R., Calcium absorption and achlorhydria, *N. Engl. J. Med.* 1985; 313:70–73.

21. Bo Linn, G.W., Davis, G.R., Buddrus, D.J., Morawski, S.G., Santa Ana, C., and Fordtran, J,S., An evaluation of the importance of gastric acid secretion in the absorption of dietary calcium, *J. Clin. Invest.* 1984; 73:640–647.

22. Vanderhoof, J.A., Young, J., Murray, N., and Kaufman, S.S., Treatment strategies for small bowel bacterial overgrowth in short bowel syndrome, *J. Pediatr. Gastroenterol. Nutr.* 1998; 27:155–160.

23. O'Keefe, S.J.D., Peterson, M.E., and Fleming, C.R., Octreotide as an adjunct to home parenteral nutrition in the management of permanent end-jejunostomy syndrome, *J. Parenter. Enteral Nutrition* 1994; 18:26–34.

24. Reichlin, S., Somatostatin, *N. Engl. J. Med.* 1983; 309:1495–1501.

25. Anthony, L,B., Long-acting formulations of somatostatin analogues, *Ital. J. Gastroenterol. Hepatol.* 1999 Oct; 31 Suppl 2:S216–218.

26. Nightingale, J.M., Walker, E.R., Burnham, W.R., Farthing, M.J., and Lennard-Jones, J.E., Octreotide (somatostatin analogue) improves the quality of life in some patients with a short intestine, *Aliment Pharmacol. Ther.* 1989; 3:367–373.

27. Kvols, L.K., Moertel, C.G., O'Connell, M.J., Schutt, A.J., Rubin, J., and Hahn, R.G., Treatment of the carcinoid syndrome: Evaluation of a long acting somatostatin analogue, *N. Engl. J. Med.* 1986; 315:663–666.

28. Baudet, S., Medina, C., Vilaseca, J., Guarner, L., Sureda, D., Andreu, J., and Malagelada, J.R., Effect of short-term octreotide therapy and total parenteral nutrition on the development of biliary sludge and lithiasis, *Hepatogastroenterology* 2002 May–Jun; 49(45):609–712.

29. O'Keefe, S.J., Haymond, M.W., Bennet, W.M., Oswald, B., and Nelson, D.K., Long-acting somatostatin analog therapy and protein metabolism in patient with jejunostomies, *Gastroenterology* 1994; 107:379–388.

30. Seydel, A.S., Miller, J.H., Sarac, T.P., Ryan, C.K., Chey, W.Y., and Sax, H.C., Octeriotide diminishes luminal nutrient transport activity, which is reversed by epidermal growth factor, *Am . J. Surgery* 1996; 172:267–271.

31. Poley, J.R. and Hofmann, A.F., Role of bile acid malabsorption in the pathogenesis of diarrhea and steatorrhea in patients with ileal resection. I. Response to cholestyramine or replacement of dietary long-chain triglycerides by medium-chain triglycerides, *Gastroenterology* 1972; 62:918–934.

32. Booth, C.C., Aldis, D., and Read, A.E., Studies on the site of fat absorption. 2. Fat balances after resection of varying amounts of small intestine in man, *Gut* 1961; 2:168–174.

33. Gruy-Kapral, C., Little, K.H., Fordtran, J.S., Meziere, T.L., Hagey, L.R., and Hofmann, A,F., Conjugated bile acid replacement therapy for short-bowel syndrome, *Gastroenterology* 1999; 116:15–21.

34. Ulshen, M.H., Dowling, R.H., Fuller, C.R., Zimmerman, E.M., and Lund, P,K., Enhanced growth of small-bowel in transgenic mice overexpressing bovine growth hormone, *Gastroenterology* 1993; 104:973–980.

35. Gomez, D.E., Segura, I.A., Aguilera, M.J., Codesal, J., Dodoceo, R., and DeMiguel, E., Comparative effects of growth hormone in large and small bowel resection in the rat, *J. Surg. Res.* 1996; 62:5–11.

36. Shulman, D.I., Hu, C.S., Ducket, G., Lavallee-Gray, M., Effects of short term-growth hormone therapy in rats undergoing 75% small intestinal resection, *J. Pediatr. Gastroenterol. Nutr.* 1992; 14:3–11.

37. Park, J.H. and Vanderhoof, J.A., Growth hormone did not enhance mucosal hyperplasia after small-bowel resection, *Scan. J. Gastroenterol.* 1996; 31:349–354.

38. Wilmore, D.W., Lacey, J.M., Soultanakis, R.P., Bosch, R.L., and Byrne, T.A., Factors predicting a successful outcome after pharmacologic bowel compensation, *Ann. Surg.* 1997; 226:288–293.

39. Scolapio, J.S., Camilleri, M., Fleming, C.R., Oenning, L.V., Burton, D.D., Sebo, T.J., Batts, K.P., and Kelly, D.G., Effect of growth hormone, glutamine and diet on adaptation in short-bowel syndrome: A randomized controlled study, *Gastroenterology* 1997; 113:1074–1081.

40. Szkudlarek, J., Jeppesen, P.B., and Mortensen, P.B., Effect of high dose growth hormone with glutamine and no change in diet on intestinal absorption in short bowel patients: A randomized, double blind, crossover, placebo controlled study, *Gut* 2000; 47:199–205.

41. Seguy, D., Vahedi, K., Kapel, N., Souberbielle, J.C., and Messing, B., Low-dose growth hormone in adult home parenteral nutrition-dependent short bowel syndrome patients: a positive study, *Gastroenterology* 2003 Feb; 124(2):293–302.

42. Drucker, D.J., Erlich, P., Asa, S.L., and Brubaker, P.L., Induction of intestinal epithelial proliferation by glucagons-like peptide 2, *Proc. Natl. Acad. Sci. USA* 1996; 93:7911–7916.

43. Scott, R.B., Kirk, D., MacNaughton, W.K., and Meddings, J.B., GLP-2 augments the adaptive response to massive intestinal resection in rat, *Am. J. Physiol.* 1998; 275:G911–921.

44. Gleeson, M.H., Bloom, S.R., Polak, J.M., Henry, K., and Dowling, R.H., An endocrine tumour in kidney affecting small bowel structure, motility, and absorptive function, *Gut* 1971; 12:773–782.

45. Rountree, D.B., Ulshen, M.H., Selub, S., Fuller, C.R., Bloom, S.R., and Ghatei, M.A., Nutrient-independent increases in proglucagon and ornithine decarboxylase messenger RNAs after jejunoileal resection, *Gastroenterology* 1992; 103:462–468.

46. Fuller, P.J., Beveridge, D.J., and Taylor, R.G., Ileal proglucagon gene expression in the rat: characterization in intestinal adaptation using in situ hybridization, *Gastroenterology* 1993; 104:459–466.

47. Brubaker, P.L., Crivici, A., Izzo, A., Ehrlich, P., Tsai, C.H., and Drucker, D.J., Circulating and tissue forms of the intestinal growth factor, glucagon-like peptide 2, *Endocrinology* 1997; 138:4837–4843.

48. Xiao, Q., Boushey, R.P., Drucker, D.J., and Brubaker, P.L., Secretion of the intestinotropic hormone glucagon-like peptide 2 is differentially regulated by nutrients in humans, *Gastroenterology* 1999; 117:99–105.

49. Jeppesen, P.B., Hartmann, B., Hansen, B.S., Thulesen, J., Holst, J.J., and Mortensen, P.B., Impaired meal-stimulated glucagon-like peptide-2 response in ileal resected short bowel patients with intestinal failure, *Gut* 1999; 45:559–563.

50. Tsai, C-H, Hill, M., Asa, S.L., Brubaker, P.L., and Drucker, D.J., Intestinal growth-promoting properties of glucagon-like peptide 2 in mice, *Am. J. Physiol.* 1997; 273:E77–84.

51. Benjamin, M.A., McKay, D.M., Yang, P.C., Cameron, H., and Perdue, M.H., Glucagon-like peptide-2 enhances intestinal epithelial barrier function of both transcellular and paracellular pathways in the mouse, *Gut* 2000; 47:112–119.

52. Chance, W.T., Foley-Nelson, T., Thomas, I., and Balasubramaniam, A., Prevention of parenteral nutrition-induced gut hypoplasia by coinfusion of glucagon-like peptide-2, *Am. J. Physiol.* 1997; 273:G559–563.

53. Ljungmann, K., Hartmann, B., Kissmeyer-Nielsen, P., Flyvbjerg, A., Holst, J.J., and Laurberg, S., Time-dependent intestinal adaptation and GLP-2 alterations after small bowel resection in rats, *Am. J. Physiol. Gastrointest. Liver Physiol.* 2001; 281:G779–785.

54. Scott, R.B., Kirk, D., MacNaughton, W.K.,and Meddings, J.B., GLP-2 augments the adaptive response to massive intestinal resection in rat, *Am. J. Physiol.* 1998; 275:G911–921.

55. Wojdemann, M., Wettergren, A., Hartmann, B., and Holst, J.J., Glucagon-like peptide-2 inhibits centrally induced antral motility in pigs, *Scand. J. Gastroenterol.* 1998; 33:828–832.

56. Jeppesen, P.B., Hartmann, B., Thulesen, J., Graff, J., Lohmann, J., Hansen, B.S., Tofteng, F., Poulsen, S.S., Madsen, J.L., Holst, J.J., and Mortensen, P.B., Glucagon-like peptide 2 improves nutrient absorption and nutritional status in short-bowel patients with no colon, *Gastroenterology* 2001; 120:806–815.

11 Pancreatic Enzyme Replacement and Bile Acid Therapy

Tyler Stevens and Darwin L. Conwell

CONTENTS

Intestinal resection has multiple adverse effects on digestion. Though the primary digestive defect is decreased absorptive surface area, a plethora of other physiologic changes occur, including rapid gastric emptying, decreased small intestinal transit time, gastric acid hypersecretion, bacterial overgrowth, and bile salt depletion.[1] Each of these individual factors may adversely affect either the breakdown or uptake of nutrients across the small intestinal mucosa. While awaiting the process of intestinal adaptation, management of short bowel syndrome involves parenteral nutrition, dietary changes, and medications that modify the individual pathophysiologic mechanisms. Bile acid therapy and pancreatic enzymes are among the specific therapies that address the maldigestive processes occurring after intestinal resection.

In this chapter, we first review the normal intraluminal digestion of fats and proteins. A discussion of the numerous causes of malabsorption occurring after intestinal resection follows, including deficiencies in bile acids and pancreatic function. We then discuss the rationale and limited available literature supporting the use supplementary bile acids and pancreatic enzymes for short bowel syndrome (SBS).

NORMAL INTRALUMINAL DIGESTION

The bulk of nutrient absorption occurs in the duodenum and proximal portion of the jejunum, where chyme mixes with biliary and pancreatic secretions. The timed secretion of these digestive fluids allows proper breakdown of fat, protein, and carbohydrate polymers into their respective monomers (i.e., fatty acids, monoglycerides, amino acids, di- and tripeptides, etc.). After breakdown of proteins and emulsification of fats, nutrients are absorbed through active and passive transport processes across the villous epithelial cell membrane.

The following is a brief description of fat and protein digestion, as this most directly influences understanding of pancreatic enzyme and bile salt supplementation in intestinal resection. For a more thorough discussion of normal digestive physiology, refer to Chapters 1 and 2.

DIGESTION AND ABSORPTION OF PROTEIN

Protein digestion is initiated in the stomach by the mechanical grinding of food and through the enzymatic effect of pepsin. During the gastric phase of protein digestion, the enzyme precursor pepsinogen is released from antral chief cells in response to vagal nerve stimulation.[2] Through exposure to gastric acid, pepsinogen is rapidly converted to the active endopeptidase pepsin. As food churns within the gastric antrum, pepsin interacts with individual peptides to begin the cleavage process. As individual food particles become smaller, coordinated gastric antral contraction and relaxation of pyloric tone allow small amounts of acid-chyme to pass the pyloric channel. The alkaline environment of the duodenum inhibits pepsin, and digestion of protein continues through the action of endogenous pancreatic enzymes.

The regulation and release of pancreatic fluid is complex.[3] Though initiated during the *gastric* phase of digestion through the action of the hormone gastrin and vagal neural input, the majority of pancreatic secretion occurs during the *intestinal phase*. In the intestinal phase, bicarbonate and enzyme-rich fluid are secreted in response to the presence of acid and digestion products in the proximal small intestine. The individual components of pancreatic fluid are modulated through complex neurohormonal control. The duodenum acts as a "sensory organ," vital for the precise timing of release of digestive hormones. The primary hormones that regulate pancreatic secretion are cholecystokinin (CCK) and secretin. Secretin principally acts on the pancreatic ductal cells to release bicarbonate for neutralization of acid chyme reaching the intestine.[4] CCK triggers pancreatic acinar cells to release enzymes for digestion of proteins and fats.

The postprandial entrance of acid-chyme into the duodenum triggers mucosal endocrine cells to release secretin into the bloodstream. Blood-borne secretin acts directly on the pancreatic ductal cells to cause secretion of bicarbonate through a second messenger. Other neural and hormonal messengers, including CCK, VIP, and acetylcholine, may amplify the secretin stimulus; this process is known as secretin-stimulus coupling (Figure 11.1).[5] As large volumes of bicarbonate rich fluid reaches the lumen, the pH of the intestinal fluid increases and secretin release is inhibited (negative-feedback inhibition).

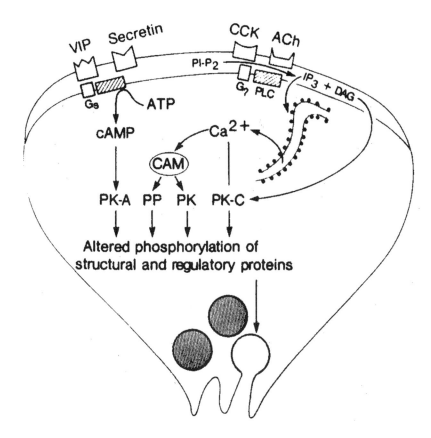

FIGURE 11.1 Schematic diagram of stimulus-secretion coupling of pancreatic acinar cell protein secretion. VIP, secretin, CCK, and ACh act independently through a second messenger to activate the release of enzymes. ACh, acetylcholine; CCK, cholecystokinin; CAM, calmodulin; DAG, diacylglycerol; PK, protein kinase; PP, protein phosphatase; VIP, vasoactive intestinal polypeptide. (Adapted from Williams, J.A., Burnham, D.B., Hootman, S.R., Cellular regulation of pancreatic secretion. In *Handbook of Physiology—The Gastrointestinal System,* Vol. 3, Forte, J., Ed., American Physiology Society, 1989; 419.)

CCK is the primary hormone responsible for pancreatic enzyme release (Figure 11.2). Duodenal enterochromaffin cells release CCK in response to the presence of proteins and fats during the intestinal phase. There is evidence that the effect of CCK on the pancreatic acinar cells is mediated both hormonally and through neural pathways.[6] CCK stimulates acinar cells zymogen granules to release digestive pro-enzymes into the pancreatic ductule. Through the cleavage of trypsinogen to trypsin by the mucosal enzyme enterokinase, trypsin functions to cleave and activate the various other pro-enzymes for digestion of protein.

Like secretin, CCK is closely regulated through a negative feedback loop.[7] Though the exact mechanism of this regulation is not completely understood, it is likely that the CCK releasing factor (CCK-RF) produced by duodenal endocrine cells is the primary molecule responsible for the release of CCK.[8] Between meals,

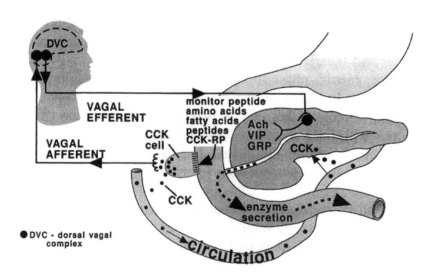

FIGURE 11.2 Intestinal phase of pancreatic enzyme secretion. CCK stimulates pancreatic enzyme secretion by both neural and hormonal pathways. (Adapted from Pandol, S.J., Pancreatic physiology and secretory testing. Reprinted from: Sleisenger and Fordtran's Gastrointestinal and Liver Disease, Feldman et al., Eds., Pandol, S.J., Raybould, H.E., Pancreatic physiology and secretory testing, p. 876, 2002, with permission from Elsevier, and the Undergraduate Teaching Project in Gastroenterology and liver disease, Alpers, D.H., Ed., The integrated response to a meal, American Gastroenterological Association, Unit 29.)

CCK-RF is hydrolyzed by gastric acid or residual trypsin. During a meal, the luminal pH increases through the secretion of bicarbonate, and trypsin is occupied with the digestion of exogenous proteins. During this period, CCK-RF levels increase within the lumen and stimulate the release of CCK, stimulating the pancreas through neurocrine and endocrine pathways. As exogenous protein is digested and absorbed, and the acid environment returns, trypsin is again available to degrade CCK-RF, leading to CCK inhibition.

Once released into the small intestine, the various pancreatic proteases act to facilitate the digestion of proteins through cleavage of specific peptide bonds (Table 11.1).[9] As proteins are cleaved by pancreatic proteases, luminal brush-border peptidases further degrade the remaining oligo-peptides into individual amino acids and di- and tripeptides. These small protein components are thus prepared for rapid assimilation into the mucosal cells through carrier-mediated transport. Amino acids are largely absorbed into the mucosal cell through co-transport with sodium, then passively diffuse across the basolateral membrane into the venous capillaries. Di- and tri-peptides are actively transported across the luminal membrane, then are cleaved intracellularly into individual amino acids.

DIGESTION AND ABSORPTION OF FATS

Fat absorption is complex and involves the coordinated activity of multiple components of the digestive system. Ingested fats such as triglycerides, phospholipids, and

TABLE 11.1
Pancreatic Proteases

Peptidase	Function
Endopeptidases	Hydrolyzes *internal* peptide bonds
Trypsin	Cleaves adjacent to basic amino acids (lysine and arginine)
Chymotrypsin	Cleaves adjacent to aromatic amino acids (phenylalanine, tryptophan, tyrosine)
Elastase	Cleaves aliphatic peptide bonds (leucine)
Exopeptidases	Hydrolyzes at the carboxy-terminal ends of peptides
Carboxypeptidase A	Cleaves at the carboxy-terminal ends of *neutral* peptides
Carboxypeptidase B	Cleaves at the carboxy-terminal ends of *basic* peptides

cholesterol are sheared within the antrum into small droplets, beginning the process of emulsification of fat (mixing with water). Gastric lipase begins the process of lipolysis within the stomach; however, the bulk of lipid digestion occurs within the intestinal phase.[10] Pancreatic enzymes and bile salts interact to digest and solubilize fats for absorption across the small intestinal mucosa. CCK is the principle hormone required for the proper timed release of bile and pancreatic lipolytic enzymes.

Bile is synthesized in the liver and consists of bile acids, bile pigments, cholesterol, and alkaline phosphatase. The primary bile acids cholic acid and chenodeoxycholic acid are synthesized by the hepatocytes, conjugated with taurine or glycine, secreted into the bile, and stored within the gallbladder. When primary bile acids reach the small intestine, some are converted by bacteria to secondary bile acids, such as lithocholic or deoxycholic acid (Figure 11.3). In the small intestine, bile acids are critical for the digestion and absorption of fats and fat-soluble vitamins. In the ileum, 95% of both primary and secondary bile acids are actively transported across the villi into the portal venous system. These bile acids return to the liver where they are recycled into the bile (enterohepatic circulation).[11] The small percentages of bile acids that are lost in the stool are replenished through daily hepatic synthesis.

The postprandial release of CCK produces two major physiologic effects pertinent to fat digestion: 1) Secretion of fat-digesting enzymes from the pancreas, and 2) stimulation of flow of bile through gallbladder contraction and sphincter of Oddi relaxation.[12] Pancreatic lipase and colipase interact to begin the breakdown of triglycerides within the duodenum. Through the postprandial "alkaline tide" of pancreatic bicarbonate secretion, bile salts emulsify dietary fat through the assembly of spherical micelles. Pancreatic lipase interacts with colipase and bile salts on the surface of the micelles to cleave triglycerides to individual fatty acids. Also in the presence of bile salts, pancreatic esterase and phospholipase A2 begin the breakdown of cholesterol and fat-soluble vitamins through the hydrolysis of ester bonds.

As fats are broken down on the surface of the micelle, the fat-soluble products of digestion (free fatty acids, cholesterol, monoglycerides) are transported through passive diffusion across the luminal membrane of the enterocyte. Within the

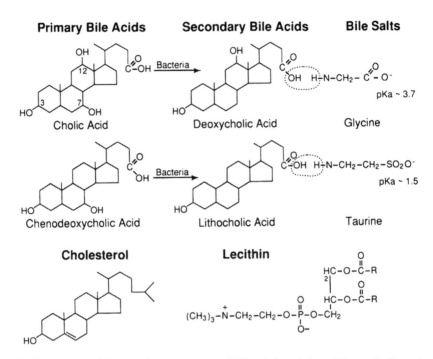

FIGURE 11.3 Principle organic components of bile. (Adapted from Johnson L, Secretion. In *Essential Medical Physiology*, 3rd ed., Johnson, L., Ed., Lippincott Williams and Wilkin, 2003, 522.)

endoplasmic reticulum, the lipid products are assembled into chylomicrons that enter lymphatic vessels and flow to the systemic circulation via the thoracic duct. The bile salts remain within the intestinal lumen and are carried to the ileum for uptake and recycling.

INTESTINAL RESECTION

MECHANISMS OF MALABSORPTION

Intestinal resection adversely affects the intraluminal digestion of nutrients through several mechanisms, depending on the site of resection (Table 11.2).[13] After extensive ileal resections with less than 100 cm of remaining jejunum, lack of absorptive surface area leads to severe malabsorption, requiring parenteral nutrition. Motility disturbances prevent adequate contact of chyme with digestive enzymes and the absorptive surface. Loss of the ileum and colon can result in rapid gastric emptying of hyperosmolar gastric contents, resulting in the dumping syndrome.[14] Extensive ileal resection can also produce rapid small bowel transit,[15,16] occurring through loss of the ileo-cecal valve, changes in the migrating motor complex,[17] and loss of gut hormones that mediate the "ileal brake" mechanism.[18] These changes lead to a high stomal output and may lead some patients to restrict their protein and fat intake.

TABLE 11.2
Mechanisms of Nutrient
Malabsorption after Intestinal
Resection

Decreased absorptive surface area
Rapid gastric emptying and dumping
Decreased intestinal transit time
Small bowel bacterial overgrowth
Bile-salt deficiency
Gastric acid hypersecretion
Impaired pancreatic function
Decreased secretion of intestinal hormones
Pancreatic enzyme inactivation by gastric acid

Small bowel bacterial overgrowth is common in SBS, particularly with loss of the ileo-cecal valve.[19] Bacterial overgrowth may impair digestion of fat by deconjugating bile acids, making them less suitable for micelle formation. Bacterial overgrowth further worsens absorption by hastening intestinal transit.

Gastric acid hypersecretion is known to occur in many patients with short bowel syndrome, depending on the site of resection. Though not completely understood, the mechanism may relate to increased gastrin levels.[20] Increased gastrin levels have been attributed to several possible mechanisms, including decreased catabolism of gastrin by the small intestine,[21] loss of gastrointestinal inhibitor proteins such as peptide YY, or stimulation of release of gastrin by bacterial effects in the intestine.[22] Gastric acid hypersecretion may produce mucosal ulceration to the further detriment of nutrient absorption.

PANCREATIC DYSFUNCTION IN INTESTINAL RESECTION

Normal pancreatic secretory physiology is disordered after intestinal resection through several mechanisms. Resection of the proximal small bowel results in a decreased density of enterochromaffin cells that secrete secretin and CCK. This results in lower postprandial levels of these hormones, decreasing both pancreatic and biliary secretion for proper digestion of nutrients.

There is evidence that severe malnutrition adversely affects pancreatic insufficiency after intestinal resection. Past studies of patients with SBS have revealed a reduced volume of pancreatic secretion and decreased enzyme output after hormonal stimulation with secretin or CCK.[23,24] More recently, Winter et al. used direct pancreatic function testing to evaluate severely undernourished patients.[25] The pancreatic enzyme outputs were significantly lower in the undernourished group compared to healthy subjects. Another study showed a similar decrease in pancreatic enzyme outputs in undernourished patients, as well as improvement in outputs after nutritional repletion.[26] Based on these studies, it is plausible that that exocrine pancreatic insufficiency may contribute substantially to maldigestion in malnourished patients with SBS.

Previous studies have also demonstrated that gastric acid inactivates exogenous pancreatic enzymes.[27] The gastric acid hypersecretion present in SBS may also contribute to the degradation or functional impairment of endogenous pancreatic enzymes. For example, it is known that pancreatic lipase is denatured at a pH of 4.0 and below.[28] Gastric acid hypersecretion combined with decreased pancreatic bicarbonate secretion may produce a more acidic duodenal lumen, leading to pancreatic enzyme inactivation. Acid within the duodenum may also stimulate increased biliary and pancreatic secretion, leading to dilution of pancreatic enzymes.

BILE-SALT DYSFUNCTION AFTER INTESTINAL RESECTION

Bile acid deficiency likewise plays a significant role in nutrient malabsorption.[29,30,31] Resection of less than 100 cm of ileum may result in a watery, secretory diarrhea due to the irritant effect of bile acids on the colonic mucosa.[32] This "bile salt" diarrhea often responds well to bile acid sequestrants, such as cholestyramine.[33] However, when greater than 100 cm of ileum is resected, the hepatic synthesis of bile acids cannot keep pace with their loss from the enterohepatic circulation and the bile acid pool becomes depleted.[34] Bile salt deficiency combined with the deconjugation of remaining bile acids by small intestinal bacteria prevents proper micelle formation, resulting in fat malabsorption as well as secretory diarrhea from fatty acids.

In summary, intestinal resection results in a spectrum of pathophysiologic changes that interferes with normal digestion, including the loss of normal biliary and pancreatic function. Medical or dietary therapy that addresses these independent factors may therefore prove efficacious in ameliorating these maldigestive processes.

BILE ACID THERAPY

The rationale for use of supplemental bile acid therapy after intestinal resection is based on bile acid deficiency as a major cause of fat and vitamin malabsorption. The purpose of bile acid supplementation at the time of oral intake or enteral feeding is to improve fat emulsification and absorption by supplementing depleted endogenous stores of bile salts. This will allow the intestinal concentration of bile acids to achieve the "critical micellar concentration" required for proper micelle formation and fat absorption.[35]

In the past, several arguments have been leveled against the use of bile acid therapy. Some have suggested that the major cause of fat malabsorption in short bowel syndrome is lack of surface area, rather than bile acid deficiency; therefore bile acid supplementation is unlikely to make a substantial impact. However, even patients with extensive resections may eventually absorb adequately through the process of intestinal adaptation. In the interim, short-term "fixes" such as bile acid supplementation may allow more timely reinstitution of enteral feeding. Another concern has been the cathartic effects of bile salts. Past experiments in which bile acids were perfused in human small[36,37] or large[38] intestine showed increased mucosal transport of water and electrolytes, which may worsen diarrhea. Finally, the use of medium chain triglycerides in enteral feeding has helped to circumvent the need for bile acids as an aid for absorption of fat, though this therapy is most effective in patients with intact colons[39] and they do not provide essential fatty acids.

Recently, a few studies have demonstrated a benefit for this therapy and have alleviated concerns about the cathartic effects of these agents. Therapeutic investigations of bile acids in short bowel syndrome began in the early 1980s through the use of ox bile supplements. A small number of case reports demonstrated efficacy of orally administered ox bile extracts in decreasing stool weight, improving steatorrhea, and enabling weight gain in patients after ileectomy and colectomy.[40,41]

More recently, Gruy-Kapral et al. investigated the use of natural conjugated bile acids and the artificial bile acid cholylsarcosine in a single patient with extensive intestinal and colonic resection, severe malnutrition, and intolerance of parenteral nutrition.[42] Cholylsarcosine is an artificial bile acid synthesized by conjugating cholic acid with the amino acid sarcosine (Figure 11.4). Cholylsarcosine is resistant to bacterial deconjugation, in theory preventing the potential cathartic effects.[43-45] In this interesting experiment, the patient received natural conjugated bile acids (desiccated ox bile extracts) and cholylsarcosine during two separate treatment periods. Metabolic balance studies, including stool fecal outputs, were performed after each treatment period. The absorption of fat increased twofold (47 to 95 grams per day) associated with a concomitant reduction in ileostomy fat output and caloric content during the natural conjugated bile acid treatment period. Furthermore, the 6 g/day dose was 75% as effective as the 12 g/day dose in improving fat absorption. Treatment with cholylsarcosine produced similar results, with marked improvement in steatorrhea at both the 6 and 12 g/day doses. Treatment with both preparations minimally increased the ileal output of water and electrolytes. The initial study was followed by a prolonged treatment period with natural bile acids (6 grams/day), resulting in a significant weight gain of 18 pounds over 4 months.

Heydorn et al. published a small case series demonstrating a similar benefit for supplemental cholylsarcosine.[46] In this study, cholylsarcosine was administered in 6 and 12 g/day doses to 4 patients with short bowel syndrome. Metabolic balance studies showed that fat absorption increased by 17 ± 3 grams per day ($p < 0.05$) for the 6-gram dose, and by 20 ± 1 grams per day ($p < 0.001$) for the 12-gram dose. The benefit of cholylsarcosine was greatest in the patient with the shortest remaining length of small intestine and most severe steatorrhea. Diarrhea worsened slightly in one patient with a remaining colon, but was unchanged in the other three patients. The authors concluded that cholylsarcosine offered a benefit of increased fat absorption but a modest gain in energy absorption.

Though supplemental bile acids seem to provide a measurable benefit in improving fat absorption, the magnitude of clinical benefit remains in question. Patients with short bowel syndrome derive most of their caloric intake from carbohydrates, which are more easily absorbed. Therefore, although fat absorption improves with bile acid therapy, only a modest benefit may be obtained in terms of total calorie absorption. In the limited available studies, the magnitude of increases in fat absorption has been relatively small. The use of synthetic bile acids such as cholylsarcosine seems equivalent to use of natural bile acids derived from ox bile. However, cholylsarcosine may have a greater role in a patient who has steatorrhea from extensive

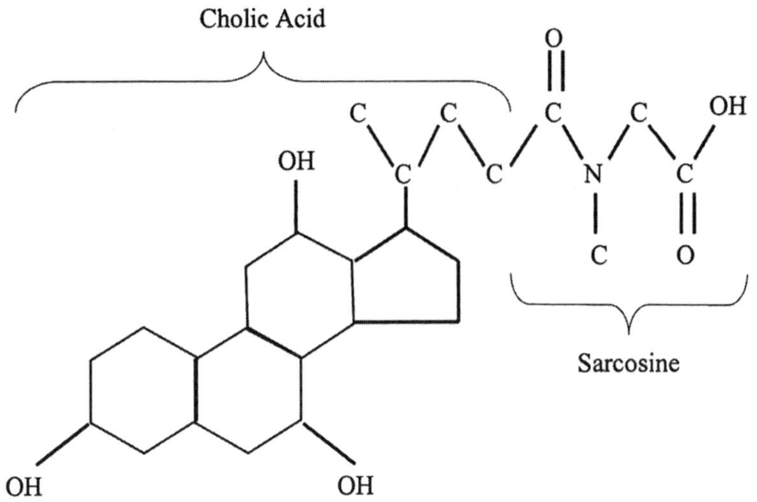

FIGURE 11.4 The chemical structure of cholylsarcosine

small intestinal resection with an intact colon; such patients may have increased bacterial deconjugation of bile acids and subsequent watery diarrhea if natural bile acid supplements are used.

Further studies in larger groups of patients are required prior to the widespread recommendation of bile acid therapy in short bowel syndrome. In the meantime, bile acid therapy may be tried in patients with severe fat malabsorption from short bowel syndrome. It appears that a dose of 6 g per day is as efficacious as higher doses for both cholylsarcosine and natural bile acids. Ideally, to ensure the benefit of this therapy in individual patients, patient weight as well as stool weight and fat quantification should be monitored before and after initiation of bile acid supplementation. High doses of bile acids may be injurious to the liver;[47] however, this complication is likely to be avoided in the setting of endogenous bile acid depletion, normal dosing, and with close monitoring of liver function tests. Taking the medications with a glass of water will minimize the previously described esophageal injury with orally administered bile acids.[48]

PANCREATIC ENZYME SUPPLEMENTATION

As stated earlier, pancreatic exocrine insufficiency and increased gastric acid adversely effects the secretion and function of pancreatic enzymes. Theoretically, supplementing pancreatic enzymes may help to overcome these pathophysiologic mechanisms, allowing improved nutrient digestion. At our institution, we have found anecdotal success in managing some short bowel syndrome patients through the

TABLE 11.3
Commonly Available Pancreatic Enzyme Preparations

Preparation	Form	Enzyme Content (USP units)		
		Lipase	Protease	Amylase
Rapid Release				
Cotazym	Capsule	8,000	30,000	30,000
Pancreatin	Tablet	12,000	60,000	60,000
Viokase	Tablet	8,000	30,000	30,000
Delayed Release				
Creon 5/10/20	Enteric-coated	5,000	18,750	16,600
	Micro-spheres	10,000	37,500	33,200
		20,000	75,000	66,400
Pancrease MT 4/10/16/20	Enteric-coated	4,000	12,000	12,000
	Micro-tablets	10,000	30,000	30,000
		16,000	48,000	48,000
		20,000	44,000	56,000
Ultrase MT 6/12/16/20	Enteric-coated	6,000	19,500	19,500
	Micro-tablets	12,000	39,000	39,000
		18,000	58,500	58,500
		20,000	65,000	65,000

USP, U.S. Pharmacopeia

stepwise introduction of pancreatic enzymes.[49] Through introduction of this therapy, many patients notice improvement in diarrhea and increased weight gain.

There is a multitude of available pancreatic enzyme formulations (Table 11.3). Preparations differ based on the enzyme content, the use of microspheres or microtablets, and the presence a coating for delayed release. Because of the rapid intestinal transit time in SBS, uncoated, "rapid release" preparations are preferable for proper enzyme delivery to the proximal small bowel.

Dosage guidelines exist for treatment of pancreatic insufficiency, formulated based on the daily requirement of lipase; however, standard dosing is not available for treatment of SBS. It is likely that lower doses are needed for SBS, as pancreatic production of endogenous enzymes is relatively preserved; however, this is highly variable. Doses of specific enzymes differ depending on the preparation. Lipase content is the most important determinant of the effectiveness of individual enzyme preparations. We typically use pancrelipase containing 8000 IU of lipase per capsule, titrating the dose from 1 to 8 capsules with meals. As with any other therapy in SBS, careful monitoring of symptoms (patient diary), stomal outputs, and stool fat quantification may be helpful in determining the individual patient benefit. Opening the individual capsules and sprinkling the microspheres on food or mixing them with enteral feeding solutions may ease the use of these medications. To mimic normal physiology, pancreatic enzymes should be taken at the time of each meal and snack. Administering the enzymes with food not only mimics normal physiologic enzyme release, but also prevents enzyme degradation by gastric acid.

Antisecretory medications are typically given as first line treatment of patients with SBS. The detrimental effect of gastric acid on pancreatic enzymes provides another rationale for administering these drugs. Studies of patients with pancreatic exocrine insufficiency evaluating concomitant antacids or H2 blockers to preserve the function of exogenous pancreatic enzymes have yielded mixed results.[50–53] The few studies evaluating proton-pump inhibitors for this purpose have likewise been conflicting.[54,55] No studies to our knowledge have addressed the benefit of supplemental antisecretory drugs with pancreatic enzymes in the context of SBS.

Though biologic plausibility and anecdotal experience suggests a benefit for exogenous pancreatic enzyme therapy in short bowel syndrome, the scientific literature on this subject is lacking. Randomized controlled trials or crossover studies incorporating metabolic balance studies before and after therapy are needed to verify the benefit of pancreatic enzymes in the treatment of SBS.

CONCLUSION

The management of maldigestion and malabsorption after extensive intestinal resection is challenging. Although the remaining bowel may ultimately adapt, more effective treatments are needed for augmenting natural digestion. While large, well-designed studies are lacking, bile acid and pancreatic enzyme supplementation make sense physiologically. Furthermore, anecdotal experience and small case-series suggest that they are beneficial in many patients. In addition, these medications are safe and well tolerated, therefore are likely worth trying in appropriate patients. It is hoped that, as future studies emerge, bile acid and pancreatic enzymes supplementation will become standardized within the therapeutic armamentarium for extensive intestinal resection.

REFERENCES

1. Westergaard H., Short bowel syndrome, *Sem. Gastrointest. Dis.*, 13, 210, 2002.
2. Samloff I.M., Pepsins, peptic activity, and peptic inhibitors, *J. Clin. Gastroenterol.*, 3, 91, 1981.
3. Whitcomb D.C., Neurohormonal control of the pancreas, in *Gastroenterology and Hepatology: The Comprehensive Visual Reference,* Vol. 8, Toskes P.P., Ed., Churchill-Livingstone, Philadelphia, 1998, chap. 1.
4. Case R. and Argent B., Bicarbonate secretion by pancreatic duct cells: mechanisms and control, in *The Exocrine Pancreas: Biology, Pathobiology, and Disease,* Go W., Gardner, J., Brooks, F. et al, Eds. Raven Press, Philadelphia, 1986.
5. Williams, J.A. et al., Stimulus-secretion coupling of pancreatic digestive enzyme secretion, *Digestion*, 58, 42, 1997.
6. Li, Y. and Owyang, C., Vagal afferent pathway mediates physiological action of cholecystokinin on pancreatic enzyme secretion, *J. Clin. Invest.*, 92, 418, 1993.

7. Louie, D.S. et al., Cholecystokinin mediates feedback regulation of pancreatic enzyme secretion in rats, *Am. J. Physiol.*, 250, G319, 1995.

8. Liddle, R.A., Regulation of cholecystokin secretion by intraluminal releasing factors, *Am. J. Physiol.*, 269, G319, 1995.

9. Farrell, J.J., Digestion and absorption of nutrients and vitamins, in *Sleisenger and Fordtran's Gastrointestinal and Liver Disease, Seventh Edition*, Feldman M. et al., Eds., Saunders, Philadelphia, 2002, chap. 88.

10. Abrams, C.K. et al., Gastric lipase: localization in the human stomach, *Gastroenterology*, 95, 1460, 1988.

11. Carey, M.C. and Cahalane, M.J., Enterohepatic circulation, in *The Liver: Biology and Pathology, Second Edition*, Arias I.M. et al., Eds., Raven Press, New York, 1988: 576.

12. Weisbrodt, N.W., Bile production and storage, in *Gastrointestinal Physiology*, Johnson L.R., Ed., Mosby, St. Louis, 1991, chap. 10.

13. Nightingale, J.M.D., The short bowel, in *Intestinal Failure*, Nightingale J.M.D., Ed., Greenwich Medical Media Ltd., London, 2001, chap. 12.

14. Nightingale, J.M.D. et al., Disturbed gastric emptying in the short bowel syndrome, *Gut*, 34, 1171, 1999.

15. Booth, C.C., The metabolic effects of intestinal resection in man, *Postgrad. Med. J.*, 37, 725, 1961.

16. Schmidt, T. et al., Effect of intestinal resection on human small bowel motility, *Gut*, 38, 859, 1996.

17. Remington, M. et al., Abnormalities in gastrointestinal motor activity in patients with short bowels: effect of a synthetic opiate, *Gastroentoerlogy*, 85, 629, 1983.

18. Neal, D.E. et al., The effect of resection of the distal ileum on gastric emptying, small bowel transit and absorption after proctocolectomy, *Br. J. Surg.*, 71, 666, 1984.

19. Vanderhoof, J.A. et al., Treatment strategies for small bowel bacterial overgrowth in short bowel syndrome, *J. Pediatr. Gastroenterol. Nutr.*, 27, 155, 1998.

20. Straus, E., Gerson, C.D., and Yalow, R.S., Hypersecretion of gastrin associated with the short bowel syndrome, *Gastroenterology*, 66, 175, 1974.

21. Becker, H.D., Reeder, D.D., and Thompson, J.C., Extraction of circulating endogenous gastrin by the small bowel, *Gastroenterology*, 65, 903, 1973.

22. Buxton, B, Small bowel resection and gastric acid hypersecretion, *Gut*, 15, 229, 1974.

23. Barbezat, G.O. and Hansen, J.D.L., The exocrine pancreas and protein-calorie malnutrition, *Pediatrics*, 42, 77, 1978.

24. Kotler, D.P. and Levine, G.M., Reversible gastric and pancreatic hyposecretion after long-term total parenteral nutrition, *N. Engl. J. Med.* 300, 241, 1979.

25. Winter, T.A. et al., Impaired pancreatic secretion in severely malnourished patients is a consequence of primary pancreatic dysfunction, *Nutrition*, 17, 230, 2001.

26. Winter, T.A. et al., The effect of severe undernutrition, and subsequent refeeding on digestive function in human patients, *Eur. J. Gastroenterol. Hepatol.*, 12, 149, 2000.

27. Heizer, W.D., Cleaveland C.R., and Iber, F.L., Gastric inactivation of pancreatic supplements, *Bull. Johns Hopkins Hosp.*, 116, 261, 1965.

28. Lankisch, P.G., What to do when a patient with exocrine pancreatic insufficiency does not respond to pancreatic enzyme substitution, *Digestion*, 20, S97, 1999.

29. Hardison, W.G.M. and Rosenberg, I.H., Bile salt deficiency in the steatorrhea following resection of the ileum and proximal colon, *N. Engl. J. Med*, 227, 337, 1967.

30. Austad, W.I., Lack, L., and Tyor, M.P., Importance of bile acids and of an intact distal small intestine for fat absorption, *Gastroenterology*, 52, 638, 1967.

31. McLeod, G.M. and Wiggins, H.S., Bile salts in small intestinal contents after ileal resection and in other malabsorption syndromes, *Lancet*, 1, 873, 1968.

32. Mekhijian, H.S., Phillips, S.F., and Hofmann, A.F., Colonic secretion of water and electrolytes induced by bile acids: perfusion studies in man, *J. Clin. Invest.*, 50, 1569, 1971.

33. Hofmann, A.F. and Poley, J.R., Role of bile acid malabsorption in the pathogenesis of diarrhea and steatorrhea in patients with ileal resection. I. Response to cholestyramine or replacement of dietary long chain triglyceride by medium chain triglycerides, *Gastroenterology*, 62, 918, 1972.

34. Hofmann, A.F., Bile acid malabsorption caused by ileal resection, *Arch. Intern. Med.*, 130, 597, 1972.

35. Hofmann, A.F. and Mysels, K.J., Bile salts as biological surfactants, *Colloids Surf.*, 30, 125, 1988.

36. Krag, E. and Phillips, S.F., Effect of free and conjugated bile acids on net water, elctrolyte and glucose movement in the perfused human ileum, J. *Lab. Clin. Med.*, 83, 947, 1974.

37. Wingate, D.L., Phillips, S.F., and Hofmann, A.F., Effect of glycine-conjugated bile acids with and without lecithin on water and glucose absorption in perfused human jejunum, *J. Clin. Invest.*, 52, 1230, 1973.

38. Mekhjian, H.S., Phillips, S.F., and Hofmann, A.F., Colonic secretion of water and electrolytes induced by bile acids: perfusion studies in man, *J. Clin. Invest.*, 50, 1569, 1971.

39. Jeppesen, P.B. and Mortensen, P.B., Colonic digestion and absorption of energy from carbohydrates and medium-chain fat in small bowel failure, *J. Parenter. Enteral Nutr.*, 23, S101, 1999.

40. Fordtran, J.S., Bunch, F., and Davis, G.R., Ox bile treatment of severe steatorrhea in an ileectomy-ileostomy patient, *Gastroenterology*, 82, 564, 1982.

41. Djurdjevic, D. et al., Ox bile treatment of severe steatorrhea in a colectomy and ileectomy patient, *Gastroenterology*, 95, 1160, 1982.

42. Gruy-Kapral, C. et al., Conjugated bile acid replacement therapy for short-bowel syndrome, *Gastroenterology*, 116, 15, 1999.

43. Schmassmann, A. et al., Cholylsarcosine, a new bile acid analogue: metabolism and effect on biliary secretion in humans, *Gastroenterology*, 104, 1171, 1993.

44. Schmassmann, A. et al., Transport, metabolism, and effect of chronic feeding of cholylsarcosine, a conjugated bile acid resistant to deconjugation and dehydroxylation, *Gastroenterology*, 98, 163, 1990.

45. Lillienau, J., Schteingart, C.D., and Hofmann, A.F., Physicochemical and physiological properties of cholylsarcosine. A potential replacement detergent for bile acid deficiency states in the small intestine, *J. Clin. Invest.*, 89, 420, 1992.

46. Heydorn, S., Jeppesen, P.B., and Mortensen, P.B., Bile acid replacement therapy with cholylsarcosine for short-bowel syndrome, *Scand. J. Gastroenterol.*, 34, 818, 1999.

47. Palmer, R.H., Bile acids, liver injury, and liver disease, *Arch. Intern. Med.,* 130, 606, 1972.

48. Hopwood, D. et al., Effects of bile acids and hydrogen ion on the fine structure of esophageal epithelium, *Gut*, 22, 306, 1981.

49. Seidner, D.L., Short bowel syndrome: etiology, pathophysiology and management, *Pract. Gastroenterol.*, 63, 2001.

50. Regan, P.T. et al., Comparative effects of antacids, cimetidine and enteric coating on the therapeutic response to oral enzymes in severe pancreatic insufficiency, *N. Engl. J. Med.*, 296, 1314, 1977.

51. Cox et al., The effect of cimetidine on maldigestion in cystic fibrosis, *J. Pediatr.*, 94, 488, 1979.

52. Staub, J.L. et al., No effect of cimetidine on the therapeutic response to oral enzymes in severe pancreatic insufficiency, *N. Engl. J. Med*, 304, 1364, 1981.
53. Lankisch, P.G. et al., Therapy of pancreatogenic steatorrhea: does acid protection of pancraetic enzymes offer any advantage? *Z. Gastroenterol.*, 24, 753, 1986.
54. Fancisco, M.P. et al., Ranitadine and omeprazole as adjuvant therapy to pancrelipase to improve fat absorption in patients with cystic fibrosis, *J. Pediatr. Gastroenterol. Nutr.*, 35, 79, 2002.
55. Heijerman, H.G., Lamers, C.B., and Bakker, W., Omeprazole enhances the efficacy of pancreatin (pancrease) in cystic fibrosis, *Ann. Intern. Med.*, 114, 200, 1991.

12 Antimicrobials and Probiotics

Jon A. Vanderhoof and Rosemary J. Young

CONTENTS

The gastrointestinal tract is populated with a wide variety of microorganisms. Approximately 300 to 400 distinct species have been identified in each individual.[1] At least 50% of these species are not culturable and are identifiable only by molecular techniques.

Most people acquire their gastrointestinal flora very early in life. Many species are acquired during the birthing process, ingested during transit through the vaginal canal.[2] For this reason, an individual's flora closely mimics that of their mother rather than that of their father. Some gradual changes in microflora occur over the succeeding weeks and months, but most of the flora remains much the same. During the aging process, the relative numbers of some species increase while others decrease.[3] An example is *bifidobacteria*, which are often present in small infants, especially breast-fed infants, and gradually decrease throughout life, especially during the later decades. Transient colonization also occurs when people are exposed to pathogenic and even some nonpathogenic bacteria. After a few weeks to months, these species usually disappear.

The lifelong consistency of the gastrointestinal flora is largely based on the recognition and tolerance of the flora by the gut immune system.[4] During the first few days of life, the gastrointestinal immune system is heavily engaged in sampling various antigens, including microorganisms present in the gastrointestinal tract, and identifying these as normal residents.[5] It is these organisms for which the immune system develops tolerance. Subsequently, they will not evoke an immune response in the gut. This recognition by the gut immune system is strain specific, and other strains of the same species and certainly other species of microorganisms will elicit an immune response if ingested subsequent to initial colonization.

Immune sampling in the gut is a complex mechanism and is the subject of intense current investigation. Numerous binding sites or receptors on the surface of the gastrointestinal organisms interact with antigen sampling cells in or below the gut epithelium in a very complex fashion.[6] In addition to identification of pathogenic or nonpathogenic bacteria, the immune system is capable of differentiating bacterial antigens from food antigens in most instances. When tolerance to bacterial or food antigens is not acquired, an allergic reaction may result, causing inflammation in the gut epithelium and underlying structures.[7] It is these reactions that are partly responsible for some of the symptoms induced by small bowel bacterial overgrowth in short bowel syndrome.[8]

NORMAL GASTROINTESTINAL FLORA

The flora in the normal gastrointestinal tract changes and increases in number proximally to distally. A variety of predominantly aerobic organisms inhabit the oral pharyngeal cavity. These organisms present in the food and other swallowed material enter the stomach, where they are intermittently subjected to the low pH of the stomach. This, in conjunction with the normal immunoglobulins present in the salivary secretions, is the first order of defense against ingested microorganisms. The low pH of the stomach and, subsequently, the exposure to bile in the proximal duodenum eliminates many of the organisms swallowed. As a result, the bacterial counts in the duodenum are relatively low, usually 10^3 per milliliter or less. Progressing through the small bowel, bacterial counts rise and a gradual transition from aerobic to anaerobic flora occurs. In the distal small bowel, 10^7–10^8 microorganisms per milliliter are not uncommon. Once across the ileocecal valve, the bacterial counts jump dramatically, where there are 10^{10}–10^{11} microorganisms per milliliter. Here, a variety of organisms, predominantly bacteroides and bifidobacteria but also strains of enterococcus and lactobacilli, and numerous others coexist with the host, helping to ferment and digest nutrients not absorbed in the small bowel and helping to modulate the immune functions of the lower gut.

Most microorganisms reside within the lumen of the gastrointestinal tract. This nutrient-rich aqueous phase is an ideal culture media for bacteria. The gut epithelium itself is lined with mucins, extensively glycosylated proteinaceous compounds that function as binding sites for many of the gut bacteria. In this sense, the mucin may function to assist or inhibit bacterial attachment to the underlying epithelium or antigen sampling cells.[9]

Once bacteria enter the small bowel, there are several normal mechanisms to prevent overgrowth of existing bacteria. The primary mechanism is peristalsis. After the stomach has emptied and most of the material is digested in the small intestine, the entire small bowel undergoes stripping motions known as migrating motor complexes, which propel the gut contents from proximal to distal, forcing the remaining nutrients and the large volumes of bacteria into the colon. When gut motility is normal and small bowel anatomy is intact, this process is usually quite effective in preventing excess bacteria from multiplying in the small bowel.

In addition, the largest fraction of immunoglobulins secreted in the human body is the secretory IgA originating in the gastrointestinal tract in dimer form, which also aids in preventing bacterial proliferation.[10] Numerous resident bacteria themselves may also produce chemicals or bacteriocins that kill or inhibit multiplication of other surrounding bacterial species.[11]

Intestinal mucus normally traps bacteria intraluminally, preventing its ability to damage the epithelial surface. Therefore, high bacterial counts may be identified but are not problematic. Enzymatic digestion of bacteria from gastric acid, pancreatic secretions, and bile acid also controls excess bacterial proliferation. The presence or absence of an ileocecal valve has been identified by some as a significant factor in controlling the bacterial load in the small bowel.[8]

SHORT BOWEL SYNDROME

In short bowel syndrome, it is not uncommon and, in fact, it is the norm for anatomic and motility abnormalities to exacerbate small bowel bacterial overgrowth.[12] Shortly after resection of a large portion of the small bowel, the gut undergoes a massive adaptation response destined to cause a deepening of the crypts and lengthening of the villi, all markedly increasing the absorptive surface area.[7] As this process progresses, there is a tendency for the small bowel lumen to dilate. This is especially true if there is any stricture formation distally, but is not uncommon even in the absence of a functional or anatomical obstruction. Concurrently, transit through the small bowel is often slowed, again as a compensatory response to increase nutrient absorption from the limited mucosal surface. The combination of gut dilatation and slower transit increases the concentration of bacteria present in the small bowel per milliliter of fluid.[13]

Dilatation of the small bowel makes peristalsis less effective or ineffective at removing gut bacteria. It is not uncommon radiographically to see to and fro flux of gastrointestinal contents in a dilated bowel when performing a small bowel radiographic study in a patient with short bowel syndrome. It is in patients with ineffective peristalsis where small bowel bacterial overgrowth is most likely to be present in such a manner as to cause symptoms. In short bowel syndrome patients with no anatomic abnormalities or gut dilatation, and radiographic or other evidence of normal or rapid transit through the small bowel, small bowel bacterial overgrowth is rarely present, at least to the extent to which it would create a problem.

Excess bacterial content of the small bowel in short bowel syndrome is not necessarily bad. In fact, it may be beneficial. Numerous macronutrients, most notably complex carbohydrates, undergo a significant amount of digestion through bacterial fermentation.[14] This normally happens to some degree in the colon. Competition with the host for micronutrients is rarely a significant problem. In fact, production of micronutrients such as vitamin B_{12} and folic acid are an important physiologic role of gut bacteria. Small bowel bacteria, when present in excessive numbers, can deconjugate bile acids, making them rapidly absorbed and unavailable for micellar solubilization.[15] The role of exacerbated bile acid deficiency-induced fat malabsorption has not been well studied but most likely plays a minimal role in the adverse effects of excess small bowel bacteria in short bowel syndrome. Excess proliferation of bacteria in the small bowel can, however, occasionally produce untoward effects particularly gas and abdominal distention.

PATHOPHYSIOLOGY

The major pathophysiology related to excess small bowel bacteria is due to the inflammatory changes that occur in the gut.[16,17] Inflammation causes reduced absorptive surface area through flattening of the villi. In addition, the absorptive surface is less effective due to damage of the brush border membrane. Inflammation is also associated with the number of cytokines and inflammatory mediators, which may disrupt or inhibit the absorptive process.[18] The cause of inflammation in small bowel bacterial overgrowth is likely multifactorial. Periodically, certain bacterial species may invade the small bowel mucosa, causing a defensive inflammatory response as one might expect. More frequently, inflammation may be an inappropriate or over-aggressive reaction to absorbed bacterial antigens. In such instances, it is not uncommon to see other evidence of immune dysregulation, including arthritis, especially large joint arthritis, which often resembles that seen with inflammatory bowel disease.[19] This finding was originally observed in patients with intestinal bypass for treatment of obesity and, at that time, was identified as a complication of small bowel bacterial overgrowth.

Another complication of small bowel bacterial overgrowth is D-lactic acidosis. Some patients are very poor metabolizers of D-lactate, the dextro isomer of lactic acid. Normally, L isomers are produced by human bacterial organisms, absorbed, and subsequently metabolized in the liver. Certain bacteria, however, may produce a combination of D and L isomers or even exclusively D isomers.[20,21] If an individual patient has an abundant flora of D-lactate-producing lactobacilli, for instance, an elevation of the serum D-lactate level may occur, which may result in a variety of central nervous system symptoms varying from poor school performance to frank coma. This is especially common in younger patients and responds dramatically to antimicrobial therapy or flushing of the small bowel contents with a balanced oral PEG solution.[22] Luminal production of alcohol through the overgrowth of alcohol-producing yeast has also been reported in short bowel syndrome, although this complication appears exceedingly rare.[23]

DIAGNOSIS

Small bowel bacterial overgrowth in short bowel syndrome should be suspected in pediatric patients when growth plateaus or the patient develops abdominal distention and a significant succussion splash on physical examination. In adults, symptoms of bloating, flatulence, and weight loss, especially if associated with loosening of the stool or more frequent stooling, should suggest this possibility. Small bowel bacterial overgrowth is virtually always present in patients with anatomic dilatation of the small bowel or delayed transit, although the relative role of the overgrowth in producing untoward symptoms is often difficult to assess.

Diagnosis of pathological small bowel bacterial overgrowth is difficult. If the organisms are predominantly hydrogen or methane producing, analysis of exhaled respiratory gases can be performed following a carbohydrate load.[24] Glucose is often utilized in this situation because it is absorbed in the small intestine. In patients with short bowel syndrome and rapid transit, it is difficult to differentiate small bowel vs. colonic production of hydrogen when using a nonabsorbable substrate such as lactulose. With lactulose, a reading reflective of an early hydrogen peak is suggestive of small bowel bacterial contamination. In addition to high D-lactate levels, other biochemical indicators such as high folate levels, metabolic acidosis, and excess indicans in the urine may occasionally suggest small bowel bacterial overgrowth.[22] Previously, culture of the small bowel fluid via endoscopy using a sterile tube was considered the gold standard to measure bacterial overgrowth, but the procedure itself is fraught with significant technical difficulties, primarily due to contamination of the specimen during its transit into and through the small bowel. Since it is known that greater than 50% of the bacterial species in the gut are not culturable, the validity of the technique comes even more into question.

The determination of excess bacteria and its correlation to symptoms is not as simple as determining if excess counts are present. Virtually all of these diagnostic techniques, however, are designed specifically to evaluate the presence of excess numbers of bacteria in the small bowel and do not determine whether or not the bacteria are doing any harm. As noted, a certain level of commensual bacteria is important, but it may be either the species type and/or an excess number that can cause inflammation and the development of symptoms. In this instance, extensive biopsies of the small bowel may give the best indication of whether or not the bacteria present are actually harmful. Inflammatory changes consisting of blunting of the villi associated with the mixed inflammatory cell infiltrate is often suggestive of pathological small bowel bacterial overgrowth if no other likely cause of small bowel mucosal injury is present. The presence of adherent or intracellular bacteria further supports the diagnosis.

TREATMENT STRATEGIES

Once pathological small bowel bacterial overgrowth has been identified, a strategy for control must be developed. The goals must be clearly identified. One should not attempt to sterilize the gastrointestinal tract.[25] Gut bacteria are important in maintaining normal gut function, normal immune function, and normal digestion of nutrients. The goal is simply to reduce the numbers of potentially pathogenic bacteria present in the lumen. As culture of the lumen will not necessarily identify which species or strains of bacteria are causing the significant problem, trial and error of antibiotic treatment is often the best means of determining appropriate therapy.

Antimicrobial therapy is usually the first modality used to treat overgrowth. Antibiotics should be given in a dosage selected to reduce the numbers of potentially pathogenic gut bacteria down to a level where they can be adequately tolerated by the host. This is often empirical and is usually initiated at somewhere around one-half of the normal dose one might give for a systemic infection. The choice of antibiotics varies greatly. Numerous different regimes are outlined in Table 12.1.

TABLE 12.1
Antibiotic Regimens In Bacterial Overgrowth

Drug	Childhood Dose	Adult Dose
Amoxicillin	25 mg/kg/d	500–1000 mg/d
Amoxicillin-clavulanic acid	20 mg/kg/d	500–1000 mg/day
Ciprofloxacin	20–30 mg/kg/d	20–30 mg/kg/d
Gentamicin	5–10 mg/kg/d	5–10 mg/kg/d
Metronidazole	20–25 mg/kg/d	20–25 mg/kg/d
Neomycin	50 mg/kg/d	1 gm/d
Tetracycline (Doxycycline)	25 mg/kg/d	25 mg/kg/d
	(5 mg/kg/d)	(5 mg/kg/d)
Trimethoprim Sulfamethoxazole		
(based on TMP component)	10 mg/kg/d	160 mg/d
Vancocin™	20 mg/kg/day	250 mg/day

Successful treatment of small bowel bacterial overgrowth will result in improved symptoms, such as better weight gain and more formed stools in a child or reduction in gas and bloating in an adult. However, once an antibiotic has been given for a long time, resistance is likely to develop. When symptoms recur, it is usually time to change the regimen using a different antibiotic preparation or dosing protocol. It may only be necessary to treat some patients for the first 5–7 days of each month or even every other week. More often, the need for antibiotics becomes chronic and continuous, and it is at this time that periodic rotation of the protocol results in the best therapeutic response. The goal is to reduce the number of bacteria to a tolerable level, and to not necessarily target and eliminate all species present.

Other therapies for controlling small bowel bacterial overgrowth include avoidance of medications that predispose to overgrowth, such as antimotility drugs (loperamide), and agents that suppress gastric acid, since gastric acid is an important defense against small bowel bacterial overgrowth. Occasionally, motility may be enhanced by prokinetics, such as cisapride or erythromycin, but these are rarely beneficial. Dilated or poorly peristaltic segments of bowel often require correction surgically through either tapering and/or lengthening procedures.[26] Placement of an ascending colostomy has also been noted to be of benefit in limited circumstances.[22] Periodic flushing of the small bowel with balanced polyethylene glycol solutions can give a transient reduction in bacterial overgrowth.[22] The bowel could be flushed 2–3 times a week to avoid the complications of overgrowth as well as obviate the need for antibiotic therapy. A large oral dose of magnesium citrate may accomplish the same purpose without requiring administration of large volumes of fluid and risking potential fluid and electrolyte disturbances.

In children, nutritional therapy to reduce bacterial proliferation includes using a high-fat, low-carbohydrate diet as most bacteria ferment only carbohydrates. Fat is not significantly metabolized by the bacteria and supplies a good calorie source for the child. High-fat formulas may be helpful if a child receives a large percentage of calories via enteral tube feeding.[27] Diets high in meat are well tolerated, even in infants.

We have occasionally had the experience with young children who experience a profound reluctance to defecate as a natural response to control the diarrhea associated with short bowel syndrome. In the absence of an ileocecal valve, extensive small bowel contamination can occur and, in this setting, encouraging the child to defecate more frequently is often successful in relieving bacterial overgrowth.

PROBIOTICS

Recently, probiotics have been popularized for the treatment and prevention of a wide variety of gastrointestinal disorders, especially infectious ones.[28] Probiotics are live human-derived organisms that, when administered to a patient, result in some beneficial health-promoting effects. Most probiotic species are either lactobacilli or bifidobacteria, or certain yeasts such as saccharomyces.

Several probiotic organisms have been shown to be useful in the treatment of viral gastroenteritis in children. These include Lactobacillus casei (subspecies rhamnosus, LGG), Lactobacillus reuterii, and Bifidobacteria bifidum.[29] Saccharomyces boulardii has been shown to be quite beneficial in antibiotic-associated diarrhea in adults, especially in C. difficile-induced diarrhea, and Lactobacillus GG has been shown to be of benefit in antibiotic-associated diarrhea in children.[30] For these reasons, and because abnormal bacterial flora are known to be present in short bowel syndrome, the use of probiotics has been suggested to be potentially beneficial in this situation.

Unfortunately, little positive evidence exists to detail any beneficial effects of probiotics in short bowel syndrome, especially in patients with small bowel bacterial overgrowth. This may be due to the fact that administration of a probiotic has very little impact in the overall number of bacteria in the gut. For example, administration of lactobacilli may result in a slight increase in total lactobacillus count and a secondary increase in the number of bifidobacteria, but overall, the total number of organisms changes little. Consequently, the beneficial effects of the probiotic are likely limited to the individual strain's effect on the gut immune system.[31] Certain other regulatory aspects of the probiotics may also be beneficial, but the concept of large numbers of probiotic bacteria blocking adhesion to the gut by potentially pathogenic organisms must be called into question because of the relatively small numbers of probiotic organisms that actually are able to grow in the gut following their administration.

The mechanism and frequency with which bacterial translocation occurs due to effects of bacterial overgrowth is not known but has been documented in both animal and human studies.[32] Human studies in intestinal permeability conditions associated with Crohn's disease[33] and animal studies in other conditions associated with altered permeability have shown some positive effects of probiotics in reducing bacterial translocation.[34,35] However, results have not consistently been replicated and warrant further study.[36]

Attar et al., in a placebo-controlled trial, compared antibiotic therapy with norfloxacin or amoxicillin-clavulanate to probiotic therapy with Saccharomyces boulardii in a small group of children with small bowel bacterial overgrowth identified by positive hydrogen breath testing.[37] He found that either antibiotic was more effective than Saccharomyces in decreasing the number of stools and reducing hydrogen production. Other probiotic products including Lactobacillus GG and other combination products have also received anecdotal attention as being effective in conditions of small bowel bacterial overgrowth, but controlled studies are lacking.[22,38]

Certain strains of bacteria appear to have anti-inflammatory properties that may be helpful in controlling the intestinal inflammation that occurs with bacterial overgrowth. These include Lactobacillus GG and Lactobacillus plantarum (species 299V).[39,40] The anti-inflammatory functions of these probiotics may have some positive beneficial effects. Trial and error is probably the best way to assess a clinical response, as there is little or no risk associated with probiotic therapy. The exception may be administration of a D-lactate-producing, probiotic bacteria in large numbers to a child who may potentially develop D-lactic acidosis.

CONCLUSION

Small bowel bacterial overgrowth is common in patients with short bowel syndrome. It occurs when the gut is dilated or motility is delayed. Excess bacteria in the gut are usually only a problem when they create an inflammatory reaction that can often be detected histologically. Antibiotic therapy is usually indicated in such instances. Probiotics may occasionally be beneficial but further controlled studies are needed.

REFERENCES

1. Evaldson, G. et al., The normal human anaerobic microflora, *Scand. J. Infect. Dis. Suppl.* 1982, 35, 9–15.
2. Mackie, R.I., Sghir, A., and Gaskins, H.R., Developmental microbial ecology of the neonatal gastrointestinal tract, *Am. J. Clin. Nutr.* 1999, 69(5), 1035S–1045S.
3. Reuter, G., The Lactobacillus and Bifidobacterium microflora of the human intestine: composition and succession, *Curr. Issues Intest. Microbiol.* 2001, 2(2), 43–53.
4. Ouwehand, A., Isolauri, E., and Salminen, S., The role of the intestinal microflora for the development of the immune system in early childhood, *Eur. J. Nutr.* 2002, 41(Suppl. 1), I32–37.
5. Cebra, J.J., Influences of microbiota on intestinal immune system development, *Am. J. Clin. Nutr.* 1999, 69 (5), 1046S–1051S.
6. Edwards, C. A. and Parrett, A.M., Intestinal flora during the first months of life: new perspectives, *Br. J. Nutr.* 2002, 88 Suppl. 1, S11–18.
7. Vanderhoof, J., *Short Bowel Syndrome in Children and Small Intestinal Transplantation*, ed., W.B. Saunders Company: Philadelphia, 1996, Vol. 43, 533–550.
8. Kaufman, S.S. et al., Influence of bacterial overgrowth and intestinal inflammation on duration of parenteral nutrition in children with short bowel syndrome, *J. Pediatr.* 1997, 131(3), 356–361.

9. Mack, D.R. et al., Probiotics inhibit enteropathogenic E. coli adherence in vitro by inducing intestinal mucin gene expression, *Am. J. Physiol.* 1999, 276(4 Pt 1), G941–950.

10. Riordan, S.M. et al., Small intestinal mucosal immunity and morphometry in luminal overgrowth of indigenous gut flora, *Am. J. Gastroenterol.* 2001, 96(2), 494–500.

11. Gorbach, S.L., Probiotics and gastrointestinal health, *Am. J. Gastroenterol.* 2000, 95(1 Suppl.), S2–4.

12. Husebye, E., The patterns of small bowel motility: physiology and implications in organic disease and functional disorders, *Neurogastroenterol. Motil.* 1999, 11(3), 141–161.

13. Madl, C. and Druml, W., Gastrointestinal disorders of the critically ill. Systemic consequences of ileus, *Best Pract. Res. Clin. Gastroenterol.* 2003, 17(3), 445–456.

14. Toskes, P.P., Bacterial overgrowth of the gastrointestinal tract, *Adv. Intern. Med.* 1993, 38, 387–407.

15. Shindo, K. et al., Deconjugation ability of bacteria isolated from the jejunal fluid of patients with progressive systemic sclerosis and its gastric pH, *Hepatogastroenterology* 1998, 45(23), 1643–1650.

16. Toskes, P.P. et al., Small intestinal mucosal injury in the experimental blind loop syndrome. Light- and electron-microscopic and histochemical studies, *Gastroenterology* 1975, 68(5 Pt. 1), 193–203.

17. Giannella, R.A., Rout, W.R., and Toskes, P.P., Jejunal brush border injury and impaired sugar and amino acid uptake in the blind loop syndrome, *Gastroenterology* 1974, 67(5), 965–974.

18. Riordan, S.M. et al., Mucosal cytokine production in small-intestinal bacterial overgrowth, S*cand. J. Gastroenterol.* 1996, 31(10), 977–984.

19. Lichtman, S.N., Bacterial overgrowth. In *Pediatric Gastrointestinal Disease*, 3rd ed., Walker W.A., D.P., Hamilton, J.R., Walker-Smith, J.A. Watkins, J.B., Eds., B.C. Decker Hamilton, Ontario, 2000, pp. 569–582.

20. Kaneko, T. et al., Fecal microflora in a patient with short-bowel syndrome and identification of dominant lactobacilli, *J. Clin. Microbiol.* 1997, 35(12), 3181–3185.

21. Bongaerts, G. et al., Lactobacilli and acidosis in children with short small bowel, *J. Pediatr. Gastroenterol. Nutr.* 2000, 30(3), 288–293.

22. Vanderhoof, J.A. et al., Treatment strategies for small bowel bacterial overgrowth in short bowel syndrome, *J. Pediatr. Gastroenterol. Nutr.* 1998, 27,(2), 155–160.

23. Dahshan, A. and Donovan, K., Auto-brewery syndrome in a child with short gut syndrome: case report and review of the literature, *J. Pediatr. Gastroenterol. Nutr.* 2001, 33(2), 214–215.

24. Riordan, S.M. et al., The lactulose breath hydrogen test and small intestinal bacterial overgrowth, *Am. J. Gastroenterol.* 1996, 91(9), 1795–1803.

25. Krueger, W.A. and Unertl, K.E., Selective decontamination of the digestive tract, *Curr. Opin. Crit. Care* 2002, 8(2), 139–144.

26. Thompson, J.S., Vanderhoof, J.A., and Antonson, D.L., Intestinal tapering and lengthening for short bowel syndrome, *J. Pediatr. Gastroenterol. Nutr.* 1985, 4(3), 495–497.

27. Bongaerts, G.P. et al., Lactobacillus flora in short bowel syndrome, *Dig. Dis. Sci.* 1997, 42(8), 1611–1612.

28. Vanderhoof, J.A. and Young, R.J., Use of probiotics in childhood gastrointestinal disorders, *J. Pediatr. Gastroenterol. Nutr.* 1998, 27(3), 323–332.

29. Szajewska, H. and Mrukowicz, J.Z., Probiotics in the treatment and prevention of acute infectious diarrhea in infants and children: a systematic review of published randomized, double-blind, placebo-controlled trials, *J. Pediatr. Gastroenterol. Nutr.* 2001, 33(Suppl. 2), S17–25.

30. Duggan, C., Gannon, J., Walker, W.A., Protective nutrients and functional foods for the gastrointestinal tract, *Am. J. Clin. Nutr.* 2002, 75(5), 789–808.

31. Vanderhoof, J.A. and Young, R.J., Allergic disorders of the gastrointestinal tract, *Curr. Opin. Clin. Nutr. Metab. Care* 2001, 4(6), 553–556.

32. Berg, R.D., Bacterial translocation from the gastrointestinal tract, Adv. Exp. Med. Biol. 1999, 473, 11–30.

33. Gupta, P. et al., Is lactobacillus GG helpful in children with Crohn's disease? Results of a preliminary, open-label study, *J. Pediatr. Gastroenterol. Nutr.* 2000, 31(4), 453–457.

34. Mangell, P. et al., Lactobacillus plantarum 299V inhibits Escherichia coli-induced intestinal permeability, *Dig. Dis. Sci.* 2002, 47, (3), 511–516.

35. Madsen, K. et al., Probiotic bacteria enhance murine and human intestinal epithelial barrier function, *Gastroenterology* 2001, 121(3), 580–591.

36. Kennedy, R. J. et al., Probiotic therapy fails to improve gut permeability in a hapten model of colitis, *Scand. J. Gastroenterol.* 2000, 35(12), 1266–1271.

37. Attar, A. et al., Antibiotic efficacy in small intestinal bacterial overgrowth-related chronic diarrhea: a crossover, randomized trial, *Gastroenterology* 1999, 117(4), 794–797.

38. Kanamori, Y. et al., Combination therapy with Bifidobacterium breve, Lactobacillus casei, and galactooligosaccharides dramatically improved the intestinal function in a girl with short bowel syndrome: a novel synbiotics therapy for intestinal failure, *Dig. Dis. Sci.* 2001, 46(9), 2010–2016.

39. Schultz, M. et al., Lactobacillus plantarum 299V in the treatment and prevention of spontaneous colitis in interleukin-10-deficient mice, *Inflamm. Bowel Dis.* 2002, 8(2), 71–80.

40. Shibolet, O. et al., Variable response to probiotics in two models of experimental colitis in rats, *Inflamm. Bowel Dis.* 2002, 8(6), 399–406.

13 Use of Trophic Substances in the Treatment of Intestinal Failure

Thomas R. Ziegler, Junqiang Tian,
Naohiro Washizawa, Menghua Luo,
Lorraine M. Leader, and
Concepción Fernández-Estívariz

CONTENTS

SHORT BOWEL SYNDROME AS AN IMPORTANT CLINICAL PROBLEM

Massive small bowel resection (SBR) is a major cause of intestinal failure in adults and children. In adults, relatively common conditions such as Crohn's disease, splanchnic ischemia, repeated abdominal operations, and trauma might require massive or repeated SBR, thus leading to SBS.[1,2] Patients with SBS exhibit chronic diarrhea and malabsorption, and varying degrees of dehydration, weight loss, protein-energy and micronutrient depletion, weakness, and decreased quality of life.[3–8] In addition, patients with SBS commonly require chronic or intermittent parenteral nutrition (PN) to prevent severe malnutrition.[1–2,7–11] Unfortunately, PN is expensive

($150,000/year) and a major quality-of-life burden for SBS patients and their families.[8] Further, PN is associated with severe complications, including electrolyte disturbances, venous thrombosis, sepsis, and liver failure. [12–14] In addition, individuals with SBS face ongoing challenges due to their underlying illnesses, including infection and oxidative stress.[2] PN-dependent SBS patients also tend to develop infection with apparently gut-derived organisms, suggesting that gut barrier function is decreased.[14] Although small bowel transplantation is showing increasing promise as a method to achieve PN independence, this procedure is associated with significant morbidity and mortality,[2] and other types of surgical procedures (e.g., bowel lengthening) and novel developments, such as growing functional neomucosa, remain experimental.[2,15] Thus, there is a critical need for better management.

Severe SBS is a particularly costly orphan disease. There are approximately 15,000 patients in the U.S. who require daily or intermittent PN after massive SBR, and approximately 1 to 2,000 new severe SBS cases appear each year.[2,7] The clinical severity and PN-dependence of SBS depends on the indications for bowel resection, the degree of malabsorption, and the location, length, and functional health of the residual bowel.[9,16–17] For example, 5-year survival rates for patents with nonmalignant SBS were approximately 50% in a large French study, similar to many types of cancer.[18] The etiology and severity of SBS and the presence or absence of residual colon appear to be important factors for prognosis.[2,18] Many patients can eventually be weaned from PN following limited SBR (e.g., > 150–250 cm of residual small bowel ± colon). However, in the absence of intensive intestinal rehabilitation, most subjects with < 150–250 cm small bowel and no colon in continuity and those with < 75 cm small bowel and with colon in continuity typically require PN for life.[2,7,15] In light of (a) the clinical importance of adult and pediatric intestinal failure, (b) the extremely high health care–related costs of SBS, and (c) the dearth of effective therapies, new therapies and an understanding of mechanisms of action are clearly needed in human SBS. Hence, over the past 20 years studies in both animal models and in patients with SBS have focused on the potential efficacy of "gut-trophic" nutrients and growth factors, given alone and in combination, as strategies to enhance residual gut function in human SBS. This chapter will summarize the results of such studies and discuss their implications for care of patients with intestinal failure due to SBS.

INTESTINAL ADAPTATION

Animal models of massive SBR (e.g., rat, mouse, and rabbit) exhibit intestinal adaptation characterized by rapid cellular hyperplasia in the mucosa of the residual small bowel, and, to a lesser extent, colon.[19–27] This growth response is associated with up-regulation of expression of several growth factors, including enteroglucagon (the precursor for glucagon-like peptide-2 [GLP-2]), and insulin-like growth factor-I (IGF-I), a mediator of GH action.[25–27] Similarly, increased gut mucosal growth indices were documented in the in-continuity small intestine or colon of patients who underwent jejuno-ileal bypass for treatment of severe obesity,[28–29] and these patients appeared to achieve adaptive improvement in gut absorptive function during the first 1–2 years after surgery, manifested by decreased diarrhea. In contrast, there have been few studies of gut growth in SBR-induced human SBS. In general, these limited studies do not demonstrate an increase in gut mucosal growth indices in human SBS in contrast to that observed in animal models[30–33] (Figure 13.1). However, SBS patients have not been studied serially and mucosal biopsies in the published reports were obtained primarily in patients with chronic SBS.[30–33] Further, possible changes in the enterocyte microvilli, which account for the majority of the small bowel surface area, have not been evaluated after SBR in humans, and little, if any, information is published on postresection responses in human residual colon. Thus, increased gut mucosal growth may occur postoperatively in SBS patients, but these data are lacking, especially during the first 2 years after SBR, when adaptive improvement in gut absorptive function is often manifested by decreased meal-associated diarrhea. Information about the regulation of gut mucosal turnover in specific gut segments and as a function of time since SBR, dietary intake changes, etc. will help to direct the design and timing of administration of trophic factors (e.g., specific nutrients and growth factors as outlined below) to augment gut mucosal growth or absorptive function in human SBS.[34–50] This information may also aid management of other disorders, such as inflammatory bowel disease (IBD), sepsis, malnutrition, and ischemia-reperfusion injury.

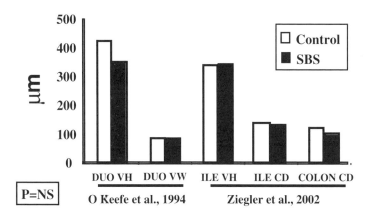

FIGURE 13.1 Lack of evidence for adaptive small bowel or colonic mucosal growth in patients with chronic SBS versus unresected control subjects. CD = crypt depth; Duo = duodenum; Ile = ileum; VH = villus height; VW = villus width. Adapted from O'Keefe, S.J., Haymond, M.W., Bennet, W.M., Oswald, B., Nelson, D.K., and Shorter, R.G., Long-acting somatostatin analogue therapy and protein metabolism in patients with jejunostomies, *Gastroenterology,* 107, 379, 1994; and Ziegler, T.R., Estivariz, C.F., Gu, L.H., Wallace, T.M., Díaz, E.E., Pascal, R.R., Bazargan, N., Galloway, J.R., Wilcox, J.N., and Leader, L.M., Distribution of H+/peptide transporter PepT1 in human intestine: up-regulated expression in the colonic mucosa of patients with short bowel syndrome, *Am. J. Clin. Nutr.,* 75, 922, 2002.)

POTENTIAL MECHANISMS OF GUT ADAPTATION

Dynamic gut mucosal cell turnover is a function of rates of cell proliferation, migration from crypt to villus, and cell death via apoptosis.[19–21,24] Animal studies suggest that all of these functions are accelerated during gut adaptation,[19,21,24] but these have not been studied in human SBS.

The most clearly defined factor to enhance mucosal cell growth is luminal food, particularly if the diet is complex as opposed to elemental.[19,51–52] Specific nutrient substrates also may be important for mucosal regeneration (e.g., zinc, vitamin B12, retinoic acid, dietary fiber, and glutamine).[27,53] Unfortunately, conventional PN does not support gut adaptation in animals, perhaps because trophic nutrients are lacking, or because apical nutrient delivery is important for enterocyte growth responses.[27] For example, the presence of luminal nutrients increases pancreatic-biliary secretion, neuronal activity, splanchnic blood flow, and mucosal levels of glutathione,[54–55] and each of these facilitate gut mucosal cell growth, either directly or indirectly.[27] Limited data in humans show that small bowel mucosal atrophy occurs in the absence of enteral nutrition, despite PN administration.[56]

The mucosa of bypassed human small bowel loops undergoes relatively little atrophy following jejunoileal bypass procedures,[57–58] presumably because systemic factors and/or local growth substances maintain growth independent of the direct effects of luminal food.[27–28,57–58] In animal models, bowel resection and enteral feeding increase expression of several peptide growth factors in residual bowel, including enteroglucagon, epidermal growth factor (EGF), and insulin-like growth factor-I (IGF-I).[24–25,27,59–61] Although only limited data are available, IGF-I mRNA[62–63] and several IGF binding proteins (IGFBPs), which modulate IGF-I action, are present in human intestine.[64–65] Receptors for GH, GLP-2, IGF-I, and KGF are present in human small bowel and colonic mucosa as well.[66–68] These data suggest that local (and systemic) growth factor action pathways may be important mediators of physiologic and pathophysiologic gut mucosal turnover and function and the potential responsiveness to exogenous administration of these agents in human SBS.

Increased expression and function of gut mucosal nutrient transporters has been demonstrated in some animal models of SBS, but this depends on the timing after resection.[23,27,69] For example, increased ileal α-glucosidase and neutral aminopeptidase activity, and sodium-glucose co-transporter expression occurs independent of changes in cell mass in the residual small bowel of small bowel-resected animals.[23,70–72] In contrast, small bowel transport of amino acids and glucose was shown to be transiently decreased after SBR in rabbit and mouse models of SBS.[69,73] Unfortunately, only minimal information is available on serial absorptive function in human SBS, although improved absorption has been reported during the first two years after massive SBR in small series or individual cases.[5,30,74–75]

The colon is critically important as a site of fluid and electrolyte absorption in SBS, and the presence of any residual colon positively influences outcome.[16,18] In addition, the colon has the capacity to absorb medium chain triglycerides (MCT) as an energy source,[17] and produces SCFA (butyrate, proprionate, acetate) from dietary carbohydrate and fiber sources; SCFA provide energy and stimulate sodium and water transport across the colonic epithelia.[3,10,76] Brush border transport of small

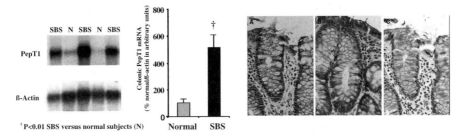

FIGURE 13.2 Up-regulated expression of steady-state PepT1 mRNA in mid-residual colonic mucosa of adults with chronic SBS versus expression in unresected, normal subjects by Northern blotting (left). Quantitative data from 5 SBS and 12 N subjects is shown in in the middle panel. Colonic PepT1 protein expression by immunohistochemistry is shown in the right panel. A = normal control subject; B = SBS patient; C = negative control section from the normal subject shown in A. (Data adapted from Ziegler, T.R., Estivariz, C.F., Gu, L.H., Wallace, T.M., Díaz, E.E., Pascal, R.R., Bazargan, N., Galloway, J.R., Wilcox, J.N., and Leader, L.M., Distribution of H+/peptide transporter PepT1 in human intestine: up-regulated expression in the colonic mucosa of patients with short bowel syndrome, *Am. J. Clin. Nutr.*, 75, 922, 2002.)

peptides is the major mechanism for accrual of protein digestion products,[77] and the transporter PepT1 plays a major role in intracellular accumulation of luminal di-tripeptides.[77–79] In the first study to show that changes in gut mucosal nutrient transporter expression may occur in human SBS, we found that PepT1 mRNA is increased in colonic mucosa of short-gut patients, possibly as an adaptive mechanism to increase di/tripeptide accrual (Figure 13.2).[33] Consistent with animal studies demonstrating colonic transport of l-amino acids,[80–82] the concentration of l-amino acids was recently shown to be high in the distal ileum of healthy adults after oral amino acid or protein loads.[83] Also, expression of the broad-spectrum amino acid transporter ATB[0+] [84–85] was up-regulated in the colonic mucosa of one patient with long-standing severe SBS.[86] Thus, elucidation of adaptive changes in nutrient trans-porters in both small bowel and colonic mucosa may help to direct new dietary management in SBS. Studies on potential growth factor-induced up-regulation of these nutrient transporters are needed.

SPECIFIC NUTRIENTS AS METHODS TO ENHANCE INTESTINAL GROWTH, REPAIR, AND ADAPTATION

Specific nutrient substrates, including linoleic acid, short-chain fatty acids (SCFA), zinc, and vitamin A, have been shown to improve gut mucosal growth responses after massive SBR in rats; in the case of zinc and vitamin A, these agents were effective compared to animals deficient in these nutrients.[27,87–90] Glutamine (Gln) is a nonessential amino acid but is utilized as a major substrate of gut mucosal epithelial cells.[91–92] Studies of catabolic animal models demonstrate beneficial effects of dietary Gln supplementation of enteral and parenteral diets enriched in either l-Gln or Gln-dipeptides on small bowel and colonic growth, repair and/or gut barrier function.[26–27,93–98] However, results of Gln supplementation have been mixed in animal models of SBS,[26–27,99–103] with some studies showing stimulation of adaptive gut mucosal growth[26,103] and others showing no effect.[99–102] The relative efficacy of enteral versus parenteral Gln on gut growth and function in SBS is not known. In vitro studies show that Gln is essential for endogenous and growth factor-stimulated intestinal epithelial cell proliferation, and this amino acid also inhibits gut epithelial cell apoptosis.[27,104–105] Furthermore, some studies in animal models of SBS suggest that the combination Gln and GH or IGF-I has additive or synergistic effects on intestinal adaptive growth following small bowel resection.[26,106] Zhou et al. found that Gln + GH resulted in an additive increase in gut glucose and palmitate absorption in resected rats.[106] Conversely, another study found that while GH improved anabolic indices in parenterally fed small bowel-resected rats, parenteral Gln + GH did not have an additive effect.[107]

Several investigations suggest that Gln or Gln dipeptide administration improves growth and/or function of human gut epithelial cells.[27,108–109] Addition of either L-Gln or the dipeptide alanyl-glutamine increased cellular proliferation in cells isolated *ex vivo* from ileal and proximal and distal colonic mucosal biopsies of healthy adults without SBS.[108] PN-dependent patients, some with SBS, given glycyl-Gln-supplementation of PN versus standard Gln-free PN, demonstrated significantly increased duodenal villus height and decreased intestinal permeability.[109] We recently found that addition of alanyl-glutamine dipeptide to PN in critically ill postsurgical patients (without SBS) markedly improved D-xylose absorption compared to abnormally low absorption in controls.[110] Taken together, these data suggest the possibility that certain nutrients may have trophic or other beneficial effects when supplemented to patients with intestinal failure, but controlled studies are needed in this area.

ADMINISTRATION OF RECOMBINANT GROWTH FACTORS IN ANIMAL MODELS OF SBS

Studies in rodent models of SBS demonstrate that administration of recombinant GH,[111–115] IGF-I,[116–119] EGF,[120–122] KGF,[123–124] GLP-2,[125–126] and leptin[127] enhance gut mucosal growth, and in some cases, absorptive function. In a recent comparative study in the rat model of 80% mid-jejunoileal resection, we found that GH, GLP-2, and KGF treatment exert modest but differential trophic effects on post-SBR bowel mucosa that are gut segment-specific.[128] These growth factors also improve intestinal repair, barrier function, and/or nutrient transport functions in models of PN, chemotherapy administration and colitis in rodents.[27,129–133] Some studies in rat models of SBS suggest that combining dietary L-Gln with IGF-I[26] or GH[134–135] provides additive effects on gut mucosal growth, but other studies conflict on this point.[107] Additional translational studies on the efficacy and mechanism(s) of action of these agents remains are needed and are the focus of several investigations.

STUDIES ON THE EFFICACY OF GH, GLP-2, GLN AND/OR MODIFIED ORAL DIET TO ENHANCE INTESTINAL REHABILITATION IN HUMAN SBS

A growing number of studies have evaluated individual nutrient supplementation, diet therapy, and recombinant growth factors, alone and in combination therapy, to enhance bowel rehabilitation in human SBS.[2–4,10,35–50] No individual nutrient supplementation, diet therapy, or growth factor has been rigorously evaluated as a therapy in human SBS. GH and GLP-2 are the only growth factors so far tested in human SBS, and both show efficacy in improving nutrient absorption.[3–4,38–39,45–49] Studies on diet therapy alone (e.g., references 34–37) are covered elsewhere in this volume. Several studies have evaluated GH treatment (0.024–0.050 mg/kg/day) as the primary active therapy[41,46] or as one of two active therapies in the trial.[4] Other studies have evaluated combination therapies with addition of GH + oral/intravenous Gln and no change in usual oral diet as the active therapy.[4,43,45] Several unblinded and double-blind trials have evaluated a form of modified oral diet + GH (0.10–0.14 mg/kg/day) + oral/intravenous Gln (30 g Gln/day).[4,38–39,42] GH was an attractive agent for SBS given its potent protein-anabolic effect,[3,10] in addition to trophic effects on bowel and ability to stimulate gut nutrient transport in animal models.[3,10] GLP-2 has potent and specific trophic effects on gut epithelial cells in various animal models, including SBS and inflammatory bowel disease, and in mucosal injury induced by chemotherapy.[67,128–130] Two recent unblinded studies have evaluated efficacy of either native GLP-2[47] or a GLP-2 analog[48] in SBS. The GLP-2 analog is synthesized with glycine substituted for alanine at position 2 to confer resistance to degradation by the enzyme dipeptidyl peptidase IV and thus prolong the half-life of this agent in the circulation.[67] However, as no agent or combination of therapies has as yet been rigorously evaluated, the true utility of all of these strategies remains controversial.[2,136]

In one of two small trials to date on Gln supplementation alone in human SBS (see the study in Reference 4, which incorporated a Gln treatment arm), Scolapio et al. performed a small, randomized, double-blind crossover study in 8 subjects with SBS.[44] The patients had a mean residual small bowel length of 102 cm (range 50–150 cm) and 6 had partial colon in continuity. All subjects were placed on a high-carbohydrate, low-fat diet for the 16 weeks of study (8 weeks during which 30 g/day [0.45 g/kg/day] of supplemental oral L-Gln powder was added to dietary liquids and 8 weeks in which polycose was given as the placebo).[44] Subjects were admitted to the hospital for 3-day efficacy studies at the end of each 8-week treatment period. Supplemental dietary Gln had no effect on duodenal villus height and crypt depth, gastric emptying, or intestinal fluid, xylose, and fat absorption in the 8 SBS patients.[44]

GH and GLP-2 are the only recombinant growth factors so far tested in human SBS, and the available data indicates efficacy of these agents to improve nutrient absorption.[3–4,38–39,42,45–46,47–48] The initial studies demonstrating the concept of "intestinal rehabilitation" in SBS patients previously dependent on PN were performed by Byrne and colleagues at Brigham and Women's Hospital in Boston in the mid-1990s.[38-39] Adults (N = 10) with chronic PN-dependent SBS were studied in the General Clinical Research Center (GCRC) during a 28-day inpatient program.[38] All subjects had full or partial residual colon in continuity, and mean jejunal-ileal length was estimated to be 37 cm (range 8–90 cm). The time on PN averaged 6 ± 1 years. Baseline studies were performed during the first 7 days, during which subjects received their usual oral diet and PN regimen, based on a preadmission 7-day dietary recall and review of nutrition support records.[38] All oral diets were prepared daily in the GCRC metabolic kitchen. During the 7-day baseline period, intestinal nutrient absorption of stool wet weight, calories, protein, fat, carbohydrate, water, and sodium was determined using classical GCRC methodology. Beginning on day 8, all 10 subjects were placed on an individualized oral diet, which was continued for 3 additional weeks until after the second nutrient absorption study during week 4. Two subjects received only the modified diet (diet control). The remaining 8 subjects received intravenous GH (0.14 mg/kg/day) + enteral/intravenous L-Gln (0.63 g/kg/day). The oral modified SBS diet was designed to provide 60% of total calories from primarily complex carbohydrate, 20% from fat and 20% from protein sources.[38] A soluble fiber supplement (apple pectin) was also added daily, the principle being to increase colonic production of short-chain fatty acids via bacterial fermentation.[27] Feedings were distributed as 6 meals/day and limited in simple sugars, oxalate, lactose, carbonated beverages, and water. Near-isotonic oral dehydration solutions (ORS) replaced most dietary liquids and were sipped throughout the day (2–3 L/day). The diet was adjusted daily based on individual food and liquid tolerance and symptoms, stool output pattern, urine output, serial blood chemistries, and other standard criteria via close monitoring by the investigators.[38] PN support was weaned as indicated by standard criteria. Absorption data from the first and fourth weeks were compared, with the patients serving as their own control. Compared to baseline absorption, the combination of modified diet + GH + Gln demonstrated markedly and significantly improved intestinal absorption of calories (from 60% to 74% of intake), protein (from 49% to 63%), carbohydrate (from 60% to 82%), water (from 46 to 65%), and sodium (from 49 to 70%); stool output also significantly decreased by 500 ml/day from baseline (all P<0.05).[38] Fat absorption did not change. No significant improvements in absorptive indices from baseline were observed in the 2 subjects treated with modified diet alone.[38] GH + Gln + diet therapy was well tolerated with the exception of mild peripheral arthralgias and edema that developed in some patients. The inpatient program outlined above was given in an unblinded manner to another group of subjects (N = 47).[39] The subjects were 25 men and 22 women dependent on PN for an average of 6 ± 1 years. Their average length of residual small bowel was 50 ± 7 cm (median + 35 cm) in those with all or partial colon (N = 43) and 102 ± 24 cm in the 4 subjects without residual colon. Attempts to wean the subjects from PN using a standardized algorithm were made after initiation of the diet/GH/Gln therapy in the GCRC setting. A total of 57% of these individuals were able to have PN discontinued over the 3 weeks of active treatment. The subjects were then maintained on the individualized diet modification and ORS with oral l-Gln (30 g/day) alone at discharge. After an average of one year, 40% of the subjects remained free of PN and an additional 40% of subjects had reduced requirements for PN, due to improved tolerance to oral diet and diminished diarrhea and malabsorption.[39] Although unblinded, these two reports demonstrated "proof of principle" in that an aggressive bowel rehabilitation program that utilizes dietary change as a key component is able to allow long-standing SBS patients formerly dependent on PN to have the need for this therapy be reduced or eliminated.

In contrast to these studies were the results of a small, double-blinded crossover study in 8 chronic SBS patients (7 with Crohn's disease) published by Scolapio et al. in 1997.[42] Unlike the studies by Byrne et al., 6 of these 8 subjects did not have a colon remnant in continuity and average length of residual small bowel was only 71 cm. During the active 21-day treatment phase, subjects consumed a high-carbohydrate, low-fat diet, but this was nonindividualized in that a set amount of calories and protein were given (1500 kcal/day and 1.0 g protein/kg/day); further subjects were not allowed to take their usual antidiarrhea medications during the study.[42] In addition to the diets, subjects received oral L-Gln (0.63 g/kg/day) mixed in dietary liquids + s.c. GH (0.14 mg/kg/day) during the active treatment phase. The control phase was an identical 21-day period in which placebo injections and polycose powder were administered. Subjects received the two treatments at home, except for 4-day balance periods in the hospital at the end of each phase. Results showed that during active treatment, absorption of sodium and potassium were modestly but significantly improved versus results during the control period, but group mean absorption of nitrogen and fat did not change.[42] Inspection of individual data, however, showed that 4 of 8 subjects improved absorption of nitrogen and fat, respectively, in some cases markedly. Thus, there were individuals with a generalized improved absorptive response in this protocol. Although duodenal crypt depth and villus height were unchanged by active treatment, gastric emptying and 2-hr ostomy output were significantly decreased.[42] Several subjects were reported to experience arthralgias, sleep disturbances, and peripheral edema while on active therapy. Thus, although this blinded study is often cited as refuting the unblinded pilot studies of Byrne et al., the results of Scolapio et al. can easily be interpreted as being positive. Further, differences in study design (oral diet, use of only oral L-Gln, antidiarrhea medication elimination, treatment in the outpatient setting) make strict comparisons between the studies difficult.

Another small, double-blinded, crossover trial in chronic SBS patients dependent on PN was published by Szkudlarek et al. in Denmark in 2000.[43] These investigators used s.c. GH (0.12 mg/kg/day) + supplemental oral (28 g/day) and IV (5. g/day) L-Gln and no specific dietary regimen was given for 28 days.[43] The placebo control consisted of saline injections and or L-alanine (30 g/day). Treatment was administered on an outpatient basis. Subjects underwent nutrient absorption and other studies at baseline, and 5 days after, the active or placebo treatments were terminated.[43] Four SBS subjects had a residual colon with a mean small bowel length of 108 cm, and 4 subjects did not have residual colon and mean residual small bowel length was 100 cm. Compared to baseline, no improvements were observed for active treatment in terms of absorption of energy, carbohydrate, fat, nitrogen, and electrolytes.[43] All subjects experienced peripheral edema and/or arthralgias, and some required diuretic and/or analgesic therapy.[43] Differences between this study and the Byrne and Scolapio studies include the lack of diet modification and the determination of nutrient absorption 5 days after active treatment ended, thus possibly obscuring an effect of GH + Gln that may have waned after active treatment was discontinued.

The same year the Scolapio study was published, Ellegard et al. published a double-blind, crossover study in 10 chronic adult SBS patients with mean jejunoileal length of 130 cm (range 90–170 cm).[41] Subjects were given either low-dose GH (0.024 mg/kg/day s.c.) or placebo for 8 weeks with a 12-week washout period and then another 8-week treatment phase. Improved body weight and lean body mass and loss of fat mass were demonstrated, but no change was noted in intestinal absorption of water, protein, or energy.[41] A recent study by Seguy et al, used a double-blind, randomized, crossover design in 12 chronic PN-dependent SBS patients with an average small bowel length of 48 cm (9 of 12 with residual colon).[46] Subjects were given an intermediate dose of recombinant GH (0.05 mg/kg/day s.c) for 21 days versus placebo injections for 21 days, separated by a one-week washout period.[46] A difference from previous studies was that the subjects received an unrestricted "hyperphagic" diet (> twofold basal metabolic rate and > 2.0 g protein/kg/day), but did follow basic SBS dietary principles. GH was well tolerated with no side effects and significantly improved lean body mass. GH treatment also significantly improved intestinal absorption of energy (+15%), nitrogen (+14%), and carbohydrate (+10%) versus placebo, and D-xylose absorption also significantly improved.[46] As in the other studies of GH therapy in SBS, plasma IGF-I concentration rose significantly; in addition, plasma Gln increased modestly with GH.[46] Of note, average oral food intake in this study was considerably higher than the studies of Byrne,[38] Szkudlarek,[43] and Scolapio,[42] in which oral diet represented 80%, 70%, and 48%, respectively, of the average intake of Seguy et al.[46] The authors concluded that one potential reason for the improved absorptive changes with low-dose GH was the increased amount of enteral nutrition, despite the lack of Gln supplementation. Further, these authors point out that large doses of L-Gln in SBS patients may themselves induce an osmotic diarrhea in some subjects.[46]

Although use of GH for SBS remains controversial, the Food & Drug Administration (FDA) approved a 4-week course of the same form of recombinant human GH for use in PN-dependent SBS in December 2003. The approval was based on a recently completed phase 3 double-blind randomized trial by the Harvard group of Drs. Byrne, Wilmore, and colleagues (Figure 13.3).[4] The design of the registration trial was based on the earlier pilot studies that suggested the efficacy of modified diet, Gln supplementation, and GH.[38–39] In the registration trial, 41 PN-dependent adult SBS subjects received either an individually modified diet supplemented with l-Gln (30 g/day) + s.c. placebo (control; N = 9), the modified diet (without Gln supplementation) + s.c. GH (0.1 mg/kg/day; N = 15) or the modified, Gln-supplemented diet + GH (N = 16), for a total of 4 weeks.[4] The treatments were started after two weeks of dietary stabilization period during which dietary intake was optimized using approaches outlined above.[38–39] The subjects were then randomized to one of the three treatment groups. After beginning the blinded study period, daily PN or intravenous (IV) fluid intake was modified using a standardized weaning algorithm. The primary endpoints were the change in total weekly PN and total intravenous fluid requirements over 4 weeks of active treatment. Results showed that diet + Gln (control) subjects exhibited an average 3.8 liter/week decrease in PN

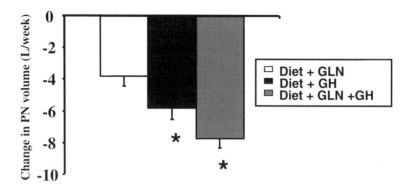

FIGURE 13.3 The decrease in parenteral nutrition (PN) requirments from baseline to week 4 of active treatment in a recent double-blind, randomized trial of diet modification with either glutamine (GLN) supplementation alone, growth hormone (GH) treatment alone, or GLN+GH in 41 adult-PN dependent SBS patients. * P < 0.05 vs. diet + GLN group. (Data adapted from Byrne, T.A., Lautz, D.B., Iyer, K.R., DiBaise, J.K., Gertner, J.M., Robinson, M.K., and Wilmore, D.W., Recombinant human growth hormone (rhGH) reduces parenteral nutrition (PN) in patients with short bowel syndrome: A prospective, randomized, double-blind, placebo-controlled study, *J. Parent. Enteral Nutr.*, 27, S17 (abstract), 2003.)

requirements, the diet + GH group had a 5.8 liter/week decrease (P = 0.043 vs. controls), and the diet + Gln + GH group exhibited a 7.7 liter/week decrease in PN needs (P = 0.001 vs. controls; NS vs. diet + GH) (Figure 13.3).

The PN calorie requirements decreased by 2661 ± 311/week in the controls, but fell to a greater extent in both GH-treated groups (-4323 ± 329 kcal/week with diet + GH and –5745 ± 369 kcal/week with diet + Gln + GH, respectively; each P < 0.05 vs. controls).[4] The days of PN infusion/week also decreased significantly in the GH-treated groups (control –2.0 ± 0.2, diet + GH –3.0 ± 0.3 and diet + Gln + GH -4.2 ± 0.2 L/week, respectively; P < 0.05 each GH group vs. controls). Some subjects in the two GH groups developed peripheral edema and arthralgias (expected adverse events), but these resolved after dose reduction; no subject dropped out of the study. Serious adverse events (SAEs) were similar between groups and were deemed unrelated to the study drug.[4] Of interest, two recent unblinded studies from two independent Chinese groups also suggest that the combination of GH + Gln improved gut nutrient absorption and decreased PN needs in patients studied in the acute phase after massive small bowel resection.[45,137]

Two studies on administration of either native GLP-2[47] or the GLP-2 analog outlined above[48] have now been published. In the first study, Jeppesen et al. gave native GLP-2 400 μg/day s.c. twice daily for 35 days to SBS patients with chronic jejunostomies and no colonic remnant.[47] This group was chosen because these authors previously demonstrated extremely low circulating levels of GLP-2 in these individuals, who lacked distal ileum and colon, the major sites of GLP-2 production in mucosal L-cells.[49] Four of the 8 subjects had required chronic PN for 4 to 14 years, with residual jejunal/ileal length averaging 82 cm; the other 4 subjects were not receiving PN and residual jejunal/ileal length averaged 106 cm. Crohn's disease was the cause of SBS in 6 of the 8 subjects. Subjects were treated at home and the oral diet was unrestricted.[47] For 72-hr nutrient absorption, body composition, gastric emptying, and distal jejunal/ileal mucosal biopsy studies, the subjects were admitted to the hospital for 5 days at baseline and again at the end of the 35-day treatment phase for absorption and other tests. Treatment with native GLP-2 significantly improved absorption of stool wet weight (from 25% to 36%), energy (from 50% to 53%), and nitrogen (from 47% to 52%).[47] Further, GLP-2 was well tolerated and increased body weight was manifested by a significant increase in lean body mass during the treatment phase, which appeared to be accounted for by the increase in energy and nitrogen absorption. Finally, although no significant changes in gut mucosal morphology occurred (despite trends toward an increase in villus height and crypt depth), gastric emptying in response to a standardized meal was significantly delayed, a known effect of GLP-2.[47] A multicenter, dose-ranging pilot study using the GLP-2 analog in PN-dependent SBS patients with jejunostomies was recently published in abstract form (48). Results in 10 subjects studied showed a significant increase in stool wet-weight absorption and a significant decrease in stool volume and energy with this agent, which was well tolerated by the patients.[48] Further, more definitive studies on the use of this agent in PN-dependent SBS are in progress.

Since the previous studies of trophic factors in SBS have been either unblinded,[38–39,45,47–48,137] used multiple therapies,[38–39,42–43,45,137] and/or had small sample sizes,[38–39,41–43,45,47–48] and employed, in some cases, uncertain dietary control,[41-43,45,137] the individual contributions of diet, GH, Gln, and GLP-2 in the therapy in human SBS still remain unclear. Moreover, the potential mechanisms of action of these agents are unknown. Thus, data are critically needed on the longer-term safety (GH and GLP-2) and efficacy (GH, GLP-2, and Gln) combined with dietary modification in subjects with severe, PN-dependent SBS. In light of the limited clinical data to date, and the suggestion of benefit from some studies, additional randomized, blinded, and controlled trials of Gln, GH, and GLP-2 alone, GH + Gln, GLP-2 + Gln, and GH + GLP-2, in the context of appropriate dietary modification, seem warranted. Data are also needed on gut mucosal mechanisms of action and to define optimal patient selection criteria (e.g., nature of residual bowel, age, underlying illnesses), timing and duration of therapy, and the specific dietary regimens most useful for individual SBS patients.

Underlying nutritional status, adherence to SBS dietary guidelines (e.g., small frequent feedings, avoidance of simple sugars, decreased intake of fat and specific food items that worsen diarrhea, use of oral rehydration solutions), and appropriate use antidiarrhea medication regimens likely has a major impact on the intestinal responses to Gln (and growth factor) treatment.[2,10] Thus, to define the true efficacy of these therapies, future clinical studies in SBS will need to carefully control for these variables. Larger, controlled clinical trials and more uniform patient selection and treatments are necessary to define the efficacy of combination or single Gln and growth factor therapy in SBS. Nonetheless, with the FDA approval of recombinant GH for use in SBS, it will be imperative that patient management using an intestinal rehabilitation team of experienced specialists be involved with use of this potent agent, that has common, but manageable side effects such as arthralgias, peripheral edema, and occasional hyperglycemia. Administration of promising therapies such as GH, GLP-2, Gln, and/or modified diet are likely to become standard-of-care in the management of patients with severe SBS.

REFERENCES

1. Vanderhoof, J.A. and Langnas, A.N., Short-bowel syndrome in children and adults, *Gastroenterology*, 113, 1767, 1997.
2. Buchman, A.L., Scolapio, J., and Fryer, J., AGA technical review on short bowel syndrome and intestinal transplantation, *Gastroenterology*, 124, 1111, 2003.
3. Byrne, T.A., Cox, S., Karimbakas, M., Veglia, L.M., Bennett, H.M., Lautz, D.B., and Wilmore D.W., Bowel rehabilitation: an alternative to long-term parenteral nutrition and intestinal transplantation for some patients with short bowel syndrome, *Trans. Proc.*, 34, 887, 2002.
4. Byrne, T.A., Lautz, D.B., Iyer, K.R., DiBaise, J.K., Gertner, J.M., Robinson, M.K., and Wilmore, D.W., Recombinant human growth hormone (rhGH) reduces parenteral nutrition (PN) in patients with short bowel syndrome: A prospective, randomized, double-blind, placebo-controlled study, *J. Parent. Enteral Nutr.*, 27, S17 (abstract), 2003.
5. Gouttebel, M.C., Aubert, B.S., Colette, C., Astre, C., Monnier, L.H., and Joyeux, H., Intestinal adaptation in patients with short bowel syndrome: Measurement by calcium absorption, *Dig. Dis. Sci.*, 34, 709, 1989.
6. Woolf, G.M., Miller, C., Kurian, R., and Jeejeebhoy, K.N., Nutritional absorption in short bowel syndrome: Evaluation of fluid, calorie, and divalent cation requirements, *Dig. Dis. Sci.*, 32, 8, 1987.
7. Howard, L., Ament. M., Fleming. C.R., Shike, M., and Steiger, E., Current use and clinical outcome of home parenteral and enteral nutrition therapies in the United States, *Gastroenterology*, 109, 355, 1995.
8. Jeppesen, P.B., Langholz, E., and Mortensen, P.B., Quality of life in patients receiving home parenteral nutrition, *Gut*, 44, 844, 1999.
9. Jeppesen, P.B. and Mortensen, P.B., Intestinal failure defined by measurements of intestinal energy and wet weight absorption, *Gut*, 46, 701, 2000.
10. Ziegler, T.R., Estívariz, C.F., Jonas, C.R., Gu, L.H., Jones, D.P., and Leader, L.M., Interactions between nutrients and peptide growth factors in intestinal growth, repair and function, *J. Parenter. Enteral Nutr.*, 23, S174, 1999.
11. Gouttebel, M.C., Saint-Aubert, B., Astre, C., and Joyeux, H., Total parenteral nutrition needs in different types of short bowel syndrome, *Dig. Dis. Sci.*, 31, 718, 1986.
12. Fukushima, T. and Ziegler, T.R., Liver Disease and Parenteral Nutrition. In Zakim, D.M., Boyer, T.D., *Hepatology: A Textbook of Liver Disease*, 4th ed., W.B. Saunders Co., Philadelphia, 1677, 2003.
13. Howard, L. and Ashley, C., Management of complications in patients receiving home parenteral nutrition, *Gastroenterology*, 124, 1651, 2003.
14. O'Keefe, S.J., Burnes, J.U., and Thompson, R.L., Recurrent sepsis in home parenteral nutrition patients: an analysis of risk factors, *J. Parent. Enteral Nutr.*, 18, 256, 1994.
15. Sax, H.C., The future for the patient with severe short gut syndrome, *Nutrition*, 16(7–8), 618, 2000.

16. Carbonnel, F., Cosnes, J., Chevret, S., Beaugerie, L., Ngo, Y., Malafosse, M., Parc, R., Le Quintrec, Y., and Gendre, J.P., The role of anatomic factors in nutritional autonomy after extensive small bowel resection, *J. Parenter. Enternal. Nutr.*, 20, 280, 1996.

17. Jeppesen, P.B. and Mortensen, P.B., Significance of a preserved colon for parenteral energy requirements in patients receiving home parenteral nutrition, *Scand. J. Gastroenterol.*, 33, 1175, 1998.

18. Messing, B., Crenn, P., Beau, P., Boutron-Ruault, M.C., Rambaud, J.C., and Matuchansky, C., Long-term survival and parenteral nutrition dependence in adult patients with the short bowel syndrome, *Gastroenterology*, 117, 1043, 1999.

19. Williamson, R.C.N., Intestinal adaptation I and II. *N. Engl. J. Med.*, 298, 1393, 1444, 1978.

20. Weser, E. and Hernandez, M.H., Studies of small bowel adaptation after intestinal resection in the rat, *Gastroenterology*, 60, 69, 1971.

21. Tang, Y., Swartz-Basile, D.A., Swietlicki, E.A., Yi, L., Rubin, D.C., and Levin, M.S., Bax is required for resection-induced changes in apoptosis, proliferation, and members of the extrinsic cell death pathways, *Gastroenterology*, 126, 220, 2004.

22. Iannoli, P., Miller, J.H., Ryan, C.K., Gu, L.H., Ziegler, T.R., and Sax, H.C., Human growth hormone induces system B transport in short bowel syndrome, *J. Surg. Res.*, 69, 150, 1997.

23. Musch, M.W., Bookstein, C., Rocha, F., Lucioni, A., Ren, H., Daniel, J., Xie, Y., McSwine, R.L., Rao, M.C., Alverdy, J., and Chang, E.B., Region-specific adaptation of apical Na/H exchangers after extensive proximal small bowel resection, *Am. J. Physiol.*, 283, G975, 2002.

24. OíBrien, D.P., Nelson, L.A., Huang, F.S., and Warner, B.W., Intestinal adaptation: structure, function, and regulation, *Sem. Pediatr. Surg.*, 10, 56, 2001.

25. Taylor, R.G., Verity, K., and Fuller, P.J., Ileal glucagon gene expression: ontogeny and response to massive small bowel resection, *Gastroenterology*, 99, 724, 1990.

26. Ziegler, T.R., Mantell, M.P., Chow, J.C., Rombeau, J.L., and Smith, R.J., Gut adaptation and the insulin-like growth factor system: regulation by glutamine and insulin-like growth factor-I administration, *Am. J. Physiol.*, 271, G866, 1996.

27. Ziegler, T.R., Evans, M.E., Fernandez-Estivariz, C., and Jones, D.P., Trophic and cytoprotective nutrition for intestinal adaptation, mucosal repair and barrier function, *Annu. Rev. Nutr.*, 23, 229, 2003.

28. Appleton, G.V., Wheeler, E.E., Al-Mufti, R., Challacombe, D.N., and Williamson, R.C., Rectal hyperplasia after jejunoileal bypass for morbid obesity, *Gut* 29, 1544, 1988.

29. Barry, R.E., Barsch, J., Bray, G.A., Sperling, M.A., Morin, R.J., and Benfield, J., Intestinal adaptation after jejunoileal bypass in man, *Am. J. Clin. Nutr.*, 30, 32, 1977.

30. Dowling, R.H. and Booth, C.C., Functional compensation after small-bowel resection in man. Demonstration by direct measurement, *Lancet*, 2, 146, 1966.

31. O'Keefe, S.J., Haymond, M.W., Bennet, W.M., Oswald, B., Nelson, D.K., and Shorter, R.G., Long-acting somatostatin analogue therapy and protein metabolism in patients with jejunostomies, *Gastroenterology*, 107, 379, 1994.

32. Porus, R.L., Epithelial hyperplasia following massive small bowel resection in man, *Gastroenterology*, 48, 753, 1965.

33. Ziegler, T.R., Estivariz, C.F., Gu, L.H., Wallace, T.M., Díaz, E.E., Pascal, R.R., Bazargan, N., Galloway, J.R., Wilcox, J.N., and Leader, L.M., Distribution of H+/peptide transporter PepT1 in human intestine: up-regulated expression in the colonic mucosa of patients with short bowel syndrome, *Am. J. Clin. Nutr.*, 75, 922, 2002.

34. Beaugerie, L., Cosnes, J., Verwaerde, F., Dupas, H., Lamy, P., Gendre, J.P., and Le Quintrec, Y., Isotonic high-sodium oral rehydration solution for increasing sodium absorption in patients with short-bowel syndrome, *Am. J. Clin. Nutr.*, 53, 769, 1991.

35. Levy, E., Frileux, P., Sandrucci, S., Ollivier, J.M., Masini, J.P., Cosnes, J., Hannoun, L., and Parc, R., Continuous enteral nutrition during the early adaptive stage of the short bowel syndrome, *Br. J. Surg.*, 75, 549, 1988.

36. Messing, B., Pigot, F., Rongier, M., Morin, M.C., Ndeindoum, U., and Rambaud, J.C., Intestinal absorption of free oral hyperalimentation in the very short bowel syndrome, *Gastroenterology*, 100, 1502, 1991.

37. Woolf, G.M., Miller, C., Kurian, R., and Jeejeebhoy, K.N., Diet for patients with a short bowel: high fat or high carbohydrate? *Gastroenterology*, 84, 823, 1983.

38. Byrne, T.A., Morrissey, T.B., Nattakom, T.V., Ziegler, T.R., and Wilmore, D.W., Growth hormone, glutamine, and a modified diet enhance nutrient absorption in patients with severe short bowel syndrome, *J. Parenter. Enteral Nutr.*, 19, 296, 1995.

39. Byrne, T.A., Persinger, R.L., Young, L.S., Ziegler, T.R., and Wilmore, D.W., A new treatment for patients with short-bowel syndrome. Growth hormone, glutamine, and a modified diet, *Annu. Surg.*, 222, 243, 1995.

40. Wilmore, D.W., Lacey, J.M., Soultanakis, R.P., Bosch, R.L., and Byrne, T.A., Factors predicting a successful outcome after pharmacologic bowel compensation, *Annu. Surg.*, 226, 288, 1997.

41. Ellegard, L., Bosaeus, I., Nordgren, S., and Bengtsson, B.A., Low-dose recombinant human growth hormone increases body weight and lean body mass in patients with short bowel syndrome, *Annu. Surg.*, 225, 88, 1997.

42. Scolapio, J.S., Camilleri, M., Fleming, C.R., Oenning, L.V., Burton, D.D., Sebo, T.J., Batts, K.P., and Kelly, D.G., Effect of growth hormone, glutamine, and diet on adaptation in short-bowel syndrome: a randomized, controlled study, *Gastroenterology*, 113, 1074, 1997.

43. Szkudlarek, J., Jeppesen, P.B., and Mortensen, P.B., Effect of high dose growth hormone with glutamine and no change in diet on intestinal absorption in short bowel patients: a randomised, double blind, crossover, placebo controlled study, *Gut*, 47, 199, 2000.

44. Scolapio, J.S., McGreevy, K., Tennyson, G.S., and Burnett, O.L., Effect of glutamine in short-bowel syndrome, *Clin. Nutr.*, 20, 319, 2001.

45. Wu, G.H., Wu, Z.H., and Wu, Z.G., Effects of bowel rehabilitation and combined trophic therapy on intestinal adaptation in short bowel patients, *World J. Gastroenterology*, 9, 2601, 2003.

46. Seguy, D., Vahedi, K., Kapel, N., Souberbielle, J.C., and Messing, B., Low-dose growth hormone in adult home parenteral nutrition-dependent short bowel syndrome patients, a positive study, *Gastroenterology*, 124, 293, 2003.

47. Jeppesen, P.B., Hartmann, B., Thulesen, J., Graff, J., Lohmann, J., Hansen, B.S., Tofteng, F., Poulsen, S.S., Madsen, J.L., Holst, J.J., and Mortensen, P.B., Glucagon-like peptide 2 improves nutrient absorption and nutritional status in short-bowel patients with no colon, *Gastroenterology*, 120, 806, 2001.

48. Jeppesen, P.B., Blosch, C.M., Lopansri, J.B., Sanguinetti, E.L., Buchman, A.L., Scolapio, J.L., Ziegler, T.R., Howard, L., and Mortensen, P.B., ALX-0600, a dipeptidyl peptidase-IV resistant glucagon-like peptide-2 (GLP-2) analog, improves intestinal function in short bowel syndrome (SBS) patients with a jejunostomy, *Gastroenterology*, 122 (suppl.), A191 (abstr.), 2002.

49. Jeppesen, P.B., Mortensen, P.B., Enhancing bowel adaptation in short bowel syndrome, *Curr. Gastroenterol. Rep.*, 4, 338, 2002.

50. Wilmore, D.W., Indications for specific therapy in the rehabilitation of patients with the short-bowel syndrome, *Best Pract. Res. Clin. Gastroenterol.*, 17, 895, 2003.

51. Levine, G.M., Deren, J.J., Steiger, E., and Zinno, R., Role of oral intake in maintenance of gut mass and disaccharide activity, *Gastroenterology*, 67, 975, 1974.

52. Brown, H.O., Levine, M.L., and Lipkin, M., Inhibition of intestinal epithelial cell renewal and migration induced by starvation, *Am. J. Physiol.*, 205, 868, 1963.

53. Swartz-Basile, D.A., Wang, L., Tang, Y., Pitt, H.A., Rubin, D.C., and Levin, M.S., Vitamin A deficiency inhibits intestinal adaptation by modulating apoptosis, proliferation, and enterocyte migration, Am. J. Physiol. Gastrointest. Liver Physiol., 285, G424, 2003.

54. Aw, T.Y., Biliary glutathione promotes the mucosal metabolism of luminal peroxidized lipids by rat small intestine *in vivo*, *J. Clin. Invest.*, 94, 1218, 1994.

55. Lash, L.H., Hagen, T.M., and Jones, D.P., Exogenous glutathione protects intestinal epithelial cells from oxidative injury, *Proc. Natl. Acad. Sci.*, 83, 4641, 1986.

56. Pironi, L., Paganelli, G.M., Miglioli, M., Biasco, G., Santucci, R., Ruggeri, E., DiFebo, G., and Barbara, L., Morphologic and cytoproliferative patterns of duodenal mucosa in two patients after long-term total parenteral nutrition: Changes with oral refeeding and relation to intestinal resection, *J. Parent. Enteral Nutr.*, 18, 351, 1994.

57. Buchan, A.M.J., Pederson, R.A., Koop, I., Gourlay, R.H., and Cleator, I.G.M., Morphological and functional alterations to a sub-group of regulatory peptides in human pancreas and intestine after jejuno-ileal bypass, *Int. J. Obes. Related Metabolic Disorders*, 17, 109, 1993.

58. Owen, D.A., Montessori, G.A., and Dykstra, R.P.J., Jejunoileal bypass and extreme adaptive mucosal hyperplasia, *Histopathology*, 20, 450, 1992.

59. Goodlad, R.A., Ghatei, M.A., Domin, J., Bloom, S.R., Gregory, H., and Wright, N.A., Plasma enteroglucagon, peptide YY and gastrin in rats deprived of luminal nutrition, and after urogastrone-EGF administration. A proliferative role for PYY in the intestinal epithelium? *Experientia*, 45, 168, 1989.

60. Ziegler, T.R., Almahfouz, A., Pedrini, M.T., Smith, R.J., A comparison of rat small intestinal insulin and IGF-I receptors during fasting and refeeding, *Endocrinology*, 136, 5148, 1995.

61. Ziegler, T.R., Mantell, M.P., Rombeau, J.L., Smith, R.J., Intestinal adaptation after extensive small bowel resection: Differential changes in growth and IGF-I system mRNAs in jejunum and ileum, *Endocrinology*, 139, 3119, 1998.

62. Han, V.K., D'Ercole, A.J., and Lund, P.K., Cellular localization of somatomedin (insulin-like growth factor) messenger RNA in the human fetus, *Science*, 236, 193, 1987.

63. Han, V.K.M., Lund, P.K., Lee, D.C., and D'Ercole, A.J., Expression of somatomedin/insulin-like growth factor messenger RNAs in the human fetus: Identification, characterization and tissue distribution, *J. Clin. Endocrinol. Metab.*, 66, 422, 1988.

64. Delhanty, P.J.D., Hill, D.J., Shimasaki, S., Han, V.K.M., Insulin-like growth factor binding protein -4, -5 and -6 mRNAs in the human fetus: localization to sites of growth and differentiation? *Growth Regulation*, 3, 8, 1993.

65. Hill, D.J. and Clemmons, D.R., Similar distribution of insulin-like growth factor binding proteins-1, -2, -3 in human fetal tissues, *Growth Factors*, 6, 315, 1992.

66. Delehaye-Zervas, M-C, Mertani, H., Martini, J-F, Nihoul-Fekete, C., Morel, G., and Postel-Vinay, M-C, Expression of the growth hormone receptor gene in human digestive tissues, *J. Clin. Endocrinol. Metab.*, 78, 1473, 1994.

67. Drucker, D.J., Biological actions and therapeutic potential of the glucagon-like peptides, *Gastroenterology*, 122, 531, 2002.

68. Estívariz C.F., Gu, L.H., Scully, S., Eli, E., Jonas, C.R., Farrell, C.L., and Ziegler, T.R., Regulation of keratinocyte growth factor (KGF) and KGF receptor mRNAs by nutrient intake and KGF administration in rat intestine, *Dig. Dis. Sci.*, 45, 736, 2000.

69. Avissar, N.E., Ziegler, T.R., Wang, H.T., Gu, L.H., Miller, J.H., Iannoli, P., Leibach, F.H., Ganapathy, V., and Sax, H.C., Growth factor regulation of rabbit sodium-dependent neutral amino acid transporter ATB^0 and oligopeptide transporter 1 mRNA expression after enterectomy, *J. Parent. Enteral Nutr.*, 25, 65, 2001.

70. Hines, O.J., Bilchik, A.J., Zinner, M.J., Skotzko, M.J., Moser, A.J., McFadden, D.W., and Ashley, S.W., Adaptation of the Na^+/glucose cotransporter following intestinal resection, *J. Surg. Res.*, 57, 22, 1994.

71. Thomson, A.B.R. and Wild, G., Adaptation of intestinal nutrient transport in health and disease, part II, *Dig. Dis. Sci.*, 42, 470, 1997.

72. Diamond, J.M. and Karasov, W.H., Adaptive regulation of intestinal nutrient transporters, *Proc. Natl. Acad. Sci. USA*, 84, 2242, 1987.

73. Sarac, T.P., Seydel, A.S., Ryan, C.K., Bessey, P.Q., Miller, J.H., Souba, W.W., and Sax, H.C., Sequential alterations in gut mucosal amino acid and glucose transport after 70% small bowel resection, *Surgery*, 120, 503, 1996.

74. Althausen, T.L., Doig, R.K., Uyeyama, K., and Weiden, S., Digestion and absorption after massive resection of the small intestine. II. Recovery of the absorptive function as shown by intestinal absorption tests in two patients and a consideration of compensatory mechanisms, *Gastroenterology*, 16, 127, 1950.

75. Weinstein, L.D., Shoemaker, C.P., Hersh, T., and Milliken, W.T., Enhanced intestinal absorption after small bowel resection in man, *Arch. Surg.*, 99, 560, 1969.

76. Nordgaard, I., Hansen, B.S., and Mortensen, P.B., Colon as a digestive organ in patients with short bowel, *Lancet*, 343, 373, 1994.

77. Adibi, S.A., Regulation of expression of the intestinal oligopeptide transporter (Pept-1) in health and disease, *Am. J. Physiol.*, 285, G779, 2003.

78. Fei, Y.J., Kanai, Y., Nussberger, S., Ganapathy, V., Leibach, F.H., Romero, M.F., Singh, S.K., Boron, W.F., and Hediger, M.A., Expression cloning of a mammalian proton-coupled oligopeptide transporter, *Nature*, 368, 563, 1994.

79. Liang, R., Fei, Y-J, Prasad, P.D., Ramamoorthy, S., Han, H., Yang-Feng, T.L., Hediger, M.A., Ganapathy, V., and Leibach, F.H., Human intestinal H^+/peptide cotransporter. Cloning, functional expression, and chromosomal localization, *J. Biol. Chem.*, 270, 6456, 1995.

80. Binder, H.J., Amino acid absorption in the mammalian colon, *Biochim. Biophys. Acta.*, 219, 503, 1970.

81. Robinson, J.W.L., Luisier, A.L., and Mirkovitch, V., Transport of amino acids and sugars by the dog colonic mucosa, *Pflugers Arch.*, 345, 317, 1973.

82. Rhoads, J.E., Stengel, A., Riegel, C., Cajori, F.A., and Frazier, W.D., The absorption of protein split products from chronic isolated colon loops, *Am. J. Physiol.*, 125, 707, 1939.

83. Gaudichon, C., Bos, C., Morens, C., Petzke, K.J., Mariotti, F., Everwand, J., Benamouzig, R., Dare, S., Tome, D., and Metges, C.C., Ileal losses of nitrogen and amino acids in humans and their importance to the assessment of amino acid requirements, *Gastroenterology*, 123, 50, 2002.

84. Sloan, J.L. and Mager, S., Cloning and functional expression of a human Na(+) and Cl(-)-dependent neutral and cationic amino acid transporter B(0+), *J. Biol. Chem.*, 274, 23740, 1999.

85. Rajan, D.P., Huang, W., Kekuda, R., George, R.L., Wang, J., Conway, S.J., Devoe, L.D., Leibach, F.H., Prasad, P.D., and Ganapathy, V., Differential influence of the 4F2 heavy chain and the protein related to $b^{0,+}$ amino acid transport on substrate affinity of the heteromeric $b^{0,+}$ amino acid transporter, *J. Biol. Chem.*, 275, 14331, 2000.

86. Zibrik, L., Dyer, J., Ellis, T., and Shirazi-Beechey, S.P., Amino acid transport in human colon in short bowel syndrome, *Gastroenterology*, 124, A31, 2003 (abstr.).

87. Kripke, S.A., De Paula, J.A., Berman, J.M., Fox, A.D., Rombeau, J.L., and Settle, R.G., Experimental short-bowel syndrome: effect of an elemental diet supplemented with short-chain triglycerides, *Am. J. Clin.. Nutr.*, 53, 954, 1991.

88. Swartz-Basile, D.A., Wang, L., Tang, Y., Pitt, H.A., Rubin, D.C., and Levin, M.S., Vitamin A deficiency inhibits intestinal adaptation by modulating apoptosis, proliferation, and enterocyte migration, *Am. J. Physiol. Gastrointest. Liver Physiol.*, 285, G424, 2003.

89. Park, J.H., Grandjean, C.J., Hart, M.H., Baylor, J.M., and Vanderhoof, J.A., Effects of dietary linoleic acid on mucosal adaptation after small bowel resection, *Digestion*, 44, 57, 1989.

90. Tappenden, K.A., Thomson, A.B., Wild, G.E., and McBurney, M.I., Short-chain fatty acid-supplemented total parenteral nutrition enhances functional adaptation to intestinal resection in rats, *Gastroenterology*, 112, 792, 1997.

91. Windmueller, H.G., Glutamine utilization by the small intestine, *Adv. Enzymol.*, 53, 210, 1982.

92. Souba, W.W., Glutamine: A key substrate for the splanchnic bed, *Annu. Rev. Nutr.*, 11, 285, 1991.

93. Alverdy, J.C., Effects of glutamine-supplemented diets on immunology of the gut, *J. Parent. Enteral Nutr.*, 14, 109S, 1990.

94. Klimberg, V.S., Salloum, R., Kasper, M., Plumley, D.A., Dolson, D.J., Hautamaki, R.D., Mendenhall, W.R., Bova, F.C., Bland, K.I., and Copeland, E.M., 3d Oral glutamine accelerates healing of the small intestine and improves outcome following whole abdominal radiation, *Arch. Surg.*, 125, 1040, 1990.

95. Fujita, T. and Sakurai, K., Efficacy of glutamine-enriched enteral nutrition in an experimental model of mucosal ulcerative colitis, *Br. J. Surg.*, 82, 749, 1995.

96. Tamada, H., Nezu, R., Imamura, I., Matsuo, Y., Takagi, Y., Kamata, S., and Okada, A., The dipeptide alanyl-glutamine prevents intestinal mucosal atrophy in parenterally fed rats, *J. Parenter. Enteral Nutr.*, 16, 110, 1992.

97. Bai, M.X., Jiang, Z.M., Liu, Y.W. Wang, W.T., and Li. D.M., Effects of alanyl-glutamine on gut barrier function, *Nutrition*, 12, 793, 1996.

98. Dugan, M.E. and McBurney, M.I., Luminal glutamine perfusion alters endotoxin-related changes in ileal permeability of the piglet, *J. Parent. Enteral Nutr.*, 19, 83, 1995.

99. Michail, S., Mohammadpour, H., Park, J.H., and Vanderhoof, J.A., Effect of glutamine-supplemented elemental diet on mucosal adaptation following bowel resection in rats, *J. Ped. Gastroenterol. Nutr.*, 21, 394, 1995.

100. Vanderhoof, J.A., Kollman, K.A., Griffin, S., and Adrian, T.E., Growth hormone and glutamine do not stimulate intestinal adaptation following massive small bowel resection in the rat, *J. Ped. Gastroenterol. Nutr.*, 25, 327, 1997.

101. Wiren, M.E., Permert, J., Skullman, S.P., Wang, F., and Larsson, J., No differences in mucosal adaptive growth one week after intestinal resection in rats given enteral glutamine supplementation or deprived of glutamine, *Eur. J. Surg.*, 162, 489, 1996.

102. Yang, H., Larsson, J., Permert, J., Braaf, Y., and Wiren, M., No effect of bolus glutamine supplementation on the postresectional adaptation of small bowel mucosa in rats receiving chow ad libitum, *Dig. Surg.*, 17, 256, 2000.

103. Satoh, J., Tsujikawa, T., Fujiyama, Y., and Banba, T., Enteral alanyl-glutamine supplement promotes intestinal adaptation in rats, *Int. J. Mol. Med.*, 12, 615, 2003.

104. Ziegler, T.R., Bazargan, N., Leader, L.M., and Martindale, R.G., Glutamine and the gastrointestinal tract, *Curr. Opin. Clin. Nutr. Metabol. Care*, 3, 355, 2000.

105. Evans, M.E., Jones, D.P., Ziegler, T.R., Glutamine prevents cytokine-induced apoptosis in human colonic epitheilial cells, *J. Nutr.*, 133, 3065, 2003.

106. Zhou, X., Li, Y.X., Li, N., and Li, J.S., Glutamine enhances the gut-trophic effect of growth hormone in rat after massive small bowel resection, *J. Surg. Res.*, 99, 47, 2001.

107. Gu, Y. and Wu, Z., The anabolic effects of recombinant human growth hormone and glutamine on parenterally fed, short bowel rats, *World J. Gastroenterol.*, 8, 752, 2002.

108. Scheppach, W., Loges, C., Bartram, P., Christl, S.U., and Richter, F., Effect of free glutamine and alanyl-glutamine dipeptide on mucosal proliferation of the human ileum and colon, *Gastroenterology*, 107, 434, 1994.

109. Van der Hulst, R.R.W., van Kreel, B.K., von Meyenfeldt, M.F., Brummer, R.J., Arends, J.W., and Souters, P., Glutamine and the preservation of gut integrity, *Lancet*, 341, 1363, 1993.

110. Ziegler, T.R., Fernandez-Estivariz, C., Griffith, D.P., Szezycki, E.E., Bazargan, N., Luo, M., Daignault, N.M., Dave, N., Bergman, G.F., McNally, A.T., Battey, C.H., Furr, C.E., Gu, L.H., Jonas, C.R., Cotsonis, G.A., Jones, D.P., and Galloway, J.R., Parenteral nutrition supplemented with alanyl-glutamine dipeptide decreases infectious morbidity and improves organ function in critically ill post-operative patients: Results of a double-blind, randomized, controlled pilot study, *J. Parent. Enteral Nutr.*, 28, S11, 2004 (abstr.).

111. Shulman, D.I., Hu, C.S., and Duckett, G., Effects of short-term growth hormone therapy in rats undergoing 75% small intestinal resection, *J. Pediatr. Gastroenterol. Nutr.*, 14, 3, 1992.

112. Gomez de Segura, I.A., Aguilera, M.J., Codesal, J., Codoceo, R., and De-Miguel, E., Comparative effects of growth hormone in large and small bowel resection in the rat, *J. Surg. Res.*, 62, 5, 1996.

113. Iannoli, P., Miller, J.H., Ryan, C.K., Gu, L.H., Ziegler, T.R., and Sax, H.C., Epidermal growth factor and human growth hormone accelerate adaptation after massive enterectomy in an additive, nutrient-dependent, and site-specific fashion, *Surgery*, 122, 721, 1997.

114. Benhamou, P.H., Canarelli, J.P., Leroy, C. et al., Stimulation by recombinant human growth hormone of growth and development of remaining bowel after subtotal ileojejunectomy in rats, *J. Pediatr. Gastroenterol. Nutr.*, 18, 452, 1994.

115. Benhamou, P.H., Canarelli, J.P., Richard, S. et al., Human recombinant growth hormone increases small bowel lengthening after massive small bowel resection in piglets, *J. Pediatr. Surg.*, 32, 1336, 1997.

116. Peterson, C.A., Ney, D.M., Hinton, P.S., and Carey, H.V., Beneficial effects of insulin-like growth factor I on epithelial structure and function in parenterally fed rat jejunum, *Gastroenterology*, 111, 1501, 1996.

117. Mantell, M.P., Ziegler, T.R., Roth, B.A., Zhang, W., Adamson, W.T., Bain, A., Chow, J.C., Smith, R.J., and Rombeau, J.L., Resection-induced colonic adaptation is augmented by IGF-I and associated with upregulation of colonic IGF-I mRNA, *Am. J. Physiol.*, 269, G974, 1995.

118. Lemmey, A.B., Martin, A.A., Read, L.C., Tomas, F.M., Owens, P.C., and Ballard, F.J., IGF-I and the truncated analogue des-(1-3)IGF I enhance growth in rats after gut resection, *Am. J. Physiol.*, 260, E213, 1991.

119. Vanderhoof, J.A., McCusker, R.H., Clark, R., Mohammadpour, H., Blackwood, D.J., Harty, R.F., and Park, J.H.Y., Truncated and native insulinlike growth factor I enhance mucosal adaptation after jejunoileal resection, *Gastroenterology*, 102, 1949, 1992.

120. Lukish, J., Schwartz, M.Z., Rushin, J.M., and Riordan, G.P., A comparison of the effect of growth factors on intestinal function and structure in short bowel syndrome, *J. Pediatr. Surg.*, 32, 1652, 1997.

121. Helmrath, M.A., Falcone, R.A. Jr. and Warner, B.W., Epidermal growth factor augments adaptation following small bowel resection: optimal dosage, route, and timing of administration, *J. Surg. Res.*, 77, 11, 1998.

122. Graham, J., Martin, G., Meddings, J.B., and Sigalet, D.L., Epidermal growth factor improves nutritional outcome in a rat model of short bowel syndrome, *J. Pediatr. Surg.*, 37, 765, 2002.

123. Johnson, W.F., DiPalma, C.R., Ziegler, T.R. et al., Keratinocyte growth factor enhances early gut adaptation in a rat model of short bowel syndrome, *Veter. Surg.*, 29, 17, 2000.

124. Yang, H., Wildhaber, B.E., and Teitelbaum, D.H., Keratinocyte growth factor improves epithelial function after massive small bowel resection, *J. Parenter. Enteral Nutr.*, 27,198, 2003.

125. Scott, R.B., Kirk, D., MacNaughton, W.K., and Meddings, J.B., GLP-2 augments the adaptive response to massive intestinal resection in rat, *Am. J. Physiol.*, 275, G911, 1998.

126. Kato, Y., Yu, D., and Schwarz, M.Z., Glucagonlike peptide-2 enhances small intestinal absorptive function and mucosal mass *in vivo*, *J. Pediatr. Surg.*, 34, 18, 1999.

127. Pearson, P.Y., O'Connor, D.M., and Schwartz, M.Z., Novel effect of leptin on small intestine adaptation, *J. Surg. Res.*, 97, 192, 2001.

128. Washizawa, N., Gu, L.K., Gu, L., Openo, K.P., Jones, D.P., and Ziegler, T.R., Comparative effects of glucagon-like peptide-2, growth hormone and keratinocyte growth factor in rats after massive small bowel resection, *JPEN*, 28, S4, 2004 (abstr.).

129. Benjamin, M.A., McKay, D.M., Yang, P.C. et al., Glucagon-like peptide-2 enhances intestinal epithelial barrier function of both transcellular and paracellular pathways in the mouse, *Gut*, 47, 112, 2000.

130. Chance, W.T., Foley-Nelson, T., Thomas, I., Balasubramaniam, A., Prevention of parenteral nutrition-induced gut hypoplasia by coinfusion of glucagon-like peptide-2, *Am. J. Physiol.*, 273, G559, 1997.

131. Farrell, C.L., Bready, J.V., Rex, K.L., Chen, J.N., DiPalma, C.R., Whticomb, K.L., Yin, S., Hill. D.C., Wiemann, B., Starnes, C.O., Havill, A.M., Lu, Z.N., Aukerman, S.L., Pierce, G.F., Thomason, A., Potten, C.S., Ulich, T.R., and Lacey, D.L., KGF protects from chemotherapy and radiation-induced gastrointestinal injury and mortality, *Cancer Res.*, 158, 933, 1998.

132. Byrne, F.R., Farrell, C.L., Aranda, R., Rex, K.L., Scully, S., Brown, H.L., Flores, S.A., Gu, L.H., Danilenko, D.M., Lacey, D.L., Ziegler, T.R., and Senaldi, G., rHuKGF ameliorates symptoms in DSS and CD4(+)CD45RB(Hi) T cell transfer mouse models of inflammatory bowel disease, *Am. J. Physiol.*, 282, G690, 2002.

133. Jacobs, D.O., Evans, D.A., Mealy, K., O'Dwyer, S., Smith, R.J., and Wilmore, D.W., Combined effects of glutamine and epidermal growth factor (EGF) on the rat intestine, *Surgery*, 108, 358, 1988.

134. Gu, Y., Wu, Z.H., Xie, J.X. et al., Effects of growth hormone (rhGH) and glutamine supplemented parenteral nutrition on intestinal adaptation in short bowel rats, *Clin. Nutr.*, 20,159, 2001.
135. Zhou, X., Li, Y.X., Li, N., Li, J.S., Glutamine enhances the gut-trophic effect of growth hormone in rat after massive small bowel resection, *J. Surg. Res.*, 99, 47, 2001.
136. Scolapio, J.S., Tales from the crypt, *Gastroenterology*, 124, 561, 2003.
137. Zhu, W., Li, N., Ren, J., Gu, J., Jiang, J., and Li, J., Rehabilitation therapy for short bowel syndrome, *Chinese Med. J.*, 115, 776, 2002.

14 Enteral Nutrition in Intestinal Failure

Douglas L. Seidner and Dhanasekaran Ramasamy

CONTENTS

The goal of enteral nutrition (EN) in intestinal failure is to provide a diet that takes advantage of the functional features of the remaining intestinal tract so that a patient's reliance on parenteral nutrition (PN) can be decreased or eliminated. One must understand the principles of nutrient and fluid absorption by the gastrointestinal tract in health and disease to be successful in this endeavor. The rationale for manipulating the diet for optimal absorption also applies when selecting the most appropriate enteral tube feeding formula for patients with intestinal failure. One must keep in mind that all patients are not candidates for manipulation of the diet or the provision of enteral tube feeding to meet these objectives. This includes patients with severe short bowel syndrome, enterocutaneous fistulas, and bowel obstruction. Other patients are unable to adhere to the demanding schedule that one must follow because of socioeconomic and psychosocial constraints. This chapter will discuss these principles and will review the various enteral feeding devices available to deliver this therapy and the complications associated with its provision.

DIGESTION AND ABSORPTION IN HEALTH AND INTESTINAL FAILURE

NORMAL GASTROINTESTINAL DIGESTION AND ABSORPTION

When the intestinal tract is intact, nearly all nutrients are absorbed within the first 150 cm of the small bowel.[1] This degree of efficiency, which is quite remarkable since the normal small bowel in an adult ranges in length from 350 cm to 600 cm,[2] depends on the presence of normal gastric and pancreaticobiliary function and the absence of mucosal disease. Distal portions of the gut are also important to preserve normal intestinal function. The distal 100 cm of ileum is required for adequate absorption of vitamin B_{12} and bile salts, the colon absorbs soluble fiber after it has been fermented by resident bacteria to form short-chain fatty acids (SCFAs), and the colon also absorbs a modest amount of sodium and water that is not usually absorbed in the small bowel. The end result is that in a healthy subject 95% of the ingested energy is absorbed to satisfy the metabolic needs of the individual. Normal gastrointestinal function is more thoroughly discussed in chapter 1.

DEFINITION AND CAUSES OF INTESTINAL FAILURE

Intestinal failure can be defined as the inability to meet nutrient and fluid requirements while consuming a regular diet. It is seen in adults following extensive intestinal resection for Crohn's disease, mesenteric ischemia, and complications of abdominal and pelvic cancer therapy and has classically been referred to as the short bowel syndrome (SBS). However, some patients who have only a modest length of small bowel removed can develop intestinal failure if there is mucosal disease of the remaining bowel; the digestive function is compromised as a result of previous gastric surgery, pancreatic insufficiency, or liver failure; or if the ileocecal valve or a large portion of the colon is resected. This underscores the importance of using functional capacity of the bowel rather than length to determine what therapy is most appropriate for a given patient.

Patients with intestinal failure often require parenteral nutrition (PN) so that they can avoid the development of malnutrition, dehydration, and electrolyte abnormalities. It is evident to clinicians who manage patients on PN that they will fall into one of two categories: those that require PN because they are unable to maintain their normal weight and hydration status and those that require intravenous fluid (IVF) and electrolytes to avoid dehydration and electrolyte abnormalities but can maintain their weight through an oral diet. Clinical observations and carefully conducted balance studies that have been performed since the advent of PN have led to a better understanding of the relationship between the anatomic and functional factors that help define intestinal failure and to discriminate between patients who will require PN or IVF versus those who can be maintained on an oral diet with or without enteral tube feeding (ETF). This information can be useful in determining how best to prescribe EN.

The most important factor that determines whether a patient will be weaned from PN is bowel length. In a large home PN program in France, Messing et al.[3] demonstrated that nearly all patients with more than 100 cm of small bowel ending in a jejunostomy could discontinue PN or IVF. They also showed that patients with as little 60 cm of jejunum anastamosed to a portion of the colon or 30 cm of small bowel with the colon and the ileocecal valve could be weaned from these therapies. These observations also underscore the important role that the colon plays in its ability to absorb sodium, water, and unabsorbed carbohydrate and how the colon and ileocecal valve increase intestinal transit time.

In a carefully performed balance study, Jeppesen and Mortensen helped define the limits of intestinal failure based on measurements of intestinal energy and wet weight absorption.[4] They compared 45 home PN-dependant patients to 44 non-PN-dependant patients with fecal losses of energy that exceeded 2 MJ/day (476 kcal /day) and found that patients who did not rely on PN or IVF had energy absorption of more than 84% of their basal metabolic rate as defined by the Harris-Benedict equation (an average energy intake of 4.9 MJ/day or 1,166 kcal/day) or wet weight absorption of more than 1.4 kg/day. PN-dependent patients absorbed less of either or both of these measures. This study also showed the importance of oral intake in defining these two groups of patients. PN-dependent patients ranged from those with 0% absorption to those with 100% absorption but an inability to consume a sufficient amount of energy. There were non-PN patients who absorbed less than half of their oral intake but were able to avoid PN by eating more than their weight-based energy or fluid requirements. This later group of patients consumed 10–24 MJ/day of energy (200%–400% of their basal metabolic rate) and 3–7 kg/day of fluid. Intestinal failure can therefore occur when there is insufficient absorption in the setting of adequate oral intake or when there is insufficient intake of food in the setting of moderately significant malabsorption.

INFLUENCE OF ALTERED INTESTINAL ANATOMY AND FUNCTION

Gastrointestinal anatomy and functional factors that favor independence from PN and IVF include the presence of the ileum (as opposed to the jejunum), ileocecal valve, and colon, the absence of mucosal disease and adequate function of the stomach, pancreas, and hepatobiliary tree. A greater degree of intestinal adaptation and a patient's willingness or ability to eat an appropriate diet will affect whether a patient will be managed with PN versus ETF or diet. Remaining bowel length and intestinal segment will be briefly discussed because these two factors are pivotal in determining whether or not enteral nutrition should be prescribed and if so what dietary modifications need to be undertaken. A complete discussion of this topic can be found in Chapters 2, 3, and 9.

1. **Bowel length:** Adults with more than 200 cm of small bowel usually tolerate an oral diet and will not require PN. Patients with > 100 cm of small bowel ending in a stoma or > 60 cm of small bowel anastamosed to the colon can almost always discontinue PN supplementation with dietary modification and medications to promote absorption and minimize intestinal secretions.[3,5] While bowel length is the most pivotal factor that will determine whether a patient can be transitioned to EN, the length of remaining bowel is often not known.

2. **Site of bowel resection:** The digestion and absorption of most nutrients occurs in the duodenum and proximal jejunum.[1] The distal 100 cm of ileum is responsible for absorption of vitamin B_{12}[6] and bile salts.[7] The normal sequence of events that occurs during this process relies on the secretion of sodium and water into the duodenum and jejunum to make chyme isotonic and the absorption of sodium and water in the ileum.[8] Contact time between nutrients and the intestinal mucosa must also be adequate. Transit time through the intestinal tract is increased by the presence of the ileum and colon.[9]

These factors lead to a more favorable outcome in patients who undergo jejunal versus ileal resection of an equal length of bowel. Compared to the jejunum, the ileum is able to absorb sodium and water more efficiently, can maintain the bile salt pool necessary for the emulsification of dietary fats, and increases transit time through the proximal gut. In addition to increasing intestinal transit time, the colon is able to absorb up to five liters of fluid each day.[10] The colon is also able to salvage nearly 4.2 MJ/d (1,000 kcal/d) of energy from unabsorbed carbohydrates and soluble dietary fiber.[11] These sugars are fermented by anaerobic bacteria in the colon to create SCFAs, which are transported via the portal circulation to the liver where they are used as fuel.[12] The colon may also be able to salvage unabsorbed di- and tripeptides that are not absorbed by the small bowel through the up-regulation of the mucosal transport protein PepT 1.[13] Small bowel absorption is generally more efficient when the ileocecal valve remains, presumably because of its effects on intestinal transit and maintenance of a more normal distribution of the intestinal flora.[14]

MEASURES OF INTESTINAL FUNCTION

Two measures of intestinal function are

1. **Clinical assessment:** Balance studies that could be used to determine whether a patient can be transitioned to enteral autonomy are generally not available in clinical practice. Intestinal function can be inferred through a variety of clinical measurements. Clinical measures that are commonly used include patient weight, upper arm anthropometry, fluid intake and output, serum electrolytes and proteins, and urinary sodium, calcium, and magnesium. While many of these measures may not be specific for intestinal function or may take time to reflect changes in nutritional status, fluid balance is easy to measure and can be closely examined to determine whether a patient will require IVF. Enteral intake must exceed stool or stoma losses by at least one liter to provide an adequate amount of fluid for urine and insensible losses.
2. **Citrulline:** Plasma citrulline may prove to be an easily obtained measure of intestinal function.[15] Citrulline is an amino acid that is the metabolic byproduct of glutamine metabolism. Glutamine, which is derived predominantly from skeletal muscle and when intestinal absorption is adequate from the diet, is converted in the enterocyte to citrulline, alanine, proline, and ornithine. The plasma concentration of citrulline has been shown to correlate with bowel length and the ability to transition from PN to EN.[15] Concentrations < 20 μmol/l correlate with permanent PN, 20–30 μmol/l correlate with transient PN use, and values above 40 μmol/l are considered normal.

IMPROVING INTESTINAL FUNCTION

Medications are essential in patients who are to be transitioned from PN to EN. Digestion can be improved with bile acid and pancreatic enzymes replacement therapy and medications that decrease gastrointestinal secretions and prolong intestinal transit time (Chapters 10 and 11). Bacterial overgrowth should be treated with antibiotics, probiotics, or surgery when anatomic abnormalities are present (Chapter 12). Immune modulating and antiinflammatory drugs can improve absorption in patients with active Crohn's disease. Trophic factors may be used in patients with marginal mucosal mass (Chapter 13).

NUTRIENT REQUIREMENTS

PROTEIN AND ENERGY REQUIREMENTS

Nutrient requirements depend on several patient characteristics, including gender, age, weight, and height.[16] Additional factors that must be considered include the patient's nutritional status, underlying disease, and metabolic condition. Several acceptable methods are available that can be used to determine nutrient requirements.[16] While predictive equations that estimate protein and energy requirements are fairly reliable in determining nutrient needs when prescribing PN, they can be expected to underestimate the EN prescription for patients with intestinal failure. Therefore, one should expect the requirements for EN to exceed levels determined by predictive equations or measurements made by indirect calorimetry.

Patients who are reasonably well are often able to regulate their oral intake to meet their protein and energy requirements. On the other hand, ETF requirements must be carefully determined for patients who are not eating well or who seem to fall short of their requirements based on a decline in their body composition or functional status. One should consider these requirements to be twofold or greater than amounts determined by conventional means. This approach is supported by balance studies that have shown that an oral intake equal to 200%–400% of the basal metabolic rate is required to maintain nutrient balance in patients with severe malabsorption.[4] In one study macronutrient absorption was 81% for protein, 61% for carbohydrate, and 54% for fat in patients with SBS who consume a hyperphagic diet of nearly twice their energy requirements.[17] In another study, macronutrient absorption was 61% for protein, 79% for carbohydrate, and 52% for fat in patients with SBS who consumed 58±14 kcal/kg/d.[18] It is important to recognize that fat absorption is least efficient and can lead to essential fatty acid deficiency in patients who otherwise absorb other nutrients adequately to maintain body composition and function.[19] As is often the case it is important to initiate a reasonable nutrient prescription, to monitor a variety of outcome measures including measures of body composition, fluid, and electrolyte balance and finally to adjust the prescription as needed to maintain the health of the patient.

Micronutrient Requirement

Severe malabsorption nearly always dictates that one prescribe fat-soluble vitamins, minerals, and electrolytes to maintain the adequacy and balance of micronutrients. Requirements have been discussed in Chapters 4 and 7. Patients may require doses that are above the DRI to maintain adequate tissue and functional levels. Multiple vitamins with minerals are given by mouth two to three times daily to patients who are not receiving PN. Vitamin B_{12} injections should be started after surgical resection of more than 100 cm of terminal ileum to avoid the development of the hematologic and neurologic consequences vitamin B_{12} deficiency.[6] Dosing is often empiric, but can be based on serum and urinary measures for some of these nutrients. Table 14.1 illustrates our approach to the care of these patients.

Fluid Requirement

A sufficient amount of fluid must be consumed and absorbed to allow for a broad range of metabolic processes, including urine production, insensible fluid loss, and gastrointestinal secretions. The wet weight absorption of more than 1.4 kg/day suggested by Jeppesen et al.[4] is usually easy to achieve in patients with a remnant colon. Patients with enterostomies who have difficulty absorbing sodium and water can benefit from oral rehydration solutions.[20,21] The utility of these formulas are discussed in Chapters 2, 4, and 9.

TABLE 14.1
Vitamins and Minerals Used for Adults with Intestinal Failure

Name	Strength Available	Typical Regimen
Vitamins		
Vitamin A	5,000–50,000 IU	5,000–10,000 IU/d
Vitamin D$_2$	25,000–50,000 IU	50,000 IU 2–3 times/wk
Liquid	8,000 IU per ml	
Capsules	50,000 IU	
Vitamin D$_3$	400, 1000	400–1000 IU
1,25[OH]$_2$ D$_3$	0.25, 0.5 mcg	0.5 mcg/d
	1mcg/mL	
Vitamin E	200, 400, 500, 800, 1000 IU	100–400 IU/d
Vitamin K	5 mg	5–10 mg/d
Minerals[a]		
Calcium carbonate	500–1500 mg (200–600 mg elemental Ca)	1,000–3,000 mg/d (Ca)
Calcium citrate	200–950 mg (200–760 mg elemental Ca)	
Calcium gluconate	500–975 (45–90 mg elemental Ca)	
Magnesium chloride[+]	535 mg (64 mg)	50–500 mg/d (Mg)
Magnesium lactate[+]	840 mg (84 mg)	
Magnesium gluconate[+]	500 mg (27 mg elemental Mg)	
Potassium chloride	10, 20, 25, 50 mEq	As needed
Potassium chloride	10% solution = 20 mEq/15mL	
	20% solution = 40 mEq/15mL	
Phosphate as sodium and potassium	250 mg (8mM) PO$_4$ (7.125 mEq each of Na + K)	250–2,000 mg/d
	250 mg (8mM) PO$_4$ (1.1 mEq K and 13 mEq Na)	
	250 mg (8mM) PO$_4$ (14.25 mEq K and 0 mEq Na)	
Sodium bicarbonate	325–650 mg	1,300–5,200 mg/d
Bicitra	1 mL = 1 mEq NaHCO$_3$	As needed
Polycitra	1 mL = 1 mEq Na+K, 1 mEq HCO$_3$	
Chromium	220 mg (50 mg)	50–150 mg/d
Copper	100–200 mcg	200–600 mcg/d
Selenium	3 mg	3–6 mg/d
Zinc sulfate	50, 100, 200 mcg	200–600 mcg/d
	66 mg (15 mg elemental Zn)	50–150 mg/d
	110 mg (25 mg elemental Zn)	
	200 mg (45 mg elemental Zn)	
	220 mg (50 mg elemental Zn)	

[a] Minerals should be taken in divided doses two or four times each day. Amounts are given as total salt and (dose of parent mineral).

[+] Take one hour before meals on an empty stomach.

ORAL INTAKE IN INTESTINAL FAILURE

The goal of dietary management in patients with intestinal failure is to minimize the symptoms associated with severe malabsorption while optimizing nutrient absorption so that reliance on PN can be minimized. Food should be consumed in small quantities and divided into five or more meals each day. Protein should be of high biologic value and carbohydrates should be complex rather than simple. The intake of concentrated sweets, especially in the form of fruit juices, should be minimized, as they tend to exaggerate the underlying osmotic diarrhea. When the colon is absent or out of continuity with the small bowel fat, lactose and oxalate restriction is not necessary.[22-24] The percentage of fat absorbed is constant over a broad range, and so the calories derived from fat increases as the amount of fat consumed is increased. Patients with an intact colon often need dietary restriction of fat and lactose to minimize any secretory and osmotic diarrhea associated with these nutrients. A detailed description of diets used in intestinal failure is provided in Chapter 9.

INTESTINAL ADAPTATION TO ENTERAL TUBE FEEDING

Adaptation of the remaining bowel starts immediately after extensive small bowel resection and continues for two or more years. This dynamic process is characterized by both structural and functional changes that are manifest as an increase in villus height, crypt depth, luminal dilation, and brush border enzyme activity.[25] Interestingly, the ileum can affect these changes to a greater degree than the jejunum. The mechanism underlying this process is influenced by numerous factors and includes the presence of luminal nutrients, pancreaticobiliary secretions, neuorhumoral signals, and adequate mesenteric blood flow.[26] The practical approach to this process has been divided into three stages: the first is the immediate postoperative period where parenteral fluid and nutrients are provided until the patient is stabilized, the second includes the gradual transition from PN to EN, and the third is the attainment of complete autonomy from PN in patients with the functional capacity to meet all of their nutrient and fluid requirements through the gut. This section will review studies that have explored the role of enteral tube feeding during intestinal adaptation.

INTESTINAL STRUCTURE AND FUNCTION WITHOUT ENTERAL NUTRITION

Luminal nutrients are necessary to maintain normal mucosal structure and function. Prior to the ability to provide nutrients as PN, studies on gastrointestinal physiology were subject to the effect of malnutrition. In one of the first studies to investigate the effect of the withdrawal of EN on the intestinal tract in rats given PN as the sole source of nutrition, Levine et al.[27] found a decrease in mucosal height, mucosal protein, and DNA content and brush border lactase activity. Other studies in animals of similar design have lent further support to these initial observations.[28-30] There is only one comparative study in humans without mucosal disease and injury. In a prospective study of eight healthy volunteers maintained on PN for 14 days,

Buchman et al.[31] showed that mucosal thickness was diminished as a result of a decrease in villus height and that intestinal permeability was increased as measured by lactulose-mannitol absorption. Interestingly, villus architecture was preserved and crypt depth was maintained. In addition, mucosal protein and nucleic acid content and lactose breath hydrogen testing was unchanged from baseline after PN. In general, these studies demonstrate the importance that luminal nutrients have in maintaining the structural integrity of the digestive tract.

INTESTINAL STRUCTURE AND FUNCTION WITH ENTERAL NUTRITION

Animal Studies

Animal studies suggest that intestinal adaptation after extensive intestinal resection is optimally promoted by using polymeric enteral formulas. Compared to a standard diet of oral rat chow, an elemental formula maintains mucosal mass in the proximal but not the distal small bowel and colon.[32] The advantage of polymeric over hydro-lyzed and elemental formulas has also been noted by Young et al., who studied a series of formulas in rats with an intact intestinal tract.[33] In a study of two-by-two design comparing an enteral formula with casein versus a casein hydrolysate to animal subject to 60% jejunoileal resection versus a sham procedure, the only adverse finding attributed to the casein hydrolysate was a decrease in leucine uptake.[34] Sucrase levels were actually increased with the casein hydrolysate while other measures of mucosal hyperplasia were unaffected. In studies comparing single nutrient infusion, disaccharides were found to stimulate mucosal growth more effec-tively than monosaccharides[35] and higher concentrations of glucose lead to an increase in intestinal mass and nutrient transport.[36] In a study comparing two enteral formula that differed only in the type of fat that they contained, the formula con-taining mostly long-chain triglycerides (LCT) showed a significantly greater increase in mucosal adaptation compared to the medium-chain triglycerides (MCT) product in animals subject to extensive small bowel resection.[37] Formulas containing LCT composed of polyunsaturated fatty acids, especially those derived from fish oil, appear to be the most effective in promoting intestinal adaptation.[38,39] Nucleotides and certain amino acids, such as glutamine, may also play a role in the process of adaptation.[40] Finally, enteral formula supplemented with pectin have been shown to improve structural measures of intestinal adaptation and colonic function following extensive intestinal resection.[41,42] The effect of pectin appears to depend on colonic fermentation since treatment with the antibiotic metronidazole diminishes the effect of pectin.[43]

Human Studies

A standard polymeric formula was compared to a free amino acid peptide formula supplemented with glutamine and arginine in the study by Buchman et al.[31] that examined the effect of PN-induced mucosal changes in humans. Following 14 days of PN as the sole source of nutrition, the healthy subjects received one of two formulas via a nasoduodenal feeding tube for 5 days. Mucosal thickness improved after either enteral formula. There was no difference in the mucosal content of protein or nucleic acids after PN or either EN formula. Intestinal permeability increased after PN and even more after EN was reintroduced but was not as greatly affected by the specialized formula. Because of the design of this study, these results may not be applicable to patients with intestinal failure. Rather, this study should encourage future investigation into the role of products designed to promote intestinal adaptation in humans.

ENTERAL NUTRITION FORMULA SELECTION AND ADMINISTRATION

FORMULA COMPOSITION

Enteral formulas are a nutritionally complete emulsion of macronutrients and micronutrients that are commercially prepared for EN. Most of these products are not palatable and are only suitable for ETF. Standard formulas provide 1 kcal/ml, are nearly isotonic, and contain intact protein, glucose polymers, and triglycerides. Specialized formulas include those with di-, tri-, and oligopeptides that may promote intestinal absorption of protein. Elemental formulas refer to those products composed of free amino acids and glucose as their source of nitrogen and carbohydrate. Formulas composed of elemental and partially hydrolyzed macronutrients and those that are concentrated and provide up to 2 kcal/ml have a tonicity of up to 700 mOsm/kg. Many standard and specialized formulas contain a mixture of LCT and MCT, while a few formulas have been supplemented with omega-3 fatty acids. A handful of products are prepared with blenderized food and a few contain lactose. Over the past decade, soluble fiber has been added to some formulas to take advantage of the beneficial effect that fiber has on colon health. Although there is a tremendous variety of commercially available formulas, there is a dearth of information regarding the use of these products in patients with intestinal failure. This section will review the literature on this topic and provide the rationale used to select the most appropriate formula for these patients.

Protein

Two controlled balance studies in adult patients with jejunostomies and up to 150 cm of small bowel provide conflicting results regarding the superiority of formula containing hydrolyzed versus whole protein. McIntyre et al. studied seven patients with SBS and found both products to be equally efficacious with regard to nitrogen, energy, micronutrient, and fluid absorption.[23] On the other hand, Cosnes et al. studied six patients with SBS and found superior nitrogen absorption with a peptide-based formula.[44] It should be noted that half of the patients in the later study suffered from radiation enteritis. In a recent study of crossover design in ten infants with SBS, an enteral formula with hydrolyzed proteins did not affect intestinal permeability, nitrogen, or energy balance when compared to a nonhydrolyzed formula.[45] Given the limitations of these studies, which includes the small number of patients studies and other differences in the composition of the formulas used, in addition to the advantages that polymeric formula have in promoting adaptation of the remaining bowel, it is recommended that polymeric products with whole protein be used in patients with intestinal failure. If a standard product is not tolerated, then a specialized product can be tried.

Carbohydrate

The carbohydrate content of standard formulas ranges from 40% to 60%. Disaccharidase deficiency that results from intestinal resection or mucosal disease is often not a problem since most products are composed of glucose polymers and nearly all are lactose free. Elemental formula should be tolerated in most adults;[23] however, the high tonicity may not be tolerated in some patients. The handful of products that contain lactose should be well tolerated in patients with jejunostomies since studies have shown good tolerance to lactose 20 g/d in this group of patients.[23,46]

Soluble fiber is fermented in the colon by anaerobic bacteria that produce the SCFAs butyrate, propionate, and acetate. SCFAs are the primary fuel of the colonocyte and have a trophic effect on colonic adaptation.[41,47] They also showed that SCFAs enhanced colonic sodium and water absorption. In patients with an intact colon, soluble fiber, along with other unabsorbed carbohydrates, can provide a significant amount of energy. In one study of patients with intestinal failure, consuming an oral diet a total of 4.2 MJ/d was salvaged by this process.[11] While formulas containing fiber would appear to be optimal for patients with intestinal failure, balance studies have not directly compared products with and without soluble fiber.

Fat

The optimal fat content for enteral formulas in intestinal failure is not known. Balance studies in patients with SBS show that fat does not need to be restricted in patients with jejunostomies.[22–24] The animal studies previously cited suggest that a moderate amount of fat from LCT should be provided to optimized intestinal adaptation.[37] LCT is also responsible for prolonging the transit through more proximal segments of the intestinal tract.[48] This phenomenon is in part the result of peptide YY that is released by the colon.[49,50] One might anticipate that formula with MCT would be ideal in all patients with intestinal failure, especially since they do not rely on pancreatic and biliary secretions for small bowel absorption. Interestingly, a recent balance study of adults with SBS suggests that products with MCT only provide benefit for patients who have their colon in continuity with the small bowel.[51] In summary, a LCT restricted formula is not needed to manage most patients with intestinal failure, particularly those with jejunostomies, and a portion of the LCT may be replaced with MCT in patients with their colon when standard formulas are not tolerated.

FORMULA SELECTION

A standard isotonic, polymeric formula containing intact proteins, glucose polymers, and a mixture of LCT and MCT should be selected under most circumstances. The

TABLE 14.2
Optimal Enteral Formula Characteristics for Intestinal Failure

Nutrient	Comment
Protein	
Whole	Protein absorption is modestly decreased in intestinal failure and whole protein is well tolerated.
Hydrolyzed	
Carbohydrate	Glucose polymers are tolerated better than mono- and disaccharides. Most formulas are lactose free.
Fat	
LCT	Most standard formulas contain a mixture of LCT and MCT. LCT promotes adaptation and prolongs intestinal transit time. MCT is most efficiently absorbed when the colon is present.
MCT	
Soluble fiber	Stimulates intestinal adaptation, improves salt and water absorption and provides energy when the colon is present.
Tonicity	Isotonic formulas minimize the secretion of water into the lumen.
Sodium chloride	Additional salt may be added to formulas to improve sodium and water absorption when jejunostomy output is high.

LCT = long-chain triglycerides, MCT = medium-chain triglycerides

product should also contain soluble fiber, especially in patients with an intact colon to improve absorptive function and to serve as a source of energy. Table 14.2 summarizes the rationale behind the selection of the most appropriate formula in patients with intestinal failure.

FORMULA ADMINISTRATION

Rate and Route of Administration

ETF can be started by continuous infusion in patients with intestinal failure during the early adaptive phase. In a retrospective study of 62 patients with SBS, ETF was begun 14 days after surgery and led to the discontinuation of PN by day 36.[52] A variety of enteral formula were used by these investigators, and in some instances, they reinfused chyme into the distal bowel to achieve independence from PN. It has been suggested that initial feeding should be limited to 600 kcal/d and should only be advanced by 300–500 kcal each day when diarrhea is controlled.[53] Most patients have compromised bowel function and should be feed using a feeding pump to allow for the gradual presentation of nutrients to the remnant bowel. Once patients attain their target rate, an attempt can be made to transition the patient to nocturnal feeding. Most patients should be fed into the stomach unless they are at high risk for aspiration due to gastric dysfunction. An oral diet can be introduced when the patient has recovered adequately from surgery.

Formula Modification to Improve Tolerance

Sodium absorption in patients with jejunostomies can only take place if the luminal sodium concentration is > 90 mmol/l while the maximal sodium absorption occurs at a concentration of 120 mmol/l.[54] Patients with high-output jejunostomies need to add sodium chloride to their enteral formula since all of the commercially prepared products have a sodium concentration of approximately 40 mmol/l. Liquid preparations of narcotic antidiarrheal medications can be added to enteral formulas to help control diarrhea. Care must be taken to ensure that proper mixing occurs when sodium chloride and medications are added to enteral products.

ORAL REHYDRATION SOLUTIONS

Oral rehydration solutions can be administered through an enteral feeding tube in patients who cannot maintain their fluid balance despite optimization of diet and medications. Occasionally this approach is used in patients who cannot tolerate these solutions when taken by mouth. They may be administered as a bolus between meals or overnight using a feeding pump. In addition, we have used these solutions rather than water to flush enteral feeding tubes to keep tubes patent. This avoids the presentation of a large amount of water to the proximal small bowel that can lead to the excess loss of sodium.

ENTERAL ACCESS DEVICES

The optimal tube-feeding route depends on the anticipated duration of therapy, the adequacy of gastric function, and the competence of the lower esophageal sphincter. Immediately following surgery, hospitalized patients should be fed through naso-gastric tubes. Patients at high risk for aspiration of gastric contents due to altered mental status, an incompetent lower esophageal sphincter with gastroesophageal reflux, or gastroparesis should have feeding placed into the third portion of the duodenum or beyond. Patients who require tube feedings for more than 30 days should consider an endoscopic, radiologic, or surgical placement of gastrostomy or jejunostomy tube.[55]

NASOGASTRIC TUBE PLACEMENT

Small-bore pliable tubes made of biologically inert materials are preferred for nasoenteric feeding. Adult patients usually tolerate a tube diameter of 8 to 10 French. This size tube easily accepts standard or viscous fiber containing formulas without difficulty whether administered by pump, gravity, or bolus administration. A standard tube length of 109 cm is sufficient for nasogastric and transpyloric placement. An x-ray of the upper abdomen should always be obtained prior to tube use. Insufflation of air into the tube and auscultation over the stomach or aspiration of gastrointestinal contents is not a reliable means to confirm intragastric placement. A study of 100 consecutive radiographs obtained after tube placement showed that 80% of the tubes were in the stomach or duodenum, 19% were in the esophagus, and 1% were in the pleural space.[56]

Transpyloric Tube Placement

Nasoenteric tubes may be placed into the stomach, duodenum, or proximal jejunum. The more distal a tube is placed beyond the pylorus, the lower the risk of enterogastric reflux and aspiration. Nasoduodenal or jejunal tube placement is far more challenging than nasogastric placement. Spontaneous transpyloric passage of feeding tubes using peristalsis can lead to successful placement in 36%–56% of weighted tubes and in 84%–92% of unweighted tubes but has the disadvantage of delaying the institution of feeding.[57] Prokinetic agents (metoclopramide, erythromycin) have been used to assist in tube placement. These medications are more likely to work if they are given before tube placement.[58] An active bedside technique for placing tubes transpylorically has been described by Zaloga and involves careful advancement of the feeding tube while rotating it clockwise around its long axis.[59] Successful tube placement using this technique ranges from 40% to 92%, with higher rates seen for trained personnel. Fluoroscopic, endoscopic, and sonographic tube placement results in proper tube placement in 85% to 95% of patients but is much more costly because of the need for expensive equipment and properly trained personnel.[60–62]

Gastrostomy Tube Placement

Percutaneous endoscopic gastrostomy (PEG) is the most frequently used method for long-term access.[63] A skin-level PEG, referred to as a "button," is popular with ambulatory patients.[64] The procedure is simple and well tolerated even in debilitated patients. An experienced clinician can place a tube in a patient with previous abdominal and/or gastric surgery. Surgical gastrostomy should be considered when access to the stomach is anticipated during a major abdominal procedure or when PEG placement cannot be done safely. Fluoroscopic placement has a lower complication rate than endoscopic or surgical tube placement.[65] The decision to use one technique over the other often depends on availability and local expertise.

Jejunostomy Tube Placement

Jejunostomy tubes are reserved for patients with abnormal gastric emptying or severe gastroesophageal reflux that increases the risk for aspiration.[66] Indications for these tubes include tracheal aspiration, severe reflux esophagitis, gastroparesis, gastric outlet obstruction, or surgical procedures of the upper gastrointestinal tract that preclude gastric feeding. Endoscopy or fluoroscopy can be used to position a small bore feeding tube through a PEG tube, resulting in a combination of two tubes often referred to as a percutaneous endoscopic gastrostomy with jejunal extension tube (PEG-JET or PEG/J).[67] PEG-JET can offer simultaneous gastric decompression with small bowel feedings through a single enterogastric stoma. Unfortunately the PEG-JET is technically difficult to place and migration back into the stomach is common.[68] True percutaneous endoscopic jejunostomy (PEJ) has been described but is not commonly performed.[69] Surgical jejunostomy is the favored method for prolonged tube placement into the small bowel and may be performed as an open or laparoscopic procedure.[70,71]

TABLE 14.3
Complications of Enteral Tube Feeding

Complication	Etiology	Prevention/Treatment
Mechanical		
Tube Malposition	↓ mental status/gag reflex; inexperienced clinician	Confirmatory x-ray
Tube Occlusion	Pills, Sucralfate; failure to flush; assessment of residual gastric volume	Flush Q4h; Papain/pancrealipase; $NaHCO_3$, Mechanical device
Inadvertent removal	Poor fixation; ↓ mental status; accidental	Tube surveillance; adequate fixation; nasal bridle
Gastrointestinal		
Abdominal distention	Ileus; bowel obstruction; constipation; formula intolerance	X-ray; rectal exam; correct cause of ileus; ↓ feeding rate or bolus
Nausea, vomiting, and regurgitation	Delayed gastric emptying from GI disease; sepsis; abdominal surgery; head injury; abnormal electrolytes, narcotics; anticholinergics	↓ Feeding rate or bolus volume; prokinetic drugs; correct underlying cause
Diarrhea	Drug induced (antibiotics, magnesium, sorbitol, etc.); C. difficile colitis; malabsorption; bacterial contamination of formula	Review medications; stool C.diff toxin; fiber containing formula; antidiarrheal meds; hydrolyzed formula; ↓ feeding rate or bolus volume
Constipation	Dehydration; fecal impaction; narcotics; inadequate fiber; inactivity	Maintain hydration; disimpaction; enemas, laxatives/stool softeners; ↓ narcotics; fiber containing formula; physical activity
Infectious		
Aspiration pneumonia	↓Mental status/gag reflex; incompetent LES; rapid infusion of formula; supine position; and causes of N/V and distention	Elevate HOB; monitor gastric residual volume; jejunal feeding with gastric decompression; treat N/V and distention
Diarrhea	C. difficile colitis; bacterial contamination of formula	Stool C.diff toxin; proper formula handling
Sinusitis	Tube blocks drainage of sinus through meatus	Small-bore feeding tube; antibiotics; drainage
Metabolic		
Fluid/Electrolyte; Acid-Base; Refeeding syndrome	Inadequate or excessive fluid or formula; underlying disease; medications; organ system failure	Calculate requirements; monitor I/O; daily weights; monitor labs; replete deficits; formula selection

COMPLICATIONS OF ENTERAL TUBE FEEDING

Patients with intestinal failure are subject to all of the recognized complications of ETF. These complications include mechanical and infectious problems associated with feeding tube placement and utilization. Whereas most patients managed with ETF do not develop metabolic or gastrointestinal complications, patients with intestinal failure are far more challenging to manage because of the diminished functional reserve of their gut. Table 14.3 illustrates many of the complications associated with ETF and suggests interventions that may be used to minimize their occurrence.

SUMMARY

Enteral nutrition in patients with intestinal failure can be performed successfully by assessing the anatomy and function of the remnant bowel. Diet modification, medications, and micronutrient supplementation along with enteral tube feeding may be required for the optimal management of patients with severe malabsorption. Nutrient requirements for EN are often greater than those provided by PN to achieve the same result. Energy needs can be two or more times greater than the basal metabolic rate, and fluid requirements can approach 7 kg/d. Isotonic, polymeric formulas composed of intact protein, glucose polymers, and a mixture of LCT and MCT can promote intestinal adaptation and supply a sufficient amount of protein and energy to meet a patient's requirements. Most patients who require ETF will ultimately need a gastrostomy tube, though other devices may be used depending on the clinical circumstances. Whenever possible complications should be anticipated so that their effect can be minimized and rapidly corrected. These efforts are important in many patients with intestinal failure to avoid or diminish their reliance on PN.

REFERENCES

1. Borgstrom, C.C. et al., Studies on intestinal digestion and absorption in the human, *J. Clin. Invest.*, 36, 1521, 1957.
2. Weser, E., Nutritional aspects of malabsorption: short gut adaptation, *Clin. Gastroenterol.*, 12, 443, 1983.
3. Messing, B. et al., Long-term survival and parenteral nutrition dependence in adult patients with short bowel syndrome, *Gastroenterology,* 117, 1043, 1999.
4. Jeppesen, P.B. and Mortensen P.B., Intestinal failure defined by measurements of intestinal energy and wet weight absorption, *Gut*, 46, 701, 2000.
5. Nightingale, J.M. et al., Jejunal efflux in short bowel syndrome, *Lancet*, 336, 765, 1990.
6. Okuda, K., Discovery of vitamin B12 in the liver and its absorption factor in the stomach: A historical review, *J. Gastroenterol. Hepatology*, 14, 301, 1999.
7. Hofmann, A.F. and Poley, J.R., Role of bile acid malabsorption in the pathogenesis of diarrhea and steatorrhea in patients with ileal resection: I. response to cholestyramine or replacement of dietary long-chain triglycerides by medium-chain triglycerides, *Gastroenterology,* 62, 918, 1972.
8. Fordtran, J.S. and Dietschy, J.M., Water and electrolyte movement in the intestine, *Gastroenterology,* 50, 263, 1966.

9. Scolapio, J.S., Camilleri, M.C., and Fleming C.R., Motility considerations in short bowel syndrome, *Digestive Diseases*, 15, 253, 1997.
10. Debongnie, J.C. and Phillips, S.F., Capacity of the human colon to absorb fluid, *Gastroenterology*, 74, 698, 1978.
11. Nordgaard, I., Hansen, B.S., and Mortensen, P.B., Importance of colonic support for energy absorption as small-bowel failure proceeds, *Am. J. Clin. Nutr.*, 64, 222, 1996.
12. Royall, D., Wolever, T.M., and Jeejeebhoy, K.N., Clinical significance of colonic fermentation, *Am. J. Gastroenterol.*, 85, 1307, 1990.
13. Ziegler, T.R. et al., Distribution of the H$^+$/peptide transporter PepT1 in human intestine: up-regulated expression in the colonic mucosa of patients with short bowel syndrome, *Am. J. Clin. Nutr.*, 75, 922, 2002.
14. Gracy M., The contaminated small bowel syndrome: pathogenesis, diagnosis, and treatment, *Am. J. Clin. Nutr.*, 32, 234, 1979.
15. Creen, P. et al., Postabsorptive plasma citrulline concentration is a marker of absorptive enterocyte mass and intestinal failure in humans, *Gastroenterology*, 119, 1496, 2000.
16. ASPEN Board of Directors, Guidelines for the use of parenteral and enteral nutrition in adults and pediatric patients, *J. Parenter. Enteral Nutr.*, 26, 9SA, 2002.
17. Woolf, G.M. et al., Nutritional absorption in short bowel syndrome: Evaluation of fluid, calorie, and divalent cation requirements, *Dig. Dis. Sci.*, 32, 8, 1987.
18. Messing, B. et al., Intestinal absorption of free oral hyperalimentation in the very short bowel syndrome, *Gastroenterology*, 100, 1502, 1991.
19. Jeppesen, P.B., Hoy C.E., and Mortensen P.B., Differences in essential fatty acid requirements by enteral and parenteral routes of administration in patients with fat malabsorption, *Am. J. Clin. Nutr.*, 70, 78, 1999.
20. Camilleri, M. et al., Balance studies and polymeric glucose solution to optimize therapy after massive intestinal resection, *Mayo Clin. Proc.*, 67, 755, 1992.
21. Lennard-Jones, J.E., Oral rehydration solutions in short bowel syndrome, *Clin. Ther.*, 12, 101, 1990.
22. Nordgaard, I., Hansen, B.S., and Mortensen, P.B., Colon as a digestive organ in patients with short bowel, *Lancet,* 343, 373, 1994.
23. McIntyre, P.B., Fitchew, M., and Lennard-Jones, J.E., Patients with a high jejunostomy do not need a special diet, *Gastroenterology*, 91, 25, 1986.
24. Marteau, P. et al., Do patients with short-bowel syndrome need a lactose-free diet? *Nutrition*, 13, 13, 1997.
25. Dowling, R.H. and Booth, C.C., Functional compensation after small bowel resection in man, *Lancet*, 2, 146, 1966.
26. Robinson, M.K., Ziegler, T.R., and Wilmore, D.W., Overview of intestinal adaptation and its stimulation, *Eur. J. Pediatr. Surg.*, 9, 200, 1999.
27. Levine, G.M. et al., Role of oral intake in maintenance of gut mass and disaccharidase activity, *Gastroenterology*, 67, 975, 1974.
28. Johnson, L.R. et al., Structural and hormonal alterations in the gastrointestinal tract of parenterally fed rats, *Gastroenterology*, 68, 1177, 1975.
29. Hosada, N. et al., Structural and functional alterations in the gut of parenterally or enterally fed rats, *J. Surg. Res.*, 47, 129, 1989.
30. Goodlad, R.A. et al., Effects of urogastrone-epidermal growth factor on intestinal brush border enzymes and mitotic activity, *Gut*, 32, 994, 1991.
31. Buchman, A.L. et al., Parenteral nutrition is associated with intestinal morphologic and functional changes in humans, *J. Parenter. Enteral Nutr.*, 19, 453, 1995.

32. Morin, C., Ling, V. and Bourassa, D., Small intestinal and colonic changes induced by a chemically defined diet, *Dig. Dis. Sci.*, 25, 123, 1980.

33. Young, E.A. et al., Comparative study of nutrional adaptation to defined formula diets in rats, *Am. J. Clin. Nutr.,* 33, 2106, 1980.

34. Vanderhoof, J.A., Effect of casein versus casein hydrolysate on mucosal adaptation following massive bowel resection in infant rats, *J. Pediatr. Gastro. Nutr.*, 3, 262, 1984.

35. Weser, E., Babbitt, J., and Vandeventer, A., Relationship between enteral glucose load and adaptive mucosal growth in the small bowel, *Dig. Dis. Sci.*, 30, 675, 1985.

36. Richter, G.C., Levine, G.M., and Shiau, Y.F., Effects of luminal glucose versus nonnutritive infusates on jejunal mass and absorption in the rat, *Gastroenterology,* 85, 1105, 1983.

37. Chen, W.J. et al., Effects of lipids on intestinal adaptation following 60% resection in rats, *J. Surg. Res.*, 58, 253, 1995.

38. Vanderhoof, J. et al., Effects of dietary menhaden oil on mucosal adaptation after small bowel resection in rats, *Gastroenterology*, 106, 94, 1994.

39. Kollman, K.A., Lien, E., and Vanderhoof, J.A., Dietary lipids influence intestinal adaptation after massive bowel resection, *J. Pediatr. Gastro. Nutr.*, 28, 41–45, 1999.

40. LeLeiko, N.S. and Walsh, M.J., The role of glutamine, short-chain fatty acids, and nucleotides in intestinal adaptation to gastrointestinal disease, *Pediatr. Clin. North Am.*, 42, 451, 1996.

41. Koruda, M.J. et al., The effect of a pectin-supplemented elemental diet on intestinal adaptation to massive small bowel resection, *J. Parenter. Enteral Nutr.*, 10, 343–50, 1986.

42. Roth, J.A. et al., Pectin improves colonic function in rat short bowel syndrome, *J. Surg. Res.*, 58, 240, 1995.

43. Aghdassi, E. et al., Colonic fermentation and nutritional recovery in rats with massive small bowel resection, *Gastroenterology*, 107, 637, 1994.

44. Cosnes, J. et al., Improvement in protein absorption with a small-peptide-based diet in patients with high jejunostomy, *Nutrition*, 8, 406, 1992.

45. Ksiazyk, J. et al., Hydrolyzed versus nonhydrolyzed protein diet in short bowel syndrome in children, *J. Pediatr. Gastro. Nutr.*, 35, 615, 2002.

46. Arrigoni, E. et al., Tolerance and absorption of lactose from milk and yogurt during short-bowel syndrome in humans, *Am. J. Clin. Nutr.*, 60, 926, 1994.

47. Ruppin, H. et al., Absorption of short-chain fatty acids by the colon, *Gastroenterology,* 78, 1500, 1980.

48. Spiller, R.C., Trotman, I.F., and Higgins, B.E., The ileal brake-inhibition of jejunal motility after ileal fat perfusion in man, *Gut,* 25, 365, 1984.

49. Pironi, L. et al., Fat induced ileal break in humans: A dose dependent phenomenon correlated to the plasma levels of peptide YY, *Gastroenterology,* 105, 753, 1993.

50. Nightingale, J.M.D., et al., Gastrointestinal hormones in short bowel syndrome. Peptide YY may be the colonic brake to gastric braking, *Gut*, 39, 267, 1996.

51. Jeppesen, P.B. and Mortensen, P.B., The influence of a preserved colon on the absorption of medium chain fat in patients with small bowel resection, *Gut*, 43, 478, 1998.

52. Levy, E. et al., Continuous enteral nutrition during the early adaptive stage of the short bowel syndrome, *Br. J. Surg.*, 75, 549, 1988.

53. Wilmore, D.W., Growth factors and nutrients in the short bowel syndrome, *J. Parenter. Enteral Nutr.,* 23, S117, 1999.

54. Lennard-Jones, J.E., Review article: practical management of the short bowel. *Aliment Pharmacol. Ther.*, 8, 563, 1994.

55. Kirby, D.F., Delegge, M.H., and Fleming, C.R., American Gastroenterological Association technical review on tube feeding for enteral nutrition, *Gastroenterology*, 108, 1282, 1995.

56. Benya, R., Langer, S., and Mobarhan, S., Flexible nasogastric feeding tube tip malposition immediately after placement, *J. Parenter. Enteral Nutr.*, 4, 108, 1990.

57. Lord, L.M. et al., Comparison of weighted vs unweighted enteral feeding tubes for efficacy of transpyloric intubation, *J. Parenter. Enteral Nutr.*, 17, 271, 1993.

58. Kittinger, J.W., Sandler, R.S., and Heizer, W.D., Efficacy of metoclopramide as an adjunct to duodenal placement of small-bore feeding tubes: a randomized, placebo-controlled, double-blind study, *J. Parenter. Enteral Nutr.*, 11, 33, 1987.

59. Zaloga, G.P., Bedside method for placing small bowel feeding tubes in critically ill patients: a prospective study, *Chest*, 100, 1643, 1991.

60. Gutierrez, E.D. and Balfe, D.M., Fluoroscopically guided nasoenteric feeding tube placement: results of a 1-year study, *Radiology*, 178, 759, 1991.

61. Patrick, P.G. et al., Endoscopic nasogastric-jejunal feeding tube placement in critically ill patients, *Gastrointest. Endosc.*, 45, 72, 1997.

62. Hernandez-Socorro, C.R. et al., Bedside sonographic-guided versus blind nasoenteric feeding tube placement in critically ill patients, *Crit. Care Med.*, 24, 1690, 1996.

63. Grant, J.P., Percutaneous endoscopic gastrostomy. Initial placement by single endoscopic technique and long-term follow-up, *Ann. Surg.*, 217, 168, 1993.

64. Ferguson, D.R. et al., Placement of a feeding button ("one-step button") as the initial procedure, *Am. J. Gastroenterol.*, 88, 501, 1993.

65. Wollman, B. et al., Radiologic, endoscopic, and surgical gastrostomy: an institutional evaluation and meta-analysis of the literature, *Radiology*, 197, 699, 1995.

66. Weltz, C.R., Morris, J.B., and Mollen, J.L., Surgical jejunostomy in aspiration risk patients, *Ann. Surg.*, 215, 140, 1992.

67. Ponsky, J.L. et al., Percutaneous approaches to enteral alimentation, *Am. J. Surg.*, 149, 102, 1984.

68. Wolfsen, H.C. et al., Tube dysfunction following percutaneous endoscopic gastrostomy and jejunostomy, *Gastrointest. Endosc.*, 36, 261, 1990.

69. Shike, M. et al., Direct percutaneous endoscopic jejunostomies for enteral feeding, *Gastrointest. Endosc.*, 44, 536, 1996.

70. Tapia, J. et al., Jejunostomy: techniques, indications, and complications, *World J. Surg.*, 23, 596, 1999.

71. Murayama, K.M., Johnson, T.J., and Thompson, J.S., Laparoscopic gastrostomy and jejunostomy are safe and effective for obtaining enteral access, *Am. J. Surg.*, 172, 591, 1996.

15 Parenteral Nutrition

Cynthia Hamilton, Ezra Steiger, and Douglas L. Seidner

CONTENTS

Parenteral nutrition is given safely and effectively due to advances in formulations, intravenous access devices, and their management and ongoing research demonstrating appropriate use of parenteral nutrition (PN) in a variety of disease states. Parenteral nutrition can, however, lead to life-threatening conditions if not properly managed. For most, PN provides a temporary medical treatment during a period of serious illness. For a few, it may become a lifetime medical treatment. Most individuals will do fairly well on lifetime PN with a reasonable life expectancy; however, some individuals may develop significant complications, including sepsis and major organ dysfunction. This chapter will present the important considerations in the safe use of parenteral nutrition in the hospital and alternate site settings.

0-8493-1803-3/05/$0.00+$1.50
© 2005 by CRC Press LLC

INDICATIONS

Parenteral nutrition is indicated for the patient with a nonfunctional or inaccessible gastrointestinal tract. Specific indications include severe malabsorption, short bowel syndrome, bowel obstruction, intestinal ischemia, hyperemesis gravidarum, severe pancreatitis, inability to place a feeding tube and high risk of aspiration.[1]

Although the benefits of nutrition support, including improved nutrition status, seem obvious, nutrition support has the potential for adverse side effects, and some studies have shown increased risks with PN. The Veterans Affairs Total Parenteral Nutrition Cooperative Study, which provided preoperative PN versus intravenous fluid and an ad lib diet to malnourished patients, reported a significant increase in the incidence of major infectious complications.[2] Only patients who were severely malnourished gained benefit from this therapy by having significantly fewer noninfectious complications following surgery. Another study by Brennan et al.[3] evaluated the use of postoperative PN versus intravenous fluid (IVF) in patients undergoing major pancreatic resection. The PN group suffered significantly more major complications and no reduction in length of stay versus the IVF group. Benefits of PN in this study were also limited to severely malnourished patients. These studies illustrate that the routine use of perioperative PN is not indicated in all patients. The American Society for Parenteral and Enteral Nutrition (ASPEN) recommends initiating nutrition support in patients with inadequate oral intake for 7–14 days or in those patients in whom inadequate oral intake is expected over a 7-to-14-day period.[1]

NUTRITION ASSESSMENT

Before initiating PN therapy, a comprehensive nutrition assessment should be performed by a registered dietitian. The rationale, goals, and techniques of nutrition assessment are discussed in Chapter 6.

A nutrition assessment should be done to determine the need for PN and define baseline nutrition status. A periodic reassessment should be performed to document improvement in the nutritional status and efficacy of therapy.

PARENTERAL NUTRITION SOLUTIONS

Parenteral nutrition formulas provide a source of intravenous macronutrients, vitamins, minerals, electrolytes, and fluid, which can be infused via central or peripheral veins. Macronutrients are provided from hypertonic dextrose (up to a 70% solution) as a source of carbohydrate (3.4 kcal/g), protein as crystalline amino acids (up to a 20% solution) (4.0 kcal/g), and lipids as soybean or soybean/safflower oil emulsions (up to a 30% emulsion) (9.0 kcal/g).[4] Typical solutions of macronutrients are shown in Table 15.1. Additional sterile water may be added to PN formulas to help meet individual fluid requirements.

Electrolytes must be added to PN formulas and are commercially available as single or multiple additives. Although general guidelines exist for electrolyte requirements, these should be individualized for each patient considering the disease state and abnormal losses.[5] (See Table 15.2.)

TABLE 15.1
Typical Parenteral Nutrition Formula (70 kg Patient)

	Central 2-1 TPN[a] Gm/kcal	Central 3-1 TPN[b] Gm/kcal	Peripheral TPN Gm/kcal
Dextrose	500/1700	350/1190	150/510
Lipids	–	57/510	132/1190
Amino Acids	100/400	100/400	100/400
Total Fluid Volume	2500 cc	2500 cc	2500 cc
Total Kcals (30 kcal/kg)	2100	2100	2100
Total Nitrogen[c]	16	16	16

[a] 250 ml of 20% lipid emulsion administered 2–3 times/week to prevent essential fatty acid deficiency

[b] 30% of nonprotein kcal as fat

[c] gm protein/6.25 = gm of nitrogen

TABLE 15.2
Daily Electrolyte Requirements for Parenteral Nutrition[5]

Electrolyte	Amount
Sodium	1-2 mEq/kg/day
Potassium	1-2 mEq/kg/day
Chloride	As needed to maintain acid-base balance
Acetate	As needed to maintain acid-base balance
Calcium	11-15 mEq/day
Magnesium	8-20 mEq/day
Phosphorus	20-40 mEq/day

Parenteral vitamins and trace elements are added daily to PN solutions. Recommendations for parenteral vitamins have been recently revised and include an increase of ascorbic acid, folic acid, thiamin, B6, and the addition of Vitamin K.[6] (See Chapter 7.) Trace elements should include: chromium, copper, manganese, zinc, and selenium.[7] (See Chapter 7.)

Medications commonly added to PN formulas include heparin, histamine-2 antagonists, and insulin. Other medications that are occasionally used include metoclopramide, octreotide, corticosteroids, and iron dextran (dextrose/amino acid solutions only).

Macronutrient stability guidelines for lipid emulsion containing PN formulas, or total nutrient admixtures (TNA), should be strictly followed to prevent the fat component from separating from the water in the solution. This instability is referred to as "cracking" and is visible as a creamy or oily layer forming at the top of the container. Infusion of an unstable PN formula can cause fat embolism with serious deleterious effects.[8] Another harmful and potentially life-threatening error in compounding PN formulas is the excessive addition of calcium and phosphorus in an amount that exceeds the solubility product for these minerals.[9]

COMPLICATIONS OF PARENTERAL NUTRITION IN THE HOSPITALIZED PATIENT

Complications associated with PN include metabolic, mechanical, and septic. Hyperglycemia is a common metabolic complication of parenterally fed patients that can be due to a variety of factors, such as stress or sepsis, excess carbohydrate, excess calories, diabetes, steroids, hypokalemia, or chromium depletion. Parenteral nutrition should be initiated at half the estimated energy or approximately 200 g of dextrose for the first 24 hours. The solution can be advanced to full calories once blood sugars and electrolytes are stable. Insulin may be given subcutaneously or added to the PN formula to control hyperglycemia. Jeejeebhoy et al.[10] reported chromium deficiency in a long-term PN patient who demonstrated glucose intolerance, weight loss, and neuropathy, which reversed with supplemental chromium. Chromium deficiency should be considered and extra chromium given when glucose intolerance is unexpected or new in a patient on PN.

Increasing PN lipid calories and decreasing dextrose calories will help control hyperglycemia. The critically ill patient who is stressed or septic may be insulin resistant, and exogenous sources of insulin are frequently necessary to control blood glucose. Blood glucose control has been shown to have an effect on outcome in critically ill patients. A prospective randomized controlled trial of 1548 ICU patients showed significantly reduced ICU deaths, hospital deaths, sepsis, and need for dialysis in patients who received insulin drips to maintain blood glucose between 80 and 110 mg% compared to controls who received insulin drips to maintain blood glucose between 180 and 200 mg%.[11]

Excessive carbohydrate administration can lead to the refeeding syndrome, which occurs in severely malnourished patients who are aggressively administered parenteral (or enteral) nutrition. It is characterized by the rapid shift of several electrolytes, including potassium, phosphorus, and magnesium from the extracellular to intracellular space along with sodium and water retention. This can result in metabolic, neuromuscular, and hematologic abnormalities, which can be life-threatening. Weinser et al.[12] reported two cases of severely malnourished patients who were infused with high-calorie PN (> 80 kcal/kg/day) and developed abnormal cardiopulmonary failure with severe hypophosphatemia. Progressive multiple organ system failure ensued and led to their deaths. Patients with severe malnutrition, significant weight loss, alcoholism, eating disorders, and cancer cachexia are at risk of refeeding syndrome. Nutrition support should be started at 20 kcal/kg and adequate protein (1.2 to 1.5 g/kg/day) and a conservative amount of carbohydrate. Electrolytes and fluid balance should be monitored very closely. Calories are increased to goal over five to seven days.[12]

Hepatobiliary complications may occur during PN administration. (See Chapter 16.) Liver function tests (LFTs) have been shown to increase by two- to threefold in patients after one to three weeks of PN and persists until cessation of PN. Liver biopsies performed in some patients are consistent with hepatic steatosis.[13,14] Lowry et al.[15] correlated excess infusion of carbohydrate and nitrogen with the degree of LFT elevation. The effect of lipid infusions has been studied in patients receiving PN infusions, which supplied 3 g/kg/day of IV fat and was associated with a higher incidence of cholestatic jaundice versus patients receiving 1 g/kg/day of IV lipids.[16,17]

Though the precise etiology of abnormal liver function during PN is unknown, cyclic PN, restriction of carbohydrate and excess lipid, avoidance of overfeeding, and early enteral stimulation may minimize the development of cholestasis, hepatic steatosis, and cholelithiasis. In the adult hospitalized patient, PN can be associated with elevations of alkaline phosphatase and hepatic enzymes, but is usually not associated with an elevated bilirubin.[14]

PARENTERAL NUTRITION IN THE HOME AND ALTERNATE SITES

Patients requiring PN may be candidates for home parenteral nutrition (HPN) or long-term PN at an alternate site such as a subacute unit, extended care facility, rehabilitation facility, or hospice. Parenteral nutrition at an alternate site may be permanent or temporary while a patient undergoes rehabilitation, wound management, or training for HPN procedures prior to discharge. Due to the complex nature of parenteral therapy, a thorough evaluation of the patient's medical condition, the patient or caregiver's level of independence and ability to learn HPN procedures, psychological and social life aspects, and medical insurance coverage is necessary. The evaluation process is best accomplished by a multidisciplinary team of experts including the physician, nurse, dietitian, psychiatrist, social worker, and case manager/discharge planner.[18]

INDICATIONS FOR LONG-TERM PARENTERAL NUTRITION

The diagnosis or indications for HPN are similar to those for hospital PN. The HPN candidate is the patient who cannot, should not, or is unable to eat adequately due to severely diminished bowel function and who no longer requires acute hospitalization.[1] Common diagnoses include inflammatory bowel disease, nonterminal cancer, ischemic bowel, radiation enteritis, motility disorders of the bowel, bowel obstruction, high-output intestinal or pancreatic fistula, celiac disease, hyperemesis gravidarium, and protein-losing enteropathy.[1] Data gathered by the North American Home Parenteral and Enteral Patient Registry (supported by the Oley Foundation and ASPEN) and obtained from Medicare indicate that approximately 19,700 patients were receiving HPN in 1987[20] and in 1992 it was estimated that 40,000 patients were receiving HPN.[21] The most prevalent diagnoses for HPN were cancer and Crohn's disease. (See Table 15.3.)

Home PN may be provided as short-term or long-term treatment. Short-term PN is most commonly used in surgical patients with a prolonged postoperative ileus

TABLE 15.3
Diagnoses of HPN Patients in North America[30]

Diagnosis	Distribution (%)
Neoplasm	28.5
Crohn's disease	17.1
Ischemic bowel	10.6
Motility disorders	8.4
Neurological disorder (swallow)	0.4
Radiation enteritis	4.3
Congenital bowel defect	3.8
Chronic adhesive obstruction	2.7
AIDS	3.1
Other	21.1

who are waiting for return of bowel function and patients with enterocutaneous fistula or temporary jejunostomy created to divert fecal stream from injured or diseased bowel who will undergo corrective surgery in the near future.[22] Oral nutrition is expected to be resumed in these patients in a few weeks to months.

Long-term PN may be required for patients following extensive intestinal resection or when intestinal disease does not permit the adequate intake or absorption of nutrients. Conditions include short bowel syndrome secondary to Crohn's disease, massive small bowel resection due to mesenteric infarction or volvulus, radiation enteritis, intestinal pseudo-obstruction, and adhesive bowel obstruction. Parenteral nutrition for these patients is often lifelong.

EVALUATION PROCESS FOR HOME PARENTERAL NUTRITION

The evaluation process for HPN begins with a physician's review of the patient's medical condition and determination that the GI tract is inadequate to maintain adequate nutrition or hydration. In addition, patients must be medically stable and able to perform all tasks necessary (or have a designated caregiver), and have a reasonable life expectancy and quality of life.[23]

PSYCHOSOCIAL EVALUATION

While a patient's medical diagnosis may indicate the need for HPN, a psychosocial evaluation is important to help determine if a patient is capable of managing this complex therapy at home. A psychiatrist and/or social worker evaluation determines mental, emotional, and cognitive abilities as well as home safety issues. Home PN has a significant impact on the patient and caregiver's lifestyle and affects patients and their families differently. The support of family, friends, religion, or community resources are necessary for successful HPN therapy. Patients on HPN may experience reduced physical strength, sleep deprivation, depression, anger, anxiety, loss of identity, loss of employment, reduced social interactions, and loss of friends.[24-27] Smith et al.[28] found HPN patients who were affiliated with a national patient education and support organization compared with those not affiliated had higher quality of life scores, less incidence of depression, and decreased incidence of catheter line sepsis.

Though no specific tool for measuring quality of life in HPN patients has been developed, two popular tools are the Short Form Profile Questionnaire 36 and the EuroQuol index. Patient responses will vary with the clinical circumstances, which lead to the need for HPN therapy. A sudden illness such as a massive bowel resection will cause a dramatic change in lifestyle and loss of quality of life compared with the patient with chronic intestinal failure who has experienced several bowel resections and bouts of dehydration and diarrhea.[29] Parenteral nutrition may provide caloric and fluid support, which may improve quality of life in this situation. It is important for health-care workers not to focus solely on physiologic problems but to also understand the psychosocial impact of HPN therapy.

EVALUATION AND PLACEMENT OF VENOUS ACCESS DEVICES

Obtaining long-term safe venous access is essential to the success of HPN. Vascular access-related problems and sepsis are major causes of rehospitalization in the HPN patient.[30] Appropriate placement, proper care, and management of vascular access devices (VAD) are mandatory to prevent complications.[31]

Commonly used VADs include implantable ports, tunneled central venous catheters such as the Hickman or Broviac, and peripherally inserted central catheters (PICCs). (See Table 15.4.) The selection of the VAD depends on several factors, such as patient preference, length of therapy, ability of the patient/caregiver to manage or care for the device, and the availability of central venous access sites for cannulation.[32] Common sites include the sublcavian, external and internal jugular

TABLE 15.4
Vascular Access Devices (VAD) used for Long-term PN[32-35]

Type	Description	Use
Implanted port	Placed under skin Requires frequent needle sticks	Long-term
Tunneled central venous catheter (Hickman, Broviac)	External device on chest wall Available with multilumens	Long-term
Peripherally inserted central catheter (PICC)	May be placed by specially trained RN Increased risk of catheter malposition and dysfunction	Short-term (less than 2 months)

veins, and less common sites such as the cephalic, saphenous, and femoral veins. A skilled surgeon or interventional radiologist with an understanding of the needs of an HPN patient is important in choosing the best access routes. Translumbar placement of vascular access devices by an experienced interventional radiologist is used when other sites are not accessible. Before catheter placement, the catheter exit site or port site should be marked at a place where the patient can readily see and care for the device.[31]

FORMULA STABILIZATION

Important to evaluating and preparing the patient for HPN is establishing a formula that meets the patient's needs for macro- and micronutrients. A nutrition assessment will help establish the caloric and protein needs of nutrition support. Calorie and protein needs may change over the course of HPN due to changes in disease, illness, or physical activity. In our experience, HPN patients required 42.3 kcal/kg and 1.8 g of amino acids/kg daily to improve nutritional status, including increased body weight and serum transferrin.[36] A goal weight should be determined with the patient and the calories of the PN solution adjusted accordingly. Any special conditions such as extraordinary fluid losses from ostomies and fistulas should be considered with appropriate fluid adjustments made of the PN solution. Trace element blood studies should be drawn for chromium, copper, manganese, selenium, and zinc with adjustments made in the PN solution. Once the fluid, electrolytes, calorie, and protein requirements are determined, cycling of the daily infusion in a stepwise fashion should begin. Infusion of HPN for only part of the day provides both metabolic and psychological benefits. A period "free" from carbohydrate infusion allows the liver to mobilize stored glycogen and may decrease the incidence of fatty liver and promote better nitrogen retention.[37,38] Allowing the patient a period of time off the PN infusion also permits a more normal lifestyle.

When cycling PN solutions it is important to proceed slowly by decreasing the infusion time by 4-hour increments over several days until the desired infusion cycle is reached (usually a 12-hour overnight cycle). The patient's ability to handle the dextrose load determines how rapidly the infusion times can be decreased. Blood sugars are maintained below 150 mg% by adding insulin or reducing dextrose calories. Tapering down the last hour of PN is done to prevent rebound hypoglycemia and in some cases tapering up over the first one or two hours may be necessary to prevent hyperglycemia. Patients should be carefully assessed during cycling for tolerance of fluid volume as well.[19]

PATIENT EDUCATION

Patient and caregiver teaching should be initiated as soon as possible. The estimated time to learn all HPN procedures varies from a few days to several weeks. Home PN teaching begins in the hospital and is generally completed in the patient's home by a homecare clinician. Home PN education should include catheter care, operation of the infusion pump, PN setup and disconnection, maintenance of intake and output records, and review of metabolic complications.[18] A variety of educational tools are used, including videos, mannequins, or vests with VADs and illustrated manuals. A study by Smith et al.[39] using interactive education materials in HPN patients showed reduced complications, including catheter-related bloodstream infections (CRBSI), reactive depression, and improved ability to problem-solve with professionals. Once the patient or caregiver has demonstrated competence in all areas of HPN patient care and monitoring, homecare visits can be decreased or discontinued.

REIMBURSEMENT

The monetary cost of HPN, while less expensive than hospital care, is still high, leading to insurance coverage and reimbursement concerns.[40] Government agencies, Medicare, and Medicaid reimburse for HPN but have explicit criteria for reimbursement. Medicare requires permanence (> 90 days therapy) and specific documentation of GI failure.[41] (See Table 15.5.) Medicaid reimbursement varies from state to state.[42]

TABLE 15.5
Medicare Guidelines for Home Parenteral Nutrition[41]

Criteria	Documentation
Massive small bowel resection	Operative report
< 5 ft of SB beyond ligament of Treitz	X-ray report
	Physician letter documenting condition and need for PN
Short bowel syndrome	
– GI losses exceed oral intake by 50%	Same as above
– urine output < 1 liter	
Bowel rest for 3 months	Same as above
– symptomatic pancreatitis	
– regional enteritis exacerabation	
– proximal enterocutaneous fistula and cannot tube feed distal to the fistula	
Mechanical bowel obstruction	Same as above
– inoperable	
Severe malnutrition with weight loss ≥10%	Nutrition Assessment report by physician or RD
Serum albumin ≤ 3.4 gm/dL	
– severe fat malabsorption	Fecal fat test report
– motility disturbance unresponsive to prokinetics	Gastric empty study or barium x-ray report
Other	
– unable to maintain weight and strength after:	Nutrition assessment report
– diet modification	Results of tests/studies
– pharmacologic interventions	List of medications
– enteral feeding (failed)	

Private medical insurance plans vary greatly and need to be carefully reviewed by a case manager or hospital discharge planner during the HPN therapy evaluation process.

DISCHARGE

The patient is ready for discharge on HPN once all documentation for insurance coverage has been provided, all other medical issues have been resolved (i.e., pain, antibiotic therapy), the patient has been evaluated as safe and emotionally competent for discharge, the permanent VAD has been placed, the PN formula has been cycled, serum electrolytes are stable, and the education process of HPN procedures has been initiated. (See Figure 15.1.) It is important to provide 24-hour/day contact phone numbers of available clinicians so when problems arise they can quickly be resolved. In addition, information on available support groups such as the Oley Foundation (800-776-OLEY, www.oley.org) and local contacts should be provided and can be most helpful to patients.

MONITORING AND MANAGEMENT OF COMPLICATIONS

Patients discharged on PN require monitoring on a regular basis to determine the effectiveness and appropriateness of therapy, ensure that nutritional goals are met and reduce the associated risks of PN. (See Table 15.6)[43] Complications associated with long-term HPN therapy include metabolic; nutrient deficiencies such as essen-

New Home TPN Patient
Preparing for Initial Discharge of Cleveland Clinic Foundation Patient

Staff Approval
↓
Order Consults:
Case Manager
Social Work
Psychiatry
Nutrition Support Vascular Access RN
Notify: Home TPN Clinician
↓
Arrange Permanent Venous Access
↓
Order Trace Elements- "serum Chromium, Copper, Selenium, Zinc,
whole blood Manganese "and "Phospholipid Fatty Acids"
↓
Stabilize Formula (electrolytes, blood sugar, fluid)
↓
Cycle Formula (goal 12 hours)
↓
Address Other Medical Issues (i.e.-meds, pain, anticoagulation)

FIGURE 15.1 Home parenteral nutrition algorithm

TABLE 15.6
Home Parenteral Nutrition Monitoring

	Daily	Weekly	Monthly	Every 6 Months
Clinical				
Intake/output	X			
Temperature	X			
Weight	X			
Urinary or blood sugar	X			
Laboratory				
Electrolytes		X	X	
BUN/Cr		X	X	
Ca, PO4,Mg		X	X	
Liver Function Tests			X	
Hgb/Hct, WBC			X	
INR			X	
Special studies				
DXA scan				Every 1–2 years
24-hour urine for Ca, Mg				X
Trace elements				X
Essential fatty acids*				X

* When fat emulsion only given 1–2x per week

tial fatty acids (EFA), trace elements; catheter-related; liver failure; and metabolic bone disease.

Metabolic complications are frequently related to fluid loss from the gastrointestinal tract or associated renal and liver disease. Patients should be taught to keep daily records of their weight, temperature, gastrointestinal losses (ostomy, fistula, diarrhea, drains), urine output, and oral intake. Major changes in these parameters may necessitate prompt medical intervention and alteration of the PN formula. (See Table 15.7.) Essential fatty acid deficiency (EFAD) can occur within days to weeks of starting PN when there is an inadequate supply of EFA. Symptoms of EFAD include dermatitis, hepatic steatosis, hemolytic anemia, and immune system compromise.[44] HPN patients not receiving IV lipids have shown significantly lower plasma levels of linoleic and linolenic acids compared to controls.[44] Supplying 500 ml of 20% IV lipids once a week was sufficient to return plasma EFA levels to normal. Case reports of trace element deficiencies have been published in the literature in long-term PN patients.[10,45,46] In addition, manganese toxicity leading to neurodysfunction has been reported.[47,48] Trace element recommendations for HPN patients include chromium, copper, manganese, zinc, and selenium.[7] Trace element levels should be checked at baseline, and every three to six months thereafter. Individual trace element additives may be required to maintain normal trace element levels.[49] Clinicians should be aware of the physical signs of vitamin and trace element abnormalities. (See Chapters 6 and 7.)

TABLE 15.7
Patient Guide to Contact Home Parenteral Nutrition Clinician

Symptom	Action Patient Should Take
Catheter breaks, cracks or leaks	Clamp catheter above problem area. Call HPN clinician to arrange repair.
Catheter has withdrawal/infusion/occlusion	Call HPN clinician to arrange for catheter restoration.
Fever, chills with PN infusion	Stop PN, immediately call HPN clinician or go to emergency room for hospital admission.
Drainage, pus, tenderness, redness at catheter exit site or along catheter tract	Call HPN clinician for proper treatment.
Chest pain, shortness of breath, loss of consiousness	Clamp catheter, call 911, lay on left side.
Pump malfunction	Check electrical source, battery. Call HPN clinician or homecare pump provider for repair/replacement.
Elevated glucose in urine or blood	Call HPN clinician for adjustment of PN infusion rate or insulin.
Low blood glucose with sweating, headache, shakiness, blurred vision	Drink juice, cola beverage or sugar water if permitted to take fluid. If oral fluid restricted take hard candy or glucose gel. Call HPN clinician for adjustment of PN infusion rate or insulin.
Increased thirst, decreased urine output Increased ostomy output, muscle cramps	Call HPN clinician with intake/output record and adjustment of PN fluid volume or additional IV hydration fluids.
Rapid weight gain, swelling of hands, feet, ankles, short of breath	Call HPN clinician for adjustment of PN fluid volume.

CATHETER-RELATED COMPLICATIONS

One of the most common and serious complications of HPN is catheter-related blood stream infections (CRBSI). This complication can lead to septic shock, endocarditis, osteomyelitis, and septic phlebitis.[50] In one large HPN experience, catheter-related sepsis was a cause of death in approximately 20% of patients who died on HPN.[51]

Guidelines have been established for the prevention of intravascular catheter-related infections and reflect the concensus of the Healthcare Infection Control Practices Advisory Committee (HICPAC) of the Centers for Disease Control and Prevention (CDC).[52] Patients presenting with fever, shaking chills, and malaise should be immediately evaluated for CRBSI. (See Figure 15.2.) Diagnostic techniques include qualitative or quantitative blood cultures or endoluminal brush technique. Greater microbe counts from the catheter versus the peripheral blood sample in the absence of another source of infection (i.e., urinary tract infection, wound, pneumonia) are indicative of CRBSI and require treatment with long-term intravenous antibiotics. Catheter removal is necessary when the patient is unstable or the infection persists while on antibiotics or is due to fungus.[53]

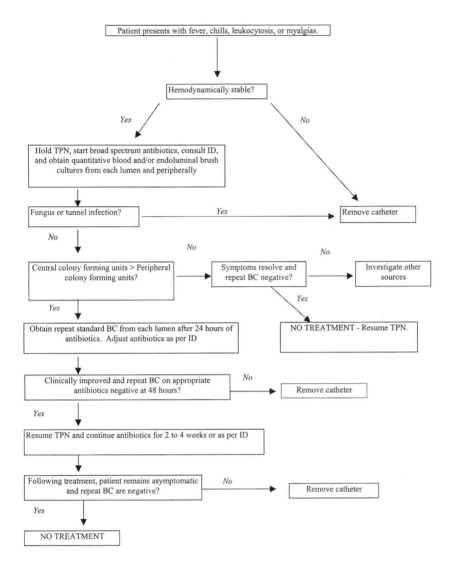

FIGURE 15.2 Algorithm for evaluation and treatment of long-term central venous access device for suspected CRBSI

Exit site infections present with drainage or redness at the catheter exit site and can usually be treated by increasing the frequency of the dressing change and the use of short-term oral or intravenous antibiotics as long as the Dacron velour cuff is not involved.[54] Subcutaneous tract or pocket infections present with local inflammation, tenderness, and purulent drainage. This type of infection generally requires removal of the catheter and treatment with systemic antibiotics.[54] (See Figure 15.3.)

Catheter occlusions associated with resistance when flushing or aspirating the catheter can be caused by a kinked or pinched catheter, retained suture, catheter clamp, or fibrin material formed at the catheter tip. A chest x-ray will help diagnose

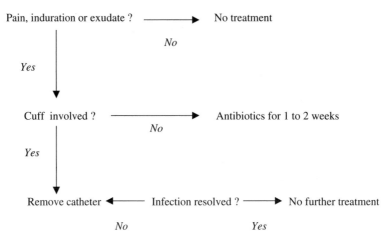

FIGURE 15.3 Algorithm for evaluation of long-term central venous access device exit site infection

a kinked or pinched catheter. Catheters occluded secondary to fibrin formation require flushing with saline or a clot dissolving agent such as tissue plasminogen activator (tPA), which can help restore catheter patency.[54]

LIVER DISEASE

Hepatic steatosis or fatty liver may occur with PN and is reversible with discontinuation of PN or alterations of the PN prescription for factors, which may contribute to liver abnormalities as previously described.[13–17] However, chronic irreversible cholestatic liver disease associated with long-term PN can lead to liver failure or even death. Significant alterations of hepatic enzymes and LFTs require evaluation to help determine the cause of liver abnormalities.

The prevalence of liver disease in long-term PN is not known but has been reported to range from 65% to 87%.[55,56] Prevention and treatment of hepatic failure in the long-term PN patient includes avoidance of carbohydrate and lipid overfeeding, cycling the PN, prevention of EFAD, and avoidance of medications known to cause liver abnormalities.[57] Metronidazole and ursodeoxicholic acid has been used in patients with PN-associated cholestasis; however, the long-term impact on liver disease is unknown.[57]

An association has been shown between plasma-free choline concentrations and hepatic steatosis in patients receiving PN.[58] Parenteral nutrition supplemented with choline has been shown to reverse hepatic steatosis and improve liver enzyme abnormalities.[59]

METABOLIC BONE DISEASE

Metabolic bone disease (MBD) is a condition of reduced total bone mass characterized by an increase in the ratio of bone resorption to bone formation. There may be normal bone mineral to bone matrix (osteoporosis) or excessive bone matrix without adequate calcification (osteomalacia). These two forms of MBD are characterized by bone or back pain, fractures with minimal or no trauma, loss of height, and evidence of low bone mineral density by dual-energy x-ray absorptiometry (DXA).[60]

Prevalence of MBD has been reported between 42 and 100%.[61,62] Several factors contributing to the development of MBD in long-term PN include inadequate provision of calcium and phosphorus,[63,64] excess amounts of amino acids,[65] excess Vitamin D,[66] and metabolic acidosis.[67] Most of these factors lead to increased urinary calcium loss. Glucocorticoids used in the treatment of inflammatory bowel diseases have also been shown to contribute to abnormal bone metabolism.[68] Early PN solutions made with casein hydrolysates contained large amounts of aluminum, which led to osteomalacia.[69–73] Parenteral solutions are now made from crystalline amino acids and contain significantly less aluminum.

Treatment of MBD in patients on long-term PN is multimodal. In patients who received HPN greater than one year with low bone mineral density given a bisphosphonate to decrease bone resorption, demonstrated increased bone mineral density in the forearm, spine, and hips.[74] Recent advances in the development of parathyroid hormone analog demonstrated significantly increased bone mineral density in postmenopausal women.[75] Its use in HPN patients with MBD has not as yet been studied.

Measures that may be used to prevent or treat MBD are to add adequate amounts of calcium, phosphorus, and magnesium; to give amino acids in the lowest dose necessary to maintain adequate protein status; and to maintain normal CO2 levels with acetate additives to prevent metabolic acidosis. A 24-hour urine for calcium and magnesium should be checked when the patient is on a stable formula to make sure normal amounts of these minerals are being excreted. Low volumes indicate an insufficient parenteral dose. A bone mineral density or DXA study should be performed and evidence of low bone mineral density should prompt review of the PN solution and a referral to an endocrinologist for treatment.[76]

TRANSITIONING NUTRITION SUPPORT

Patients may be transitioned from PN to oral or enteral nutrition or IVF once the GI tract has regained partial or full functional capacity. The patient transitioning from PN to oral intake should demonstrate sufficient calorie and fluid intake, maintenance of stable weight, adequate urine output, and stable blood electrolytes. Intake and output records, calorie counts, and blood chemistries can be used to help determine discontinuation of the PN.

The patient who has a functional GI tract but cannot take oral nutrition is a candidate for enteral nutrition. A gastric or small bowel feeding tube is placed, and standard polymeric formulas are used for full digestion and absorption capacity and hydrolyzed formulas for impaired absorptive capacity of the GI tract. The enteral formula is begun at a slow rate of 25 to 50 cc/hr and advanced to meet full caloric support as tolerance is demonstrated. The PN is concomitantly decreased as the enteral formula is increased.

Some patients may demonstrate the ability to absorb nutrients but not adequate fluids. Intravenous fluids may be needed daily to prevent dehydration or replace losses from fistulas or ostomies. These patients may benefit from a thorough evaluation of the GI tract with potential for intestinal rehabilitation. Adjustment of the diet, oral fluids, and bowel medications may be of further help in reducing the need for daily IVFs.

CONCLUSION

Parenteral nutrition can provide all of a patient's known nutrient requirements for days, months, or years at a time. Its safe use requires an in-depth knowledge of macro and micronutrient needs and carefully monitoring the patient at periodic intervals. An important element in the safe application of PN to patient care is maintaining prolonged and safe vascular access. A multidisciplinary team of physicians, dietitians, pharmacists, nurses, and other clinicians are important to assure the success of any PN program and minimize costs.[77,78]

REFERENCES

1. ASPEN Board of Directors, Guidelines for the use of parenteral and enteral nutrition in adult and pediatric patients, *J. Parenter. Enteral. Nutr.*, 26, 18SA, 2002.
2. The Veterans Affairs Total Parenteral Nutrition Cooperative Study Group, Perioperative total parenteral nutrition in surgical patients, *N. Engl. J. Med.*, 325(8), 525, 1991.
3. Brennan, M.F. et al., A prospective randomized trial of total parenteral nutrition after major pancreatic resection for malignancy, *Ann. Surg.*, 220(4), 436, 1994.
4. Mirtallo, J.M., Parenteral formulas, in *Clinical Nutrition, Parenteral Nutrition*, 3rd ed., Rombeau, J.L. and Rolandelli, R.H., Eds., W.B. Saunders Company, Philadelphia, 2001, 118–139.
5. ASPEN Board of Directors, Guidelines for the use of parenteral and enteral nutrition in adult and pediatric patients, *J. Parenter. Enteral Nutr.* 26, 22SA, 2002.
6. Food and Drug Administration, Parenteral Multivitamin Products; Drugs for Human Use; Drug Efficacy Study Implementation; Amendment: Federal Register, April 20, 65(77), 21200, 2000.
7. ASPEN Board of Directors, Guidelines for the use of parenteral and enteral nutrition in adult and pediatric patients, *J. Parenter. Enteral Nutr.*, 26, 23SA, 2002.
8. Barber, J.R., Miller, S.J., and Sacks, G.S., Parenteral feeding formulations, in *The Science and Practice of Nutrition Support,* Gottschlich, M.M., Ed., Kendall/Hunt Publishing Company, Dubuque, 2001, 251–268.
9. National Advisory Group on Standards and Practice Guidelines for Parenteral Nutrition, ASPEN Board of Directors, Safe practices for parenteral nutrition formulations, *J. Parenter. Enteral Nutr.*, 22(2), 49, 1998.
10. Jeejeebhoy, K.N. et al., Chromium deficiency, glucose intolerance, and neuropathy reversed by chromium supplementation, a patient receiving long-term parenteral nutrition, *Am. J. Clin. Nutr.*, 30, 531, 1997.
11. Van Den Berghe, G. et al., Intensive insulin therapy in critically ill patients, *N. Engl. J. Med.*, 345(19), 1359, 2001.

12. Weinser, R.L. and Krumdieck, C.L., Death resulting from overzealous total parenteral nutrition: the refeeding syndrome revisited, *Am. J. Clin. Nutr.*, 34, 393, 1980.
13. Grant, J.P. et al., Serum hepatic enzyme and bilirubin elevations during parenteral nutrition, *Surg. Gynecol. Obstet.*, 145, 573, 1977.
14. Lindor, K.D. et al., Liver function values in adults receiving total parenteral nutrition, *J.A.M.A.*, 241(22), 2398, 1979.
15. Lowry, S.F. and Brennan, M.F., Abnormal liver function during parenteral nutrition. Relation to infusion excess, *J. Surg. Res.*, 26, 300, 1979.
16. Salvian, A.J. and Allardyce, D.B., Impaired bilirubin secretion during TPN, *J. Surg. Res*, 28, 547, 1980.
17. Allardyce, D.B., Cholestasis caused by lipid emulsions, *Surg. Gynecol. Obstet.*, 154, 641, 1982.
18. Hamilton, C. et al., Home nutrition support, in *The Cleveland Clinic Foundation Nutrition Support Handbook*, Parekh, N. and DeChicco, R.L., Eds., The Cleveland Clinic Foundation, Cleveland, OH, 2004.
19. Hammond, K.A., Szeszycki, E., and Pfister, D., Transitioning to home and other alternate sites, in *The Science and Practice of Nutrition Support, A Case-Based Core Curriculum,* Gottschlich, M.M., Ed., the American Society for Parenteral and Enteral Nutrition, Kendall/Hunt Publishing Company, Dubuque, IA, 2001, 701–729.
20. The Oley Foundation, North American Home Parenteral and Enteral Nutrition: Patient Registry. Annual Report with Outcome Profiles 1985–1992. American Society for Parenteral and Enteral Nutrition, Silver Springs, MD, 1994.
21. Howard, L. et al., Current use and clinical outcome of home parenteral and enteral nutrition therapies in the United States, *Gastroenter.*, 109, 355, 1995.
22. Oakley, J.R. et al., Catastrophic enterocutaneous fistulae: The role of home hyperalimentation, *Cleveland Clinic Quart.*, 46(4), 136, 1979.
23. Barrera, R., Nutritional support in cancer patients, *J. Parenter. Enteral Nutr.*, 26(5), S63, 2002.
24. Gulledge, A.D. et al., Psychosocial issues of home parenteral and enteral nutrition, *Nutr. Clin. Prac.*, 2 (5), 183, 1987.
25. Jeppesen, P.B., Landholz, E., and Mortensen, P.B., Quality of life in patients receiving home parenteral nutrition, *Gut*, 44, 844, 1989.
26. Smith, C.E., Quality of life in long-term total parenteral nutrition patients and their family caregivers, *J. Parenter. Enteral Nutr.*, 17(6), 501, 1993.
27. Malone, M., Longitudinal assessment of outcome, health status, and changes in lifestyle associated with long-term home parenteral and enteral nutrition, *J. Parenter. Enteral Nutr.,* 26(3), 164, 2002.
28. Smith, C.E. et al., Home parenteral nutrition: Does affiliation with a national support and educational organization improve patient outcomes? *J. Parenter. Enteral Nutr.*, 26(3),159, 2002.
29. Howard, L.J., Length of life and quality of life on home parenteral nutrition, *J. Parenter. Enteral Nutr.*, 26(5), S55, 2002.
30. Oasis Annual Report, Home Nutrition Support, Patient Registry, Oley Foundation/ASPEN, 1989.
31. Steiger, E., Obtaining and maintaining vascular access in the home parenteral nutrition patient, *J. Parenter. Enteral Nutr.*, 26(5), S17, 2002.
32. Orr, M.E., Vascular access device selection for parenteral nutrition, *Nutr. Clin. Prac.*, 14(4), 172, 1999.
33. Tokars, J.I. et al., Prospective evaluation of risk factors for bloodstream infection in patients receiving home infusion therapy, *Ann. Int. Med.*, 131(5), 340, 1999.

34. Duerksen, D.R. et al., Peripherally inserted catheters for parenteral nutiriton: A comparison with centrally inserted catheters, *J. Parenter. Enteral Nutr.,* 23(2), 85, 1999.

35. Moureau, N. et al., Central venous catheters in home infusion care: outcomes analysis in 50,470 patients, *J. Vasc. Interv. Radiol.,* 13, 1009, 2002.

36. Matarese, L.E. et al., Body composition changes in cachetic patients receiving home parenteral nutrition, *J. Parenter. Enteral Nutr.,* 26(6),366, 2002.

37. Maini, B. et al., Cyclic hyperalimentation: An optimal technique for preservation of visceral protein, *J. Surg. Res.,* 20, 515, 1976.

38. Matuchansky, C. et al., Cyclic (nocturnal) total parenteral nutrition in hospitalized adult patients with severe digestive diseases, *Gastroenter.,* 81, 433, 1981.

39. Smith, C.E. et al., Clinical trial of interactive and videotaped educational interventions reduce infection, reactive depression, and rehospitalization for sepsis in patients on home parenteral nutrition, *J. Parenter. Enteral Nutr.* 27(2), 137, 2003.

40. Wateska, L.P., Sattler, L.L., and Steiger, E., Costs of a home parenteral nutrition program, *J.A.M.A.,* 244(20), 2303, 1980.

41. Palmetto Government Benefits Administrators, LLC. Region C Durable Medical Equipment Regional Carrier Supplier Manual Autumn/1998. Chapter 63: General Parenteral and Enteral Nutrition Therapy, 63:1–5.

42. Reddy, P. and Malone, M., Cost and outcomes analysis of home parenteral and enteral nutrition, *J. Parenter. Enteral Nutr.,* 22, 302, 1998.

43. ASPEN Board of Directors, Standards for Home Nutrition Support, *Nutr. Clin. Prac.,* 14(3), 151, 1999.

44. Jeppesen, P.B., Hoy, C., and Mortensen, P.B., Essential fatty deficiency in patients receiving home parenteral nutrition, *Am. J. Clin. Nutr.,* 68, 126, 1998.

45. Fleming, C.R. et al., Selenium deficiency and fatal cardiomyopathy in a patient on home parenteral nutrition, *Gastroenter.,* 83, 689, 1982.

46. VanRij, A.M. et al., Selenium deficiency in total parenteral nutrition, *Am. J. Clin. Nutr.,* 32, 2076, 1979.

47. Masumoto, K. et al., Manganese intoxication during intermittent parenteral nutrition: report of two cases, *J. Parenter. Enteral Nutr.,* 25(2), 95, 2001.

48. Takagi, Y. et al., On-off study of manganese administration to adult patients undergoing home parenteral nutrition:new indices of *in vivo* manganese level, *J. Parenter. Enteral Nutr.,* 25(2), 87, 2001.

49. Kelly, D.G., Guidelines and available products for parenteral vitamins and trace elements, *J. Parenter. Enteral Nutr.,* 26(5), S34, 2002.

50. Krzywda, E.A., Andris, D.A., and Edmiston, C.E., Catheter infections: Diagnosis, etiology, treatment, and prevention, *Nutr. Clin. Prac.,* 14(4),178, 1999.

51. Scolapio, J.S. et al., Survival of home parenteral nutrition-treated patients: 20 years of experience at the Mayo Clinic, *Mayo Clin. Proc.,* 74, 217, 1999.

52. O'Grady, N.P. et al., Guidelines for the prevention of intravascular catheter-related infections, *Federal Registry,* August 9, 1, 2002.

53. Raad, I.I. and Hanna, H.A., Intravascular catheter-related infections, *Arch. Intern. Med.,* 162, 871, 2002.

54. Grant, J., Recognition, prevention, and treatment of home total parenteral nutrition central venous access complications, *J. Parenter. Enteral Nutr.,* 26(5), S21, 2002.

55. Cavicchi, M. et al., Prevalence of liver disease and contributing factors in patients receiving home parenteral nutrition for permanent intestinal failure, *Ann. Intern. Med.,* 132, 525, 2000.

56. Seidner, D.L. et al., Liver failure is uncommon in adults on home TPN, *J. Parenter. Enteral Nutr.*, 27(1), S3 abstract, 2003.

57. Buchman, A., Total parenteral nutrition-associated liver disease, *J. Parenter. Enteral Nutr.,* 26(5), S43, 2002.

58. Buchman, A.L. et al., Choline deficiency: A cause of hepatic steatosis associated with parenteral nutrition that can be reversed with an intravenous choline chloride supplementation, *Hepatology,* 22, 1399, 1995.

59. Buchman, A.L. et al., Choline deficiency causes reversible hepatic abnormalities in patients receiving parenteral nutrition: proof of a human choline requirement: a placebo-controlled trial, *J. Parenter. Enteral Nutr.*, 25(5), 260, 2001.

60. Lipkin, E.W., Metabolic bone disease, in *Parenteral Nutrition,* 3rd ed., Rombeau, J.L. and Rolandelli, R.H., Eds., W.B. Saunders, New York, 2001, 157–171.

61. Hurley, D.L. and McMahon, M.M., Long-term parenteral nutrition and metabolic bone disease, *Endocrinol. Metab. Clin. N.A.*, 19, 113, 1990.

62. Pironi, L. et al., Prevalence of bone disease in patients on home parenteral nutrition, *Clin. Nutr.*, 21, 289, 2002.

63. Sloan, G.M., White, D.E., and Brennan, M.F., Calcium and phosphorus metabolism during total parenteral nutrition, *Ann. Surg.*, 197, 1, 1983.

64. Wood, R.J. et al., Reduction of total parenteral nutrition-induced urinary calcium loss by increasing the phosphorus in the total parenteral nutrition prescription, *J. Parenter. Enteral Nutr.*, 10, 188, 1986.

65. Bengoa, J.M. et al., Amino acid induced hypercalciuria in patients on total parenteral nutrition, *Am. J. Clin. Nutr.*, 38, 264, 1983.

66. Verhage, A.H., Cheong, W.K., Allard, J. et al., Increase in lumbar spine bone mineral content in patients on long-term parenteral nutrition with Vitamin D supplementation, *J. Parenter. Enteral Nutr.*, 19, 431, 1995.

67. Karton, M.A. et al., D-lactate and metabolic bone disease in patients receiving long-term parenteral nutrition, *J. Parenter. Enteral Nutr.*, 13, 132, 1989.

68. Abitbol, V. et al., Metabolic bone assessment in patients with inflammatory bowel disease, *Gastroenterology,* 108, 417, 1995.

69. Klein, G.L. et al., Bone disease associated with total parenteral nutrition, *Lancet*, 2, 1041, 1980.

70. Klein, G.L. et al., Aluminum loading during total parenteral nutrition, *Am. J. Clin. Nutr.*, 35, 1425, 1982.

71. Vargas, J.H. et al., Metabolic bone disease of total parenteral nutrition: course after changing from casein to amino acids in parenteral solutions with reduced aluminum content, *Am. J. Clin. Nutr.*, 48, 1070, 1988.

72. Lidor, C. et al., Successful high-dose calcium treatment of aluminum-induced metabolic bone disease in long-term home parenteral nutrition, *J. Parenter. Enteral Nutr.,* 15, 202, 1991.

73. Lipkin, E.W., Ott, S.M., and Klein, G.L., Heterogeneity of bone histology in parenteral nutrition patient, *Am. J. Clin. Nutr.,* 46, 673, 1987.

74. Haderslev, K.V. et al., Effect of cyclical intravenous clodronate therapy on bone mineral density markers of bone turnover in patients receiving home parenteral nutrition, *Am. J. Clin. Nutr.*, 76, 482, 2002.

75. Neer, R.M. et al., Effect of parathyroid hormone (1-34) on fractures and bone mineral density in postmenopausal women with osteoporosis, *N. Engl. J. Med.*, 344, 1434, 2001.

76. Hamilton, C., Parenteral nutrition-associated metabolic bone disease, *Support Line,* 25(5), 7, 2003.

77. Fisher, G.G. and Opper, F.H., An interdisciplinary nutrition support team improves quality of care in a teaching hospital, *J.A.D.A.*, 96, 176, 1996.

78. Ochoa, J.B. et al., Long-term reduction in the cost of nutritional intervention achieved by a nutrition support service, *Nutr. Clin. Prac.,* 15, 174, 2000.

16 PN-Associated Hepatobiliary and Renal Disease

Alan L. Buchman

CONTENTS

Although several of the components of PN were developed in the 1940s and 1950s, it was not until the early 1970s that a significant number of patients began to receive long-term PN that consisted of solutions containing dextrose, amino acids, lipid, and electrolytes. This therapy became a lifesaving modality for patients with insufficient intestinal absorptive surface area or impaired intestinal motility, sufficient to cause *intestinal failure*. This therapy allowed patients who would previously have died from the sequella of malnutrition live nearly as long as those with normally functioning intestines. However, the association of PN use and numerous complications was reported. One of the earliest described complications was liver disease.

THE PREVALENCE AND CLINICAL SIGNIFICANCE OF PN-ASSOCIATED LIVER DISEASE

The development of PN-associated cholestasis was initially described in an infant in 1971.[1] Another early report described an elevation in serum hepatic aminotransferase concentrations that developed within 10–14 days of beginning PN.[2] Robertson et al. reported that 88.5% of 26 adult patients with normal pre-PN serum aspartate aminotransferase (AST) and alanine aminotransferase (ALT) developed elevations in both during PN, although the serum bilirubin concentration remained normal.[3] There was a gradual rise in both AST and ALT, with peak at week four followed by a gradual decline back to baseline. Serum alkaline phosphatase became elevated as well, although PN-associated metabolic bone disease could have accounted for this observation.[4] Other studies described the incidence of liver enzyme abnormalities to occur between 25 and 100%.[5] Often heterogenous patient populations were included such as postoperative patients, patients with burns, malignancies, and inflammatory bowel disease, making the association with PN directly often tenuous at best. Many of these retrospective observations were made at a time when patients were routinely provided with 45–50 kcal/kg/day or more. Dextrose overfeeding may cause significant liver abnormalities, namely steatosis.[6] In addition, elevations in serum hepatic aminotransferase concentrations are both nonspecific and insensitive indicators of hepatic pathology during PN,[7] although more recent studies have indicated the AST begins to increase more significantly after 10 weeks of PN; the total serum bilirubin concentration may increase slightly as well.[8]

The prevalence of PN-associated liver disease is much greater in infants than in older children or in adults. The reported prevalence varies between 15 and 85%, depending on the study. In the largest series, Sondheimer et al. reported that cholestasis developed in 65% of infants after less than 2 months on PN; 13% developed hepatic failure within 6 weeks of beginning PN.[9]

Little data exist on actual liver function during PN. Rodent studies have indicated PN may be associated with increased oxidative drug metabolism,[10] and it appears PN stimulates the cytochrome P450 system in humans.[11,12] However, no long-term data are available. Antipyrine clearance was reduced in a small group of patients that received short-term PN, although these patients were also critically ill.[13]

Cavicchi et al. from Paris found an incidence of PN-associated chronic cholestasis of 55% of patients after 2 years in a group of 90 patients with no known liver disease prior to PN.[14] They defined an elevation as serum aspartate aminotransferase (AST), alanine aminotransferase (ALT), or alkaline phosphatase > 1.5X the upper limit of normal of > 6 months. The percentage increased to 64–72% in those who received PN for at ≥ 4–6 years. "Complicated" liver disease (defined as portal hypertension, biopsy-proven portal fibrosis or cirrhosis, serum bilirubin concentration > 3.5 mg/dl, or hepatic encephalopathy), developed in 26% of patients after 2 years, 39% after 4 years, and 50% after 6 years of PN. Hepatic failure accounted for 22% of the deaths in these patients. Chan et al., reviewing the Beth Israel Deaconess Hospital experience of home PN, found the incidence of endstage liver disease related to PN was 15% in their home PN patient population over the last 23 years.[15]

HISTOLOGIC ABNORMALITIES

In adult patients the dominant histologic finding is steatosis.[16] Both micro- and macrovesicular steatosis is present. Periportal distribution is characteristic, with extension to a centrilobular or even panlobular distribution as fat deposition increases. Although usually asymptomatic, massive steatosis may be associated with painful hepatomegaly. The condition may progress to steatohepatitis, fibrosis, cirrhosis, and hepatic failure.[15,17–21] PN-associated hepatic steatosis may also progress to canalicular cholestasis and later to include bile duct proliferation, portal fibrosis, and cirrhosis.[17,22] In young children, more specifically infants as well as some adults, the predominant histologic finding is cholestasis, with minimal steatosis. Ballooned hepatocytes, Kupffer cell hyperplasia, persistent extramedullary hematopoiesis, bile duct plugging, and intrahepatic cholestasis are characteristic.

PATHOGENESIS OF PN-ASSOCIATED LIVER DISEASE

Although it is likely an unknown inciting event must occur to initiate this chain of events, it appears progressive liver disease requires the presence of steatosis. It remains unclear if the cholestasis that develops in infants and some adults has the same etiology as for steatosis. Several factors have been implicated in the pathogenesis of PN-associated liver disease. However, there are little data to support most of these theories in humans. Potential etiologies can be divided into three categories: the underlying disease for which PN was required, nutrient deficiencies, and nutrient toxicities.

UNDERLYING DISEASE

Crohn's disease, malignancy, celiac sprue, and radiation therapy are associated with hepatic serum aminotransferase abnormalities.[23–26] It has been proposed that bacterial translocation, most commonly found in patients with intestinal obstruction and motility disorders, may be associated with hepatic abnormalities. However, bacterial translocation has not been associated with hepatic injury in humans.[27] Bacterial 7-α dehydroxylation of chenodeoxycholic acid to form lithocholic acid has been presumed to have hepatotoxic effects in the neoate, resulting in cholestasis. Although there are no human data to support this theory, studies in the guinea pig suggest that neonatal animals are actually more resistant to the effects of lithocholic acid on the liver than adults.[28]

Patients who require long-term PN may develop liver disease for any of the reasons that non-TPN patients develop liver disease. These include hepatitis B and C, autoimmune hepatitis, primary biliary cirrhosis, Wilson's disease, and other primary hepatic diseases as well as extrahepatic biliary obstruction. For infants, this also includes neonatal hepatitis and biliary atresia. Degree of prematurity, increased number of infections, surgical procedures, and blood transfusions are risk factors for the development of PN-associated liver disease in the neonate.[29] in addition, the biliary secretory system in preterm neonates may be underdeveloped, as suggested by the decreased bile salt pool and decreased rate of bile salt synthesis.[30] Cholesterol synthesis and hepatic lipogenesis are significantly increased in patients with severe malabsorption, regardless of whether PN is used.[31]

MALABSORPTION AND NUTRIENT DEFICIENCIES

Those patients with the least residual intestine and/or residual colon following enterectomy are at greatest risk for the development of liver disease.[14,21,32] Cambrier et al. found that patients with < 150 cm residual small intestine had a risk of developing PN-associated liver disease that was 3.2 times increased than those with > 150 cm residual intestine.[32] In addition, these investigators found that patients who had colon resections were at significantly increased risk for developing hepatic dysfunction while on PN. These patients have the most severe malabsorption, but also require the most PN.

Deficiencies in several different nutrients have been proposed to cause hepatic abnormalities. These include essential fatty acids, protein, carnitine, choline, vitamin E, and selenium. Hepatic steatosis develops in severe protein malnutrition (Kwashiorkor) because of decreased very low density lipoprotein synthesis.[33] Hepatic triglyceride excretion is thus impaired. Deficiency of linoleic acid, the only truly essential fatty acid for humans, is associated with hepatic steatosis.[34] Biochemical essential fatty acid deficiency may develop within 2 weeks of the beginning of lipid-free PN and is diagnosed on the basis of either a decreased plasma linoleic acid concentration or an elevation in the serum triene:tetrene ratio to > 0.4.[35] One or two months of lipid-free PN are required before hepatic abnormalities become evident.[36] Essential fatty acid deficiency may also occur in patients with profound steatorrhea prior to the institution of PN. There are no data to support the theory that either vitamin E and/or selenium deficiency cause hepatic steatosis. Carnitine is a quaternary amine that is required for transport of long-chain triglycerides across the inner mitochondrial membrane for oxidation. It is normally synthesized from lysine and methionine, two amino acids supplied in TN. Serum carnitine concentrations decrease to approximately 50% of normal after about 3 weeks of PN,[37] although carnitine deficiency during TPN has not been demonstrated.[38,39] Sequella of carnitine deficiency generally do not develop until serum carnitine concentrations approach approximately 10% of normal.[40] Bowyer et al. demonstrated that elevations in serum hepatic aminotransferase concentrations were unrelated to plasma carnitine concentrations.[41] In addition, these investigators found that intravenous carnitine supplementation in PN patients failed to decrease either serum hepatic aminotransferase concentrations or hepatic steatosis despite normalization of plasma carnitine concentrations.[42]

Some 90% of patients who require long-term PN have low-plasma free choline concentration. In addition, an inverse relationship between plasma-free choline concentration and AST and ALT abnormalities has been described in humans.[43] Initial studies using choline-supplemented TPN have resulted in resolution of hepatic steatosis in humans, suggesting hepatic steatosis associated with PN is caused by choline deficiency.[44–46] Choline is normally synthesized from methionine contained in the PN solution. However, the transsulfuration pathway in the liver, from which choline and other metabolic products of methionine are synthesized, appears to exhibit deficient function when presented with intravenously infused nutrients.[47,48]

Enterally consumed nutrients are absorbed via the portal circulation and are transported to the liver, where they undergo hepatic first pass metabolism. On the other hand, intravenously infused nutrients enter the circulation at the right side of the heart and only later to the liver. The route of nutrient assimilation appears to affect nutrient metabolism. This observation appears to explain why choline is not synthesized from PN-containing methionine to any significant degree.

The amino acid taurine is not added to adult PN solution, but has become a routine addition to neonatal TPN. It is thought to stimulate bile acid secretion.[49] Although initial studies suggested taurine supplementation leads to a decreased incidence of cholestasis,[50] more recent data have questioned this observation.[51,52]

NUTRIENT TOXICITIES

Several nutrients provided in PN may be hepatotoxic in excessive amounts. The maximum rate of glucose oxidation in humans is 5–7 m/kg/minute.[53,54] Infusion of dextrose in excess of this rate is associated with development of hepatic steatosis and abnormal serum hepatic aminotransferase concentrations. During excess dextrose infusion, the portal insulin:glucagon ratio is increased in rodent models,[55] and the addition of glucagon to PN (without lipid emulsion) decreased the portal insulin:glucagon ratio and prevented the development of hepatic steatosis.[56] Insulin increases hepatocellular carbohydrate uptake and stimulates carbohydrate storage as fat. Glucagon inhibits fatty acid synthesis and stimulates export of hepatic fatty acids. In humans however, glucagon infusion is associated with hyperglycemia, intestinal dysmotility, nausea and vomiting. Mucosal hypoplasia also develops in rats that receive exogenous glucagon.[57] Excessive carbohydrate infusion also leads to increased production of both acetyl CoA carboxylase and fatty acid synthetase activity, the rate-controlling enzymes for hepatic fatty acid synthesis.[58,59]

Lipid overload syndrome, resulting when > 2.5 g/kg/day of lipid emulsion is infused, may result in hepatic steatosis.[60,61] In addition, two retrospective studies have suggested that infusion of lipid emulsion at a level > 1.0 g/kg/day may be associated with increased risk for hepatic dysfunction.[14,15] There are also significant levels of plant sterols (phytosterols) in lipid emulsions.[62] Although phytosterol concentrations are elevated in patients that receive lipid emulsion, no association with hepatic abnormalities has been demonstrated in humans.

Vileisis et al. found that increased amino acid infusion (3.6 g/kg/day versus 2.3 g/kg/day) was associated with increased incidence and severity of cholestasis in preterm infants.[63] However, this observation may have been related to aluminum contamination given that protein hydroysate solutions were the basis for the amino acid solutions.

Hepatic steatosis developed in rats that received PN containing the preservative sodium bisulfate in the amino acid formulation.[2] Grant et al. found tryptophan decomposed in the presence of the sodium bisulfate preservative and sunlight.[2] Sodium bisulfate is still used as a preservative in some amino acid formulas.

Serum and red blood cell manganese concentrations are elevated in patients who receive long-term PN, and it is has been suggested that manganese toxicity results in the development of cholestasis. However, given that virtually all manganese is biliary excreted, excretion also decreases when bile flow is decreased. Therefore, it is difficult to prove that manganese has a primary role in the development of PN-associated liver disease, and it is more likely the increased manganese concentrations are observed are related to decreased biliary excretion.[64] Prior to 1985, amino acid solutions were derived from casein hydrolysate, which had significant aluminum contamination. Although studies in rodent PN models have revealed that significant aluminum contamination may result in development of cholestasis,[65,66] there is relatively little aluminum contamination in current PN formulations.[67]

Moss et al. studied PN in a rabbit model.[68] They observed that rabbits that received standard PN with lipids had subjective decreased bile flow and balloon degeneration of hepatocytes and eosinophilic infiltration of the portal triads. These findings were subjectively similar in rabbits that ate chow, but also received intravenous methionine. Although studies have not confirmed a toxicity from excessive methionine in humans, methionine concentrations are generally elevated in patients that receive long-term PN[69] as there appears to be a block in normal methionine metabolism to important metabolic products such as choline, as described above.

PREVENTION AND TREATMENT OF PN-ASSOCIATED LIVER DISEASE

Most importantly, oral intake should be maximized and PN minimized. Dextrose overfeeding should be avoided, with maximum energy provided at 40 kcal/kg/day for nutritional replenishment in adults (25–30 kcal/kg/day for maintenance). Once energy and protein stores have been repleted in the undernourished patient, PN energy support should be decreased to maintenance levels. Lipid emulsion should be provided as an integral part of PN to prevent essential fatty acid deficiency. For this, lipid emulsion should supply a minimum of 4–8% of total calories. However, lipid emulsion is an integral part of the energy composition of PN. It is especially useful in the fluid-restricted patient because the concentration of lipid emulsion is 2 kcal/ml (versus 1.1 kcal/ml for the maximal dextrose concentration) and is also useful in the hyperglycemic patient. Substitution of 33% of dextrose calories by lipid emulsion reduced serum insulin concentration by 50% and has been associated with significant improvement in serum hepatic aminotransferase concentrations.[70] This may be related to a decrease in the portal vein insulin:glucagon ratio. However, the maximal daily infusion of lipid emulsion should not exceed 2.5 g/kg/day (and possibly 1.0 g/kg/day) because of increased risk for chronic hepatic toxicity. Amino acids should be provided at a minimum level of 0.8 g/kg/day (0.6 g/kg/day for renal failure in the absence of dialysis and in cases of hepatic encephalopathy), and a maximum level of 1.7–2.0 g/kg/day. Cycling of PN to an overnight infusion has also been associated with fewer hepatic abnormalities.[71]

Metronidazole has been used to treat PN-associated liver disease in humans based on the theory that bacterial translocation is associated with hepatic derangements.[72] However, there is little evidence that bacterial translocation is associated with hepatic derrangements in humans. Retrospective studies have suggested benefit from the use of metronidazole in patients with PN-associated liver disease. However, careful review of the data indicates that many of the patients evaluated had Crohn's disease, in whom hepatic derangements are common;[23] metronidazole is an accepted treatment for Crohn's disease. Furthermore, the patients that received metronidazole also received an excessive amount of carbohydrate, which as discussed above, leads to hepatic steatosis and serum hepatic aminotransferase abnormalities. Another study suggested metronidazole could be considered for the prevention of PN-associated liver disease.[73]

Ursodeoxycholic acid has been used in both adults and children to treat PN-associated cholestasis. In adult patients, the available data consist of a single case report,[74] and a separate series of nine patients.[75] In neonates, there have been two open-labeled studies and one retrospective review.[76–78] Cocjin et al. reported that the serum total bilirubin concentration decreased in a small group of neonates who received ursodeoxycholic acid (15–45 mg/kg/day) in an unblinded study.[76] However, the infants still remained severly cholestatic. Spagnuolu et al. reported that ursodeoxycholic acid at a dose of 10 mg/kg t.i.d. for 48–575 days decreased jaundice in 5 of 7 neonates and serum hepatic aminotransferse abnormalities in 6 of 7 patients, although enteral feeding had also begun.[77]

At the present time, there is no role for carnitine supplementation.[38–42]

Choline-supplemented PN is undergoing investigational studies for the treatment and prevention of PN-associated liver disease. It is not as yet commercially available. Two placebo-controlled clinical trials, one using lecithin (phosphatidylcholine), have shown that PN-associated hepatic steatosis resolves and serum hepatic aminotransferase abnormalities significantly improve with choline supplementation, and steatosis recurs when choline is discontinued.[44,46]

For patients who develop cirrhosis or in whom hepatic failure is impending, combined liver/small bowel transplantation is the only viable alternative.[79] There are a few cases of successful isolated small bowel transplantation in patients with PN-associated liver disease who have no evidence of fibrosis or cirrhosis on liver biopsy.[80] If the serum bilirubin concentration becomes elevated, the TPN formula should be reviewed to ensure neither excessive dextrose nor lipid emulsion is being infused. The patients medication regimen should also be reviewed to exclude the possibility of medication-induced cholestasis. In the absence of necessary changes in the PN prescription, a search for extrahepatic obstruction should be undertaken. This required either noninvasive imaging techniques such as magnetic resonance cholangiopancreatography (MRCP) or endoscopic cholangiopancreatography (ERCP). The latter allows for therapeutic intervention to remove stones and debris from the common bile duct and evaluate/biopsy other abnormalties, including the possibility of sclerosing cholangitis and cholangiocarcinoma, both associated with inflammatory bowel disease, as well as other biliary abnormalities. If there is no evidence of extrahepatic cholestasis, liver biopsy should be performed to exclude other forms of liver disease, including primary biliary cirrhosis. PN-associated liver disease is a diagnosis of exclusion, and in the absence of any other etiology for liver disease, the patient should be referred to a liver/small bowel transplant center. Although PN-associated cholestasis may spontaneously improve for reasons that remain obscure and a transplant not be deemed necessary, PN-associated liver disease may be rapidly progressive once the serum bilirubin concentration becomes elevated.

The mortality in patients waiting for a combined liver/small bowel transplant is significantly greater than for those waiting solely for a liver transplant.[81] Therefore, it is important to refer patients for transplant evaluation early.

BILIARY ABNORMALITIES ASSOCIATED WITH PN USE

ACALCULOUS CHOLECYSTITIS

The first case of PN-associated acalculous cholecystitis was reported in 1972.[82] In the absence of sufficient oral intake, there is a diminished release of cholecystokinin (CCK), which results in decreased gallbladder contractility.[83] Bile stasis and increased bile lithogenecity appear to be contributing factors, although the exact pathogenesis remains unknown.[84,85]

CALCULOUS CHOLECYSTITIS

The association between cholelithiasis and PN was first described by Whitington and Black in 1980.[86] Preterm infants developed gallstones after 30–60 days of PN. Subsequently, Pitt et al. found symptomatic gallstones developed in 40% of their home PN patients, including in 25% who did not have ileal resections or Crohn's disease.[87] Messing et al. have shown that approximately 50% of patients developed biliary sludge after 4–6 weeks of PN and nil per os, 100% of patients developed biliary sludge after 6 weeks of TPN and nil per os.[88] Sludge resolved in all patients following 4 weeks of enteral or oral refeeding. Although the lithogenicity of bile is not increased during TPN,[89–91] the calcium bilirubinate concentrate is approximately doubled,[92,93] and calcium bilirubinate stones predominate.[94] The primary risk factor for the development of biliary sludge and subsequent lithiasis is stasis.[91,94] This results from incomplete gallbladder contraction, as indicated above.[95] The observation that most stones are of calcium bilirubinate origin suggests the possibility that chronic bacterial biliary infection may be a contributing factor in sludge and stone development.[96]

TREATMENT AND PREVENTION OF BILIARY TRACT ABNORMALITIES

Prevention of gallstones and acalculous cholecystitis primarily involves methods to induce gallbladder contraction. The easiest, safest, and least expensive of these modalities is to maximize oral food intake. Continuous enteral feeding, however, fails to stimulate CCK release to a significant degree, and therefore is also associated with biliary sludge formation, the leading risk factor for cholelithiasis.[97] Injection of CCK may simulate meal-induced CCK release and stimulate gallbladder contraction,[98] but not all studies have shown efficacy,[88,99] and side effects, including nausea and abdominal pain, have been described.[98,99] Rapid amino acid infusion also appears to stimulate gallbladder contraction, but is not a practical therapy.[100,101] In addition, the effect of bolus amino acid infusion on gallbladder contraction is lost when the infusion continues for more than two hours.[102] Some investigators have recommended prophylactic cholecystectomy,[103] although that is not a universal practice.

PN-ASSOCIATED NEPHROPATHY

Long-term parenteral nutrition has been associated with a decline in the glomerular filtration rate (GFR) greater than that expected on the basis of increasing age alone.[104–107] Renal tubular damage has also been shown.[105,107] Although the etiology has not been conclusively elicited, it appears that excessive chromium in the TPN solutions,[104,108] the number of catheter-related infections experienced,[105] and possibly increased endogenous oxalate production may play a role.[109] Studies in a rodent PN model indicate that significant amount of chromium deposits in the kidneys and is associated with tubular abnormalities.[108] Glomerular hypertrophy may develop following chronic, excessive protein intake,[110] although no correlation between increased amino acid infusion and a decline in GFR has been observed. The inverse relationship between the number of catheter infections and GFR may reflect chronic immune complex deposition in the kidneys, although the reason for this relationship is not clear. Although no cases of PN-associated renal failure have been reported, it would take at least 35 years of long to precipitate renal failure in the absence of other renal abnormalities.[105] It has been suggested that sufficient chromium is contained in PN solutions as a contaminant and therefore, supplemental chromium should not be added.[106] Because chromium-associated renal abnormalities may be irreversible, no improvement in GFR was observed, however, with short-term follow-up in children who had chromium removed from their PN solutions.[106] There are no other specific interventions known at the present time to treat or prevent PN-associated nephropathy.

CONCLUSION

PN-associated liver disease is one of the most common, and certainly the most significant complication of long-term PN. It appears the cause is more likely related to one or more nutrient deficiencies in PN solutions rather than a toxicity, although more investigation is clearly needed in this. PN-associated hepatic failure is, in this author's opinion, the one legitimate indication for combined liver/small intestinal transplantation. More data are necessary before it can be concluded that isolated intestinal transplant is the most appropriate option for significant PN-associated liver disease in the absence of fibrosis. Ongoing studies with choline-supplemented PN both to treat and prevent PN-associated liver disease are eagerly awaited.

PN-associated biliary disease arises primarily from altered bile-acid enterohepatic circulation and can largely be prevented by encouraging oral food intake.

PN-associated renal disease is a recently recognized complication. The etiology is not entirely clear, although both humans and rodent studies strongly suggest a role for excessive chromium supplied in the PN solutions. The clinical significance of these observations is probably most important in patients with coexisting nephorpathy as well as those patients who require PN for many years.

REFERENCES

1. Penden, V.H., Witzleben C.L., and Skelton, M.A., Total parenteral nutrition, *J. Pediatr.*, 78, 180, 1971.
2. Grant, J. et al., Serum hepatic enzyme and bilirubin elevations during parenteral nutrition, *Surg. Gynecol. Obstet.*, 145, 573, 1977.
3. Robertson, J.F.R., Garden, O.J., and Shenkin, A., Intravenous nutrition and hepatic dysfunction. *JPEN*, 10, 172, 1986.
4. Klein, G.L. et al., Bone disease associated with total parenteral nutrition, *Lancet* ii, 1041, 1980.
5. Quigley, E.M.M. et al., Hepatobiliary complications of total parenteral nutrition, *Gastroenterology* 104, 286, 1993.
6. Lowry, S.F. and Brennan, M.F., Abnormal liver function during parenteral nutrition: relation to infusion excess, *J. Surg. Res.*, 26, 300, 1979.
7. Sax, H.C. et al., Hepatic steatosis in total parenteral nutrition: failure of fatty infiltration to correlate with abnormal serum hepatic enzyme levels, *Surgery*, 100, 697, 1986.
8. Clark, P.J., Ball, M.J., and Kettlewell, M.G.W., Liver function tests in patients receiving parenteral nutrition, *JPEN*, 15, 54, 1991.
9. Sondheimer, J.M., Asturias, E., and Cadnapaphornchai, M., Infection and cholestasis in neonates with intestinal resection and long-term parenteral nutrition, *J. Pediatr. Gastroenterol.*, 27, 131, 1998.
10. Knodell, R.G. et al., Effects of parenteral and enteral hyperalimentation on hepatic drug metabolism in the rat, *J. Pharmacol. Exp. Ther.*, 22, 589, 1984.
11. Pantuck, E.J. et al., Stimulation of oxidative drug metabolism by parenteral refeeding of nutritionally depleted patients, *Gastroenterology*, 89, 241, 1985.
12. Pantuck, E.J. et al., Effects of parenteral nutrition regimens on oxidative drug metabolism, *Anesthesiology*, 60, 534, 1984.
13. Ross, L.H. et al., Hepatoxic effects of parenteral nutrition upon the *in vivo* kinetics of antipyrine. *Surg. Forum*, 34, 34, 1983.
14. Cavicchi, M. et al., Prevalence of liver disease and contributing factors in patients receiving home parenteral nutrition for permanent intestinal failure, *Ann. Intern. Med.*, 132, 525, 2000.
15. Chan, S. et al., Incidence, prognosis, and etiology of end-stage liver disease in patients receiving home total parenteral nutrition, *Surgery*, 126, 28, 1999.
16. Buchman, A.L. and Ament, M.E., Liver disease and total parenteral nutrition, In Zakim, D., and Boyer, T.D., Eds., *Hepatology, a Textbook of Liver Disease*, 3rd ed., Philadelphia: W.B. Saunders, 1992, 1810.
17. Craig, R.M. et al., Severe hepatocellular reaction resembling alcoholic cirrhosis after massive small bowel resection and prolonged total parenteral nutrition, *Gastroenterology*, 79, 131, 1980.
18. MacDonald, G.A. et al., Lipid peroxidation in hepatic steatosis in humans is associated with hepatic fibrosis and occurs predominately in acinar zone 3, *J. Gastroenterol. Hepatol.*, 16, 599–606, 2001.
19. Rabeneck, L., Freeman, H., and Owen, D., Death due to TPN-related liver failure (abstr), *Gastroenterology*, 86, 1215, 1984.
20. Bowyer, B.A. et al., Does long-term home parenteral nutrition in adult patients cause chronic liver disease? *JPEN*, 9:11, 1985.

21. Stanko, R.T. et al., Development of hepatic cholestasis and fibrosis in patients with massive loss of intestine supported by prolonged parenteral nutrition, *Gastroenterology*, 92, 197, 1987.

22. Cohen, C. and Olsen, M.M., Pediatric total parenteral nutrition, *Arch. Pathol. Lab Med.*, 105, 152, 1981.

23. Dew, M.J., Thompson, H., and Allan, R.N., The spectrum of hepatic dysfunction in inflammatory bowel disease, *Q. J. Med.*, 48, 113, 1979.

24. King, P.D. and Perry, M.C., Hepatotoxicity of chemotherapy, *Oncologist*, 6, 162, 2001.

25. Soiffer, R.J. et al., Hepatic dysfunction following T-cell-depleted allogeneic bone marrow transplantation, *Transplantation*, 52, 1014, 1991.

26. Dickey, W., McMillan, S.A., and Collins, J.S., Liver abnormalities associated with celiac sprue. How common are they, what is their significance, and what do we know about them? *J. Clin. Gastroenterol.*, 20, 290, 1995.

27. Riordan, S.M., McIver, C.J., and Williams, R., Liver damage in human small intestinal bacterial overgrowth, *Am. J. Gastroenterol.*, 93, 234, 1996.

28. Lewittes, M., Tuchwebr, B., Weber, A. et al., Resistance of the sucking pig to lithocholic acid-induced chostasis, *Hepatology*, 4, 486, 1984.

29. Drongowski, R.A. and Coran, A.G., An analysis of the factors contributing to the development of total parenteral nutrition-induced cholestasis, *JPEN*, 13, 586, 1989.

30. Watkins, J.B. et al., Bile salt metabolism in the human premature infant, *Gastroenterology*, 69, 706, 1975.

31. Cook, G.C. and Hutt, M.S.R., The liver after kwashiorkor, *Br. Med. J.*, 3, 454, 1967.

32. Chambrier, J., Lemann, M., Vahedi, M. et al., Chronic cholestasis in patients supported by prolonged parenteral nutrition (abstr), *JPEN*, 22, S16, 1998.

33. Cachefo, A. et al., Stimulation of cholesterol synthesis and hepatic lipogenesis in patients with severe malabsorption, *J. Lipid Res.* (in press).

34. Reif, S. et al., Total parenteral nutrition-induced steatosis: reversal by parenteral lipid emulsion, *JPEN*, 15, 102, 1991.

35. Holma, R.T., The ratio of the trienoic:tetrenoic acid in tissue lipids as a measure of essential fatty acid requirements, *J. Nutr.*, 70, 405, 1960.

36. Langer, B. et al., Prolonged survival after complete bowel resection using intravenous alimentation at home, *J. Surg. Res.*, 15, 226, 1973.

37. Hahn, P., Allardyce, D.B., and Frohlich, J., Plasma carnitine levels during total parenteral nutrition of adult surgical patients, *Am. J. Clin. Nutr.*, 36, 569, 1982.

38. Dahlstrom, K.A. et al., Low blood and plasma carnitine levels in children receiving long-term parenteral nutrition, *J. Pediatr. Gastroenterol. Nutr.*, 11, 375, 1990.

39. Moukarzel, A.A. et al., Carnitine status of children receiving long-term total parenteral nutrition: a longitudinal prospective study, *J. Pediatr.*, 120, 759, 1992.

40. Karpati, G. et al., The syndrome of systemic carnitine deficiency: clinical, morphologic, biochemical and pathologic features, *Neurology*, 25, 16, 1975.

41. Bowyer, B.A. et al., Plasma carnitine levels in patients receiving home parenteral nutrition, *Am. J. Clin. Nutr.*, 43, 85, 1986.

42. Bowyer, B.A. et al., L-carnitine therapy in home parenteral nutrition patients with abnormal liver tests and low plasma carnitine concentration, *Gastroenterology*, 94, 434, 1988.

43. Buchman, A.L. et al., Low plasma free choline is prevalent in patients receiving long term parenteral nutrition and is associated with hepatic aminotransferase abnormalities, *Clin. Nutr.*, 12, 33, 1993.

44. Buchman, A.L. et al., Lecithin supplementation causes a decrease in hepatic steatosis in patients receiving long term parenteral nutrition, *Gastroenterology*, 102, 1363, 1992.

45. Buchman, A.L. et al., Choline deficiency: a cause of hepatic steatosis associated with parenteral nutrition that can be reversed with intravenous choline chloride supplementation, *Hepatology*, 22, 1399, 1995.

46. Buchman, A.L. et al., Choline deficiency causes reversible hepatic abnormalities in patients during parenteral nutrition: proof of a human choline requirement; a placebo-controlled trial, *JPEN*, 25, 260, 2001.

47. Steginck, L.D. and Besten, L.D., Synthesis of cysteine from methionine in normal adult subjects: effect of route of alimentation, *Science*, 178, 514, 1972.

48. Chawla, R.K. et al., Plasma concentrations of transsulfuration pathway products during nasoenteral and intravenous hyperalimentation of malnourished patients, *Am. J. Clin. Nutr.*, 43, 219, 1986.

49. Okamoto, E. et al., Role of taurine in feeding the low-birth-weight infant, *J. Pediatr.*, 104, 936, 1984.

50. Desai, T.K. et al., Taurine supplementation and cholestasis during bone marrow transplantation (abstr), *Gastroenterology*, 104, A616, 1993.

51. Cooke, R.J., Whitington, P.F., and Kelts, D., Effects of taurine supplementation on hepatic function during short-term parenteral nutrition in the premature infant, *J. Pediatr. Gastroenterol.*, 3, 234, 1984.

52. Snyder, J. et al., TPN cholestasis in neonates: results of randomized, double-blind study of amino acid composition (abstr), *Gastroenterology*, 124, A30, 2003.

53. Burke, J.F. et al., Glucose requirements following burn injury. Parameters of optimal glucose infusion and possible hepatic and respiratory abnormalities following excessive glucose intake, *Ann. Surg.*, 190, 274, 1990.

54. Lowry, S.F. and Brennan, M.F. Abnormal liver function during parenteral nutrition: relation to infusion excess, *J. Surg. Res.*, 26, 300, 1979.

55. Blue, P.R., Burnes, J.U., and Kelly, D.G., Long-term parenteral nutrition (TPN)-associated hepatobiliary dysfunction: are there predisposing factors (abstr)? *Gastroenterology*, 84, 1203, 1989.

56. Li, S. et al., Addition of glucagon to total parenteral nutrition (TPN) prevents hepatic steatosis in rats, *Surgery*, 104, 350, 1988.

57. Rudo, N.D., Rosenberg, J.H., and Wissler, R.W., The effects of partial starvation and glucagon treatment on intestinal villus morphology and cell migration, *Proc. Exp. Soc. Exp. Biol. Med.*, 152, 277, 1976.

58. Chang, S. and Silvis, S.E., Fatty liver produced by hyperalimentation of rats, *Am. J. Gastroenterology*, 62, 410, 1974.

59. Kaminski, D.L., Adams, A., and Jellinek, M., The effect of hyperalimentation on hepatic lipid content and lipogenic enzyme activity in rats and man, *Surgery*, 88, 93, 1980.

60. Salvian, A.J. and Allardyce, D.B., Impaired bilirubin secretion during total parenteral nutrition, *J. Surg. Res.*, 28, 547, 1980.

61. Allardyce, D.B., Cholestasis caused by lipid emulsions, *Surg. Gynecol. Obstet.*, 154, 641, 1982.

62. Clayton, P.T. et al., Phytosterolemia in children with parenteral nutrition-associated cholestatic liver disease, *Gastroenterology*, 105, 1806, 1993.

63. Vileisis, R.A., Inwood, R.J., and Hunt, C.E., Prospective controlled trial of parenteral nutrition-associated cholestatic jaundice: effect of protein intake, *J. Pediatr.*, 96, 893, 1980.
64. Masumoto, K. et al., Manganese intoxication during intermittent parenteral nutrition: report of two cases, *JPEN*, 25, 95, 2001.
65. Klein, G.L. et al., Hepatic abnormalities associated with aluminum loading in piglets, *JPEN*, 11, 293, 1987.
66. Klein, G.L. et al., Aluminum associated hepatobiliary dysfunction in rats: relationship to dosage and duration of exposure, *Pediatr. Res.*, 23, 275, 1988.
67. Klein, G.L., The aluminum content of parenteral solutions: current status, *Nutr. Rev.*, 49, 74, 1991.
68. Moss, R.L. et al., Methionine infusion reproduces liver injury of parenteral nutrition cholestasis, *Pediatr. Res.*, 45, 664, 1999.
69. Chawla, R.K. et al., Plasma concentrations of transulfuration pathway products during nasoenteric and intravenous hyperalimentation of malnourished patients, *Am. J. Clin. Nutr.*, 42, 577, 1985.
70. Meguid, M.M. et al., Ameiloration of metabolic complications of conventional total parenteral nutrition, *Arch. Surg.*, 119, 1294, 1984.
71. Mani, A. et al., Cyclic hyperalimentation: an optimal technique for preservation of visceral protein, *J. Surg. Res.*, 20, 515, 1976.
72. Capron, J.P. et al., Metronidazole in prevention of cholestasis associated with total parenteral nutrition, *Lancet*, 26, 446, 1983.
73. Lambert, J.R. and Thomas, S.M., Metronidazole prevention of serum liver enzyme abnormalities during total parenteral nutrition, *JPEN*, 9, 501, 1985.
74. Lindor, K.D. and Burnes, J., Ursodeoxycholic acid for the treatment of home parenteral nutrition-associated cholestasis, *Gastroenterology*, 101, 250, 1991.
75. Beau, P. et al., Is ursodeoxycholic acid an effective therapy for total parenteral nutrition-related liver disease, *J. Hepatol.*, 20, 240, 1994.
76. Cocjin, J. et al., Ursodeoxycholic acid therapy for total parenteral nutrition-associated cholestasis (abstr), *Gastroenterology*, 104, A615, 1993.
77. Spagnuolo, M.I. et al., Ursodeoxycholic acid for treatment of cholestasis in children on long-term total parenteral nutrition: a pilot study, *Gastroenterology*, 111, 716, 1996.
78. Levin, A. et al., Parenteral nutrition-associated cholestasis in preterm neonates: evaluation of ursodeoxycholic acid treatment, *J. Pediatr. Endocrin. Metab.*, 12, 549, 1999.
79. Buchman, A.L., Scolopio, J., and Fryer, J., Technical review of the treatment of short bowel syndrome and intestinal transplantation, *Gastroenterology*, 124, 1111, 2003.
80. Sudan, D.L. et al., Isolated intestinal transplantation for intestinal failure, *Am. J. Gastroenterol.*, 95, 1506, 2000.
81. Fryer, J. et al., Mortality in candidates waiting for combined liver-intestine transplants exceeds that for other candidates waiting for liver transplants, *Liver Transpl.*, 9, 748, 2003.
82. Anderson, D.L., Acalculous cholecystitis — a possible complication of parenteral hyperalimentation. Report of a case, *Med. Ann. of DC*, 41, 448, 1972.
83. Gullick, H.D., Roentgenologic study of gallbladder following non-biliary tract surgery, *Ann. Surg.*, 151, 403, 1960.

84. Flati, G. et al., Role of cholesterol and calcium bilirubinate crystals in acute postoperative acalculous cholecystitis, *Ital. J. Surg. Sci.,* 14, 333, 1984.

85. Deitch, E.A. and Engel, J.M., Acute acalculous cholecystitis, *Am. J. Surg.,* 142, 472, 1984.

86. Whitington, P.F. and Black, D.D., Cholelithiasis in premature infants treated with parenteral nutrition and furosemide, *J. Pediatr.,* 97, 647, 1980.

87. Pitt, H.A. et al., Increased risk of cholelithiasis with prolonged parenteral nutrition, *Am. J. Surg.,* 145, 106, 1983.

88. Messing, B. et al., Does total parneteral nutrition induce gallbladder sludge formation and lithiasis? *Gastroenterology,* 84, 1012, 1983.

89. Doty, J.E. et al., Cholecystokinin prophylaxis of parenteral nutrition-induced gallbladder disease, *Ann. Surg.,* 201, 76, 1985.

90. Messing, B. et al., Gallstone formation during total parenteral nutrition: a prospective study in man, *Gastroenterology,* 86, 1183, 1984.

91. Doty, J.E. et al., The effect of intravenous fat and total parenteral nutrition on biliary physiology, *JPEN,* 8, 263, 1984.

92. Allen, B. et al., Sludge is calcium bilirubinate associated with bile stasis, *Am. J. Surg.,* 141, 51, 1981.

93. Pitt, H.A. et al., Parenteral nutrition induces calcium bilirubinate gallstones, *Gastroenterology,* 84, 1274, 1983.

94. Lee, S.P., Maher, K., and Nicholls, J.F., Origin and fate of biliary sludge, *Gastroenterology,* 94, 170, 1988.

95. Cano, N. et al., Ultrasonographic study of gallbladder motility during total parenteral nutrition, *Gastroenterology,* 91, 313, 1986.

96. Stewart, L. et al., Pigment gallstones form as a composite of bacterial microcolonies and pigment solids, *Ann. Surg.,* 206, 242, 1987.

97. Mashako, M.N.K. et al., The effect of artificial feeding on cholestasis, gallbladder sludge and lithiasis in infants: correlation with plasma cholecystokinin levels, *Clin. Nutr.,* 10, 320, 1991.

98. Sitzman, J.V. et al., Cholecystokinin prevents parenteral nutrition induced biliary sludge in humans, *Surg. Gynecol. Obstet.,* 170, 25, 1990.

99. Apelgren, K.N., Willard, D.A., and Vargish, T., TPN alters gallbladder responsivity to cholecystokinin, *JPEN,* 12S, 115, 1988.

100. De Boer, S.Y. et al., Effect of intravenous glucose on intravenous amino acid-induced gallbladder contraction and CCK secretion, *Dig. Dis. Sci.,* 39, 268, 1994.

101. Zoli, G. et al., Promotion of gallbladder emptying by intravenous amino acids, *Lancet,* 341, 1240, 1993.

102. Kalfarentzos, F. et al., Gallbladder contraction after administration of intravenous amino acids and long-chain triacylglycerols in humans, *Nutrition,* 7, 347, 1991.

103. Manji, N. et al., Gallstone disease in patients with severe short bowel syndrome dependent on parenteral nutrition, *JPEN,* 13, 461, 1989.

104. Moukarzel, A.A. et al., Renal function of children receiving long-term parenteral nutrition, *J. Pediatr.,* 119, 864, 1991.

105. Buchman, A.L. et al., Serious renal impairment is associated with long-term parenteral nutrition, *JPEN,* 17, 438, 1993.

106. Moukarzel, A.A. et al., Excessive chromium intake in children receiving total parenteral nutrition, *Lancet,* 339, 385, 1992.

107. Boncompain-Gerard, M. et al., A. Renal function and urinary excretion of electrolytes in patients receiving cyclic parenteral nutrition, *J. Parenteral Ent. Nutr.,* 24, 234, 2000.

108. Buchman, A.L. et al., Organ heavy-metal accumulation during parenteral nutrition is associated with pathologic abnormalities in rats, *Nutrition*, 17, 600, 2001.
109. Buchman, A.L., Moukarzel, A.A., and Ament, M.E., Excessive urinary oxalate excretion occurs in long-term TPN patients both with and without ileostomies, *J. Am. Coll. Nutr.*, 14, 24, 1995.
110. Luippold, G. et al., Dopamine D2-like receptors and amino acid-induced glomerular hyperfiltration in humans, *Br. J. Clin. Pharmacol.*, 51, 415, 2001.

17 Prevention of Short Bowel Syndrome in Crohn's Disease

Victor Fazio and Massarat Zutshi

CONTENTS

The effect of reduction in the functional length of small intestine below a critical length required for minimal effective absorption results in intestinal failure and has been termed the short bowel syndrome. In recent years Crohn's disease accounts for more than 50% of the cases of short bowel syndrome in adults.[1] In the U.K. it accounts for at least 40% of the adult patients on home parenteral nutrition (HPN).[2]

Multiple resections due to recurrence and complications contribute to the short bowel syndrome and are important in the surgical considerations of Crohn's disease.[2] However, these patients have a better nutritional prognosis after the initial year than those in whom the predisposing cause is ischemia or radiation enteritis. This may be due to a better adaptive response or a remission of the disease.[3]

Survival rates have improved markedly with HPN; however, it comes with a high cost (over $100,000 a year), and catheter-related problems for which patients are frequently hospitalized as well. In patients with an anticipated long-term survival, about 20% of patients with intestinal failure develop cholestatic liver disease.[4]

PATHOPHYSIOLOGY

Short bowel syndrome occurs as a result of decreased effective absorptive area leading to malabsorption and steatorrhea, coupled with decreased transit time, causing water and electrolyte loss. Multiple resections in a short period of time for obstructive complications of fistulizing disease, or intra-abdominal sepsis that require extensive resections to control sepsis, are factors that aid in the progression to short bowel syndrome.

The small intestine serves as the main organ for nutrient absorption. This is effected in the normal bowel by increasing the transit time to allow maximal absorption. Slowing the intestinal motility is under hormonal and neural control. Intestinal contents normally take 1/3 of the time to traverse the jejunum and proximal ileum and take the remaining 2/3 of the total transit time to traverse the ileum.[5] The ileocecal valve plays a role in controlling the entry of the intestinal contents into the colon and also prevents the bacterial colonization of the small intestine. The presence of the ileocecal valve after resections for Crohn's disease is therefore an important factor in the pathophysiology of intestinal failure. The duodenum and jejunum are the main areas for absorption of carbohydrates, proteins, and fat along with absorption of water, calcium, folate iron, magnesium, and phosphate. Bile salts and vitamin B_{12} are also absorbed in the ileum. Resections of the jejunum have lesser impact on absorption as the ileum adapts to take over its function; however, large resections of the ileum result in a shortened transit time and increased malabsoption. Minor resections of the ileum result in decreased bile salt reabsorption. However, major resections of more than 100 cms in an adult cause a severe depletion of bile salts, as the production of bile salts by the liver cannot keep pace with the loss in feces. This causes decreased absorption of long-chain fatty acids and fat-soluble vitamins, leading to steatorrhea, which adds to the diarrhea. Jejunostomy closure with anastomosis of the colon (jejunocolic anastomosis) adds the functional equivalent of 25–30 cms of small intestinal length. Restoration of continuity in patients with a potential to develop intestinal failure[6] is clearly desirable. Colonic deconjugation of bile salts results in the production of free bile acids that causes the secretion of water and adds to the diarrhea by decreasing the transit time. The colon is the site of sodium and water absorption, and the presence of an intact colon is an important factor in the pathophysiology of the short bowel. A normally functional colon in the absence of a normally functional small intestine adds the equivalent of about 50 cms of small intestine in its absorptive function. This allows the absorption of about 504 Kcal of carbohydrates from short-chain fatty acids in a day.[7] Colon preservation is therefore important in maintaining electrolyte balance and aids in carbohydrate metabolism. Patients with an intact colon adapt more readily than do patients with a jejunostomy.[1] However, the colon is also the region where oxalates are absorbed, and this contributes to the formation of kidney stones. This can be prevented with the oral administration of high doses of calcium (2.4-3.6 g/day of elemental Ca),[8] which bind to oxalates and prevent their absorption. Gallstones that are composed of calcium bilirubinate, and not cholesterol, are also formed when ileal length is compromised.[9]

Short bowel syndrome is characterized by diarrhea, nutritional deficiencies, steatorrhea, and malabsorption. Renal calculi, gallstones, and hypersecretion of acid are common accompaniments. Treatment is usually with parenteral nutrition, though surgical solutions may be considered. The best treatment, however, is anticipation and prevention.

THE PROCESS OF ADAPTATION

Limited resections of the small intestine have little or no impact on absorptive capacity, as the small bowel adapts with a slight increase in length and hypertrophy of the villi in enterocyte number and crypt depth, and increased number of transporters per cell increasing the absorptive surface.[8] The overall functional result is increased nutrient and fluid absorption. This is also seen in the colon, whereby absorption of water and electrolytes and compensatory procedures for energy production are increased.[10] However, when the effective length is reduced by 75% or more, nutritional supplementation is necessary for survival.

Massive resections are followed by profuse diarrhea that lasts for 3–4 months after which the period of adaptation starts. Diarrhea is lessened, as is stool volume, and electrolytes and water absorption are improved.[10] This phase lasts about 1–3 years and ends with maximal adaptation. Patients may be controlled with oral enteral feedings or may require parenteral nutrition (PN). An increase in transit time has been seen after the first 3 years, with a reduction of 70% in the parenteral nutrition requirement.

Factors that affect adaptation include luminal nutrition, glutamine, short-chain fatty acids, triglycerides and polyamines, pancreatic secretions, gut hormones, and humoral factors.[11] Prolonged use of PN and NPO status in the early phase prevents this adaptive response and should be avoided or withdrawn as soon as possible.

INDICATIONS FOR SURGERY IN CROHN'S DISEASE

Crohn's disease is a panenteric disease and recurrence is common. Endoscopic evidence of recurrence is seen in about 70% of patients at 1 year and in 85% of patients at 3 years.[12] Reports indicate that 39% of patients with ileocecal disease, 34% of patients with colonic diseases, and 26% with small bowel disease will face recurrence at 5 years. The rates of reoperations have been reported at 25% after 5 years, 45% after 10 years, and 55% after 15 years of disease onset.[13]

Surgery in Crohn's disease is not curative but is the primary treatment for the complications of the disease. It is also an alternative for disease control when medical treatment has failed to control symptoms or produces disabling side effects. Surgery may be required if symptoms progress when medical therapy is tapered off or for complications of the medical therapy itself. These include systemic hypertension, cushingoid features, cataracts, glaucoma, myopathy, peptic ulcer, osteoporosis, and aseptic necrosis of the head of the femur.[14]

The most common indication for surgery is intermittent or acute or persistent obstruction. Obstruction is usually due to strictures of the small bowel.[15] Other indications include septic complications like perforations, inflammatory masses; abscesses that could be intra-abdominal, pelvic, or perineal; anastomotic leaks; and fistulae. Failure to thrive, hemorrhage, intestinal cancer, and fulminant colitis with or without toxic megacolon are additional indications. Surgery in Crohn's disease is directed to relieve the indications mentioned above rather than to cure the disease.

GOALS OF SURGERY IN CROHN'S DISEASE

Resection of the small bowel is considered the procedure of choice for all complications, which are an inherent part in the history of the disease. Since surgery is not curative, patients undergo multiple surgeries during the course of the disease. Prevention of malabsorption should therefore play a major role in the planning of an elective procedure in these patients. Every patient undergoing surgery should be viewed as a potential candidate to develop malabsorption in the future, and younger patients should be considered at special risk.

It is important to recognize preoperatively what course the disease will take depending on the symptoms and type of disease. The disease phenotype representing a lesion requiring a resection will manifest with symptoms of obstruction or perforation. These are the patients that will return with recurrent symptoms requiring

---

TABLE 17.1
Goals of Surgery in Crohn's Disease

Minimize intestinal loss, especially small bowel
- Identify diseased areas
- Don't resect because disease is present
- Short vs. long (wide) resection
- Strictureplasty, multiple vs. resection
- Salvage out-of-circuit normal bowel
- Preserve colon
- Repair target area in fistulae vs. excision

Maintain function
- Use of high jejunostomy/diversion
- Total parenteral nutrition

Daily recurrence
- Maintenance with medical therapy

---

frequent or multiple surgeries. Minimizing resection should therefore be of paramount importance in these patients. The patients presenting with an inflammatory disease phenotype respond better to a medical management, and surgery should be deferred until obstructive symptoms are manifested.

GENERAL PRINCIPLES

The most important factor in prevention of short bowel syndrome is to practice bowel conservation to minimize the loss of intestinal length, especially of the small intestine (Table 17.1). This starts with operative recognition of Crohn's disease or its recurrence, which could be a difficult process when viewed from the external surface. However, it takes some experience to decide which area can be left behind as an uninvolved margin. Gross evidence such as fat wrapping, fat deposition in the mesentery, and corkscrew appearance of the subserosal vessels is easy to visualize. In order to make a decision as to the extent of involvement, the technique of mesenteric palpation for indurated versus soft mesenteric margins provides a good estimate.[16,17] The mesenteric margin of the bowel becomes palpable as the palpating fingers move away from the disease (Figure 17.1).

The thick mesentery with enlarged lymph nodes and fat deposition in Crohn's disease should also be carefully handled. Slipped vessel ties causing a hematoma in the mesentery can result in resection of valuable small bowel. Each part of the small

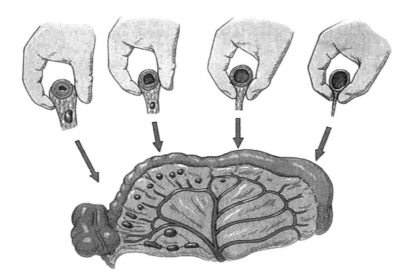

FIGURE 17.1 When resection is required, the extent of the Crohn's disease must be defined. Resection lines may be guided by palpation of the mesenteric margin of the bowel wall. As the palpating fingers are moved away from the disease, the mesenteric margin of the bowel becomes palpable when normal intestine is reached. (From Fazio V.W., *Inflammatory Bowel Disease*, 5th ed., W.B. Saunders, Philadelphia, PA, 1999. With permission.)

intestine that can be preserved at each subsequent surgery will go a long way in prevention of malabsorption. Use of serial overlapping clamps and suture ligation while dividing the mesentery prevents retractions of blood vessels and subsequent hematoma formation.[17]

Timing of a surgical procedure is a key factor in minimizing unnecessary resection. In the early postoperative period, adhesions will not only pose a problem of more time taken to enter the abdomen,[18] but also increase the chance of inadvertent trauma to the bowel. Surgery should be avoided for at least 3–6 months after an initial laparotomy to avoid encountering massive dense adhesions that could result in an inadvertent enterotomy and lead to unnecessary resection and sepsis.[19] Matted loops of bowel are best managed by delivering the mass outside the abdomen before dissection to minimize contamination. Serosal injury is repaired and the abdomen is irrigated before closure.

Another goal in surgery is to prevent recurrence and to prolong this recurrence-free period, thereby allowing intestinal adaptation. A higher risk of recurrence occurs with perianal disease, and obstructive and perforative symptoms. The role of side-to-side versus end-to-side and stapled versus hand-sewn anastomosis needs prospective evaluation, though some studies suggest lower recurrence rates with the wide side-to-side anastomosis.[20]

Fistulae are a common occurrence and should be managed surgically only if symptomatic. Uncomplicated fistulae (enteroenteric) are treated medically unless there is some obstructive pathology.[15,21] Repair rather than resection of target organ preserves bowel unless associated with an abscess, in which case a limited resection rather than an extensive one is of immense value. This is of special importance when the target organ is the colon, and we have already stressed the importance of preserving the colon.

TECHNIQUES TO PREVENT/MINIMIZE THE DEVELOPMENT OF SHORT BOWEL SYNDROME

BOWEL CONSERVATION

Bowel conservation applies to both small intestine as well as colonic resection where enhancement of absorptive surface is desirable. Early literature[22] indicated that wide margins, that is, excision beyond macroscopic and microscopic evidence of involvement by Crohn's disease with wide (several inches) clearance, was desirable to reduce recurrence rates. The majority view in current times is that a wide excision is not necessary.[16] We have reported no advantage regarding recurrence by complication rates of performing a wide or extensive excision, and caution should be used when resecting small intestine as bigger is not necessarily better.[16] A limited resection of a 2 cm margin has been shown to be as effective as a wider 12 cm one.[23] Intestine should not be resected simply because disease is present, and the presence of apthous ulcers is not indicative of disease requiring excision. The site of bowel resection should be 1–2 cm from the clinically obvious limit of involvement.[13]

Avoidance of Resection in Selected Patients

The patients who are vulnerable to short bowel syndrome are those who have had previous resections, those who have jejunoileitis, and those who present with a long segment of small bowel involvement. Strictureplasty has emerged as an attractive and effective option. Minimal surgery has proven efficacy, and various studies have shown no difference in recurrence rates between resections and strictureplasty.[24] Short strictures less than 10 cm can be treated with a Heineke-Mikulicz type of a strictureplasty (Figure 17.2) and strictures greater than 10 cm can be dealt with a Finney type of strictureplasty (Figure 17.3) or an isoperistaltic side-to-side stricture-plasty or a combination of a Finney/Heinke-Mikulicz strictureplasty.[25–27] Multiple short strictures can be treated with a combination of both the types of strictureplasty.

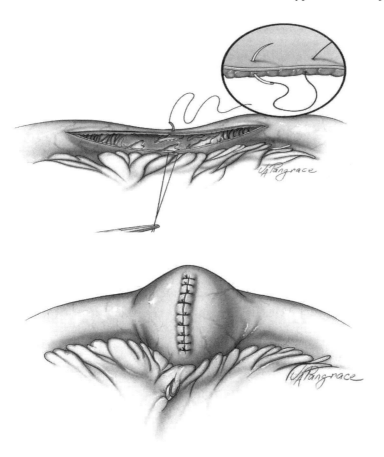

FIGURE 17.2 Heineke-Mikulicz strictureplasty.

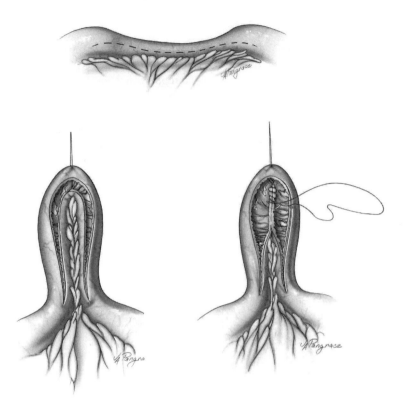

FIGURE 17.3 Finney strictureplasty.

Ileocecal recurrent Crohn's disease may be amenable to a strictureplasty as well. There are reports of the use of strictureplasty[28] during an initial resection instead of an ileocecal resection. Michelessi[29] has described the use of an isoperistaltic side-to-side anastomosis as an alternative to Finney strictureplasty to prevent diverticular formation and possible bacterial overgrowth, and a modification has been described by Pogglioli et al,[28] to overcome stricturing at the ends of the anastomosed segment. Long recurrent strictures can be treated with transection of the stricture at the midline and a side-to-side anastomosis with this technique.

AVOIDANCE OF OUT-OF-CIRCUIT (NORMAL) SMALL BOWEL OR COLON

Salvage procedures should be considered to bring back into the circuit normal intestine that has been excluded from the mainstream. An example of this is to salvage usable bowel distal to an ileostomy or colostomy that may have been created to divert the fecal stream.

Bypassing intestine is generally avoided and any intestine that is out of circuit and that cannot be kept under surveillance is best resected to reduce cancer risk[30] and future resection.

Avoidance of a Right Hemicolectomy for Ileocecal or Terminal Ileal Disease

The right colon is frequently not involved in Crohn's disease, and its preservation will add to the anatomic length of residual colon, enhancing water and electrolyte preservation. Likewise, although ileorectal anastomosis is technically easier than an ileodescending or ileosigmoid anastomosis, preservation of as much as of the remaining colon as possible will offer a similar benefit. Intraoperative colonoscopy is useful in determining the desirable level of anastomosis and conserving the length of bowel to be resected.

Do Not Resect Bowel Just Because Crohn's Disease Is Present

The presence of uncomplicated Crohn's disease is not considered an indication to resect bowel. There is little benefit in resection of small bowel unaffected by obstruction or sepsis compared to medical treatment alone. Similarly if endoscopic evaluation suggests a quiescent or inactive disease for Crohn's colitis, and surgery is being done primarily for small bowel complications, preservation of the colon is desirable.

Of the factors that affect recurrence, the ones that can be attributed to surgery are the resection margins, the type of operation, and the indications for surgery.[13] Microscopic evidence of disease at the resected margin is not indicative of higher recurrence rates of disease or of reoperations in the future,[31] compared with normal margins. The presence of apthoid ulcers is not a contraindication for an anastomosis. Intestine affected by gross macroscopic ulceration, fistulae, and strictures should not be used in an anastomosis. The use of frozen sections during surgery has not proven to be an effective indicator of recurrence and is of limited predictive or prognostic value.[32] Other factors that affect recurrences are the preoperative length of the diseased segment[33] and luminal factors as the disease is controlled when fecal diversion is performed and recurs after intestinal continuity is restored.

Segmental Resection vs. Total Colectomy

There is a considerable debate on whether segmental resection is associated with a lower recurrence rate versus total colectomy and ileorectal anastomosis. There has been no randomized controlled trial that has addressed this issue. However, a commonly held view[34] is that by conserving colon absorptive function a segmental resection is preferable in patients vulnerable to dehydration and diarrhea, especially in older patients or those patients who have had previous small bowel resection.

Chemoprophylaxis to Delay Recurrence

Prophylactic drug therapy is especially indicated in patients who have had multiple surgeries or aggressive fistulizing disease. The aim of therapy is to reduce the postoperative recurrence or delay the onset of recurrence. In patients who undergo an ileocecal resection, an endoscopic evaluation at 6–12 months is a good predictor of postoperative recurrence[35] and suggests benefits from prophylactic therapy. It has been hypothesized that altering the bacterial flora with antibiotics could decrease postoperative recurrence. Metronidazole 20 mg/kg/day has been shown to reduce the severity of endoscopic recurrence and the clinical relapse rate in one study[36] when compared with a placebo. However, long-term benefit has not been shown.

Mesalamine in doses of 2.0–2.4 g/day has been shown to reduce postsurgical recurrences by 13.1%.[37,38] Conventional corticosteroids are too toxic for long-term prophylactic therapy, and budesonide, a nonsystemic analog has been shown to reduce recurrence only for 6–9 months in doses of 6 mg/day.[39] For the patient with the obstructive phenotype, treatment with metronidazole in doses of 750–1000 mg/day[15] is better tolerated and effective. Fistulizing disease is especially prone to recurrences and infection, and antibiotics like ciprofloxacin and metronidazole may be valuable in disease control. A pilot study[40] has shown that concomitant and long-term azathioprine/6-mercaptopurine therapy can prolong the effect of initial inflix-imab therapy on fistula closure. In patients who have undergone surgery for failure of medical therapy, more rigorous therapy with immunosuppressants may be indicated. A dose of 50 mg of 6-mercaptopurine is effective in reducing relapse rates after resection.[41] Other innovative therapies include nutritional supplements and special diets that have shown to reduce recurrences, but relapses are higher on discontinuation of these diets.

SMOKING CESSATION

Smoking has a direct relationship with the status of the disease in Crohn's disease patients.[42–44] It is the most common factor in implicated recurrence, and patients should be encouraged to give up smoking.

THE ROLE OF THE HIGH DIVERTING JEJUNOSTOMY

Creation of a high diverting jejunostomy in situations where large segments of bowel are of questionable viability or have multiple skip areas in patients with major protein malnutrition is a useful option. This buys time to allow intestinal healing, allows for nutritional replacement with HPN, and prevents further resection of potentially salvageable[45] bowel. Proximal diverting jejunostomy is of special value in cases of small bowel perforation and complex fistulae formation. Another group of patients who benefit from a high jejunostomy along with HPN are those who have multiple fistulae with severe peritoneal reaction, often in a patient with a frozen abdomen where any kind of intervention could have catastrophic results[35] from a massive resection.

PREVENTION AND TREATMENT OF POSTOPERATIVE SEPSIS

The most frequent sequel to surgery in Crohn's disease, especially emergency surgery, is postoperative sepsis. This is often due to anastomotic breakdown and abscess formation. Abscesses are treated primarily with CT guided or percutaneous drainages and antibiotics.[46] Abscesses not amenable to CT guided drainage usually require surgery.

Postoperative sepsis may be minimized by reinforcing suture lines especially strictureplasty sites. After lysis of adhesions, one looks and repairs serosal tears as they occur. Such patients may benefit from omental wrapping of the anastomosis.[20]

PREOPERATIVE MANAGEMENT

Patients who present for surgery are to be assessed for their nutritional condition. Most studies have shown a high incidence of complications in nutritionally compromised patients.[26] Patients with low serum protein levels have a higher rate of postsurgical complications. Preoperative PN may have benefit in the malnourished patient whose absorption is compromised. Apart from serum protein measurements, a complete blood count to estimate leukopenia and anemia in the more chronically ill patients provides useful parameters and should be normalized before undertaking an elective procedure. Other preoperative assessments could include grip strength and anergy testing.

EARLY ENTERAL FEEDING

Early enteral feeding promotes intestinal adaptation. Prolonged use of parenteral nutrition in the early phase prevents this adaptive response. Hence postsurgical prolonged HPN with limited enteral nutrition may be detrimental to induction of intestinal adaptation. This may be necessary as a bridge to restoration of continuity with or without resection, when dense adhesions have subsided.

CONCLUSION

Short bowel syndrome is probably the most severe and feared complication of surgery for Crohn's disease. Bowel conservation operations are now standard procedures. Cessation of smoking should be encouraged in all patients. Benefits of resection are weighed against anticipated sequelae. Close collaboration with the gasteroenterologist and nutritional team is required in outlining the strategic goals and tactics to achieve them. A cost-effective medical therapy toward reducing recurrence rates with few complications of the therapy will be an option that all surgeons will be looking for the future for the management of relapses and complications of Crohn's disease.

REFERENCES

1. Nightingale, J. and Lennard-Jones, J.E., The short bowel syndrome: what's new and old? *Dig. Dis.,* 1993, 11,12–31.
2. Agwunobi, A.O., Carlson, G.L., Anderson, I.D., Irving, M.H., and Scott, N.A., Mechanisms of intestinal failure in Crohn's disease, *Diseases of Colon Rectum,* 2001, 11(12), 1834–1837.

3. Thompson, J.S., Inflammatory disease and outcome of short bowel syndrome, *Am. J. Surg.*, Dec. 2000, 180(6), 551–555.

4. Thompson, J.S., Langnas, A.N., Pinch, L.W., Kaufman, S., Quigley, E.M., and Vanderhoof, J.A., Surgical approach to short-bowel syndrome, *Ann. Surg.*, 222(4), 600–607.

5. Summers, R.W., Kent, T.H., and Osborne, J.W., Effects of drugs, ileal obstruction and irradiation on gastrointestinal propulsion, *Gasteroenterology*, 1970, 59, 731—739.

6. Carbonnel, F. et al., The role of anatomic factors in nutritional anatomy after small bowel resections, *JPEN*, 1996, 20, 275–280.

7. Nightingale, J., The short-bowel syndrome, *European J. Gastroenterology Hepatology*, 1995, 7(6), 514–520.

8. Buchman, A.L. and Sellin, J., in *Clinical Management of Short-Bowel Syndrome*, Advanced Therapy of Inflammatory Bowel Disease, chap. 102.

9. Pitt, H.A. et al., Ileal resection induced gallstones: Altered bilirubin or cholesterol metabolism? *Surgery*, 1984, 96, 154–162.

10. Earnest, D.L., in *Physiologic Consequences of Surgical Treatment for Inflammatory Bowel Disease*, Therapy, chap. 39.

11. Booth, I.W. and Lander, A.D., Short bowel syndrome, *Balliere's Clinical Gasteroenterology*, 1998, 12(4) 739—774.

12. Rutgeerts, P., Geboes, V.G., Beyls, J., Kettemans, R., and Hiele, M., Predictability of the postoperative course of Crohn's disease, *Gasterenterology*, 1990, 99; 956—963.

13. Borley, N.R., Mortensen, N.J., and Chaudry, M., in *Recurrence After Abdominal Surgery for Crohn's Disease*, Warren, B.F. et al., Eds., 2002.

14. Kornbluth, A., Sachar, D., and Salomon. Crohn's Disease, in *Gasterointestinal and Liver Disease*, Sleisenger and Fordtran, Eds., chap. 101.

15. Schraut, W.H., The surgical management of Crohn's disease, *Gastroenterol. Clin. N. Am.*, 2002, 31, 255–263.

16. Fazio, V.W. and Marchetti, F., Recurrent Crohn's disease and resection margins, bigger is not better, *Advances in Surgery*, 199, 32, 135–169.

17. Delaney, C.P. and Fazio, V.W., Crohn's disease of the small bowel, *Surgical Clinics of North America*, 2001, 81(1), 137–158.

18. Coleman, M.G., McLain, A.D., and Moran, B.J., Impact of previous surgery on time taken for incision and division of adhesions during laparotomy, *Diseases of Colon Rectum*, September 2000, 43(9), 1297–1299.

19. Laureti, S., Fazio, V.W., O'Riordain, M.G., Gramlich, T., Petras, R., Secic, M. and Balliet, J., Time course of adhesions formation and ease of re-operation after abdominal surgery: an experimental study, the Cleveland Clinic Foundation, Cleveland, OH.

20. McLeod, R. et al., Prophylactic mesalamine treatment decreases postoperative recurrence of Crohn's disease, *Gastroenterology* 1995, 106, 404—413.

21. Fazio, V.W., Fistulizing Crohn's disease, *Falk 122 International Symposium on IBD*, chap. 32, 245–255.

22. Krause, U., Ejerblad, S., and Bergman, L., Crohn's disease. A long term study of the clinical course in 186 patients, *Scand. J. Gastroenterlogy*, 1985, 20(4), 516–524.

23. Fazio, V.W., Marchetti, F., and Church, J.M., Effect of resection margins on the recurrence of Crohn's disease in the small bowel, a randomized controlled trial. *Ann. Surg.*, 1996, 224(4), 563–573.

24. Braegger, C., Thomas, A., Bishop, W.P., Haber, B.A., Lichtman, S.N., and Shneider, B.L., Postsurgical recurrences in Crohn's disease, why, when and how to prevent them, *J. Pediatr. Gastroenterol. Nutr.*, 2002, 30(5), 557–559.

25. Poggioli, G., Pierangeli, S., Laureti, S., and Ugolini, F., Review article: Indication and type of surgery in Crohn's disease, *Aliment Pharmacol. Ther.*, 2002, 16 (Suppl. 4), 59–64.
26. Fazio, V.W., When to resect and when to do strictureplasty for Crohn's disease of the small intestine — a review, *Falk 123 — VI International Symposium on IBD*, chap. 21, 173–87.
27. Dietz, D.W., Laureti, S., Strong, S.A., Hull, T.L., Church, J., Remzi, F.H., Lavery, I.C., and Fazio, V.W., Safety and long-term efficacy of strictureplasty in 314 patients with obstructing small bowel Crohn's disease, *J. Am. Coll. Surg.*, 2001, 192(3), 330–338.
28. Poggioli, G., Laureti, S., Pierangeli, F., and Ugolini, F., A new model of strictureplasty for multiple and long stenoses in Crohn's ileitis, *Diseases of the Colon and Rectum* 2003, 46(1) 127–130.
29. Michelassi, F., Hurst, R.D., Melis, M., Rubin, M., Cohen, R., Gasparitis, A., Hanauer. S.B., and Hart, J., Side-to-side isoperistaltic strictureplasty in extensive Crohn's disease: a prospective longitudinal study, *Ann. Surg.*, 2000, 232(3), 401–408.
30. Greenstein, A.J., Sachar, D.B. et al., Cancer in Crohn's disease after diversionary surgery, *Am. J. Surgery*, 1978, 135, 86—90.
31. Wolff, B.G., Resection margins in Crohn's disease, *British J. of Surgery*, 2001, 88, 771–772.
32. Heymann, T.M. et al,, Prediction of early symptomatic recurrence after intestinal resection in Crohn's disease, *Ann. Surg.*, 1993, 218, 294–299.
33. D'Haens, G., The length of recurrent ileitis after ileocolonic resection correlates with presurgical extent of Crohn's disease, *Gasteroenterology*, 1993, 104, A692.
34. Strong, S.A. and Fazio, V.W. in *The Surgical Management of Crohn's Disease in Inflammatory Bowel Disease*, 5th ed., Kirsner J.B. and Hanauer, S.B., Eds., W.B. Saunders Company, Orlando, FL, 1997.
35. Oakley, J.R., Steiger, E., Lavery, I.C., and Fazio, V.W., Catastrophic enterocutaneous fistulae, the role of home hyperalimentation, *Cleveland Clinic Q.* 46(4), Winter 1979, 133–6.
36. Rutgeerts, P. et al., Controlled trial of metronidazole treatment for prevention of Crohn's recurrence after ileal resection, *Gasteroenterology*, 1995, 108: 1617—1621.
37. Camma, C. et al., Mesalamine in the maintainance of treatment of Crohn's disease: A meta-analysis adjusted for confounding variables, *Gasteroenterology* 1997, 113, 1465–1473.
38. McLeod, R. et al., Prophylactic mesalamine treatment decreases postoperative recurrence of Crohn's disease, *Gasteroenterology*, 1995, 106, 404—413.
39. Hellers, G. et al., Oral budesonide for prevention of postsurgical recurrence in Crohn's disease, *Gasteroenterology*, 1999, 116, 294–300.
40. Ochsenkuhn, T., Goke, B., and Sackman, M., Combining Infliximab with 6- Mercaptopurine/Azathioprine for fistula therapy in Crohn's disease, *Am. J. Gasterenterology* 1997, 8, 2022–2025.
41. Harrison, J. and Hanauer, S.B., Medical treatment of Crohn's disease. *Gasteroenterolog. Clin. N. Am.*, 2002, 31, 167–184.
42. Cosnes, J. et al., Smoking cessation and the course of Crohn's disease, an intervention study, *Gasteroenterology* 2001, 120(5), 1093—1099.
43. Yamamoto, T. and Keighley, M.R., Smoking and disease recurrence after operation for Crohn's disease, *British J. of Surgery* 2000, 87(4) 398—404.

44. Pico, M.F. and Bayless, T.M., Tobacco consumption and disease duration are associated with fistulizing and structuring behavior in the first 8 years of Crohn's disease, *Am. J. Gasteroenterology* 2003, 98(2), 363—368.
45. Mulholland, M.W. and Delaney, J.P., Proximal diverting jejunostomy for compromised small bowel, *Surgery*, 1983, 93(3), 443-447.
46. Garcia, C., Persky, S., Bonis, P., and Topazian, M., Abcesses in Crohn's disease, outcome of medical versus surgical treatment, *J. Clin. Gastroenterol.*, 2001, 32(5), 409–412.

18 Surgery for Intestinal Failure

Kishore R. Iyer and Margaret Richard

CONTENTS

Intestinal failure is simply defined as failure of the intestine to adequately perform its primary function of nutrient and fluid absorption. This in turn results in a failure to meet the individual's caloric needs via the enteral route and also causes fluid and electrolyte imbalances, frequently requiring parenteral compensation. Such a simplistic definition avoids the inherent problems in attempting to define short bowel syndrome. While the latter term is intuitive, there is considerable disagreement as to what exactly is "short." This problem is further compounded by limited available data on normal bowel length at different ages in the normal population, difficulties in measurement of bowel length, the influence of the site of resection on outcome, and finally, the considerable individual differences in outcomes among patients with apparently similar gut lengths.[1-5] It is for these reasons that we prefer the term *intestinal failure* to short bowel syndrome.

The term *intestinal failure* includes the clinical subset of patients who have a functional problem in the face of normal or at least adequate gut length, as often seen in congenital idiopathic pseudo-obstruction of childhood. Since the problems faced by this latter patient population are very similar to patients who have short bowel syndrome, it appears best to consider short bowel syndrome as a specific form of intestinal failure due to a true inadequacy of gut length to support normal bowel function.

Historical surgical attempts at improving intestinal function following massive bowel resection were met with limited success.[6] All the procedures enumerated by Cywes were designed to delay intestinal transit and included vagotomy and pyloroplasty, recirculating small bowel loops, antiperistaltic gastric tubes, reversed small bowel segments, and pouch formation.[7] In a series of carefully designed animal studies, Budding and Smith confirmed that recirculating loops were of no clinical value.[7] They observed that the simplest procedure of creating an ileal reversed segment appeared to produce the best outcome but was still associated with significant complications, under their experimental conditions. They concluded that "clinical application of corrective surgical procedures in the treatment of massive resection of the small intestine seems justified only when dietary and medical measures fail to keep the patient in satisfactory condition"; this fundamental observation is just as valid today.[7] The experimental success achieved by pre-ileal and pre-jejunal transposition of the colon in puppies with 90% small intestinal resection has seen only limited clinical application.[8,9] Of these historic attempts at surgical salvage of the native remnant intestine, segmental reversal of the small intestine continues to be employed in carefully selected, adult patients with short bowel syndrome.[10] Further progress in the surgical management of intestinal failure awaited the landmark development of parenteral nutrition (PN) as a safe and routinely applicable technology.[11–17]

The effects of massive intestinal resection have been studied extensively by many groups.[3,18–23] Collectively, these physiological processes initiate the process of adaptation and are discussed in detail in Chapter 1 of this book. Viewed teleologically, adaptation has a structural component that increases available surface area for nutrient absorption, and at the same time, there is a functional increase in various enzymatic and hormonal processes that increase the intestinal capacity for nutrient absorption and digestion, as shown in Figure 18.1. Though a discussion of adaptation is beyond the scope of this chapter, certain key observations are worthy of note:[24]

1. Over time, the residual intestine dilates and lengthens.
2. Patients who undergo jejunal resection adapt much better than patients who undergo ileal resection.

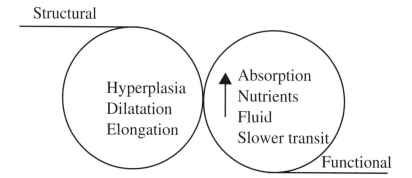

FIGURE 18.1 Structural and functional components of intestinal adaptation.

3. The adaptive process depends on luminal nutrition, pancreatobiliary secretions, and various gut hormones and mediators.
4. The time taken for adaptation is unknown, but may be even longer than 2 years in some cases.

The medical management of patients with intestinal failure is complex and the subject of detailed discussion elsewhere in this book. We believe it is labor-intensive, time-consuming, and best undertaken by an experienced multidisciplinary team that includes gastroenterology, nutrition, and surgical expertise early in the care to ensure optimal outcomes. Such an approach allows graded application of care. Goals of therapy evolve over time, from the early resuscitation, to optimization of parenteral and enteral nutrition, to prevention of complications of parenteral nutrition in the long term. In this approach, only a small subset of patients will require surgical intervention, and an even smaller group of patients will fail all conservative modalities of treatment and become candidates for intestinal transplantation.

ROLE OF THE SURGEON IN MANAGEMENT OF INTESTINAL FAILURE

We believe that the surgeon with an interest in intestinal failure and nutrition is a key member of the multidisciplinary team caring for the patient with intestinal failure. It is not in the patient's best interest for the role of the surgeon to be defined purely in terms of the technical abilities but rather to see the surgeon as the person who carries the responsibility, ideally in partnership with a gastroenterologist, for the long-term well-being of the patient. Viewed in this light, the role of the "intestinal failure" surgeon starts from reducing the severity of or even preventing the development of intestinal failure and continues with the provision of secure long-term venous access and employing strategies for autologous gut salvage in selected cases. Finally, when all conservative attempts fail to prevent or reverse the occurrence of life-threatening complications of PN, such as the development of liver disease or loss of venous access, the surgeon should play a pivotal role in determining failure of conservative therapies and the need for transplantation. Even in this late stage of the disease, the surgeon, now in concert with the intestinal transplantation program, can help optimize the care of the patient to allow the best possible outcome from intestinal transplantation.

PRINCIPLES OF EARLY SURGICAL MANAGEMENT

Very little data are available on the prevention of intestinal failure. Unpublished personal experience and limited available literature suggest that a high index of concern for the imminent development of short bowel syndrome, and a conservative approach to potential intestinal catastrophes, may allow prevention of intestinal failure and indeed improve outcomes in some cases.[25-31] The role of strictureplasties and conservative surgical strategies in Crohn's disease are covered in Chapter 17). A few fundamental principles that may have wider application are worthy of mention.

When the potential risk of development of short bowel syndrome is considered to be high, early adoption of a conservative strategy to minimize additional and preventable loss of bowel is mandatory. Such an approach relies on preservation of bowel of doubtful viability with adoption of planned "second-look" laparotomy.[32] We have adopted the "clip and drop back" technique described by Grosfeld and coworkers in the presence of compromised bowel, with excellent results.[29] Use of a silastic mesh to close the abdomen in these instances facilitates rapid reentry into the abdomen while preserving the fascio-aponeurotic layers for subsequent closure. At the same time, the mesh can serve to provide additional abdominal domain to reduce the risks of abdominal compartment syndrome secondary to ischemia-reperfusion. In the most extreme instances, the entire bowel can be exteriorized in a "silo" fashioned from a silastic sheet as frequently practiced for management of large gastroschisis, allowing the bowel to gradually return into the peritoneal cavity mainly under the influence of gravity.

Irrespective of etiology, once the patient is adequately resuscitated and stabilized, the surgical priority becomes restoration of intestinal continuity. Recruitment of distal unused intestine often facilitates reabsorption of fluid and electrolytes or in the case of the ileum, bile salts, and is an important first step toward adaptation. Prevention of disuse mucosal atrophy with restoration of luminal flow and of trophic factors is an important prerequisite for the process. There is growing appreciation of the colon's ability to salvage undigested carbohydrates by bacterial breakdown into short-chain fatty acids that can directly enter the portal circulation as energy sources. We strongly believe that as a general rule, stomas should be avoided if at all possible in patients with intestinal failure. Apart from the obligatory loss of bowel length inherent in creation (and reversal) of any stoma, clinical experience suggests that patients with difficult-to-manage and poorly placed stomas may be at significant additional risk of catheter-related infections while on long-term PN. Proximity of the catheter to the stoma site may play a role. Disadvantages and complications of early stoma closure are few but deserve attention. Unreabsorbed bile salts in the colon may stimulate an osmotic diarrhea with severe perineal irritation that requires meticulous skin protection. The diarrhea frequently requires dietary restrictions as reported in about 60% of patients without a stoma, as opposed to dietary restrictions in only 33% of patients with a stoma, reported by Nguyen et al.[33] Nevertheless, barring patients with high end-jejunostomies and/or patients with no distal bowel other than recto-sigmoid, as well as patients with functional disorders such as congenital pseudo-obstruction, we regard closure of any preexisting stomas as an important early step in the overall surgical management.

DEFINITIVE SURGICAL MANAGEMENT

Surgical options in long-term patients with intestinal failure fall into four general categories:

1. Operations to correct slow transit

2. Operations to improve intestinal motility — dilated bowel
   a. Imbrication
   b. Tapering enteroplasty
   c. Longitudinal Intestinal lengthening and tailoring (Bianchi)
   d. Transverse Intestinal lengthening (Kimura and Georgeson)
   e. STEP procedure

3. Operations to slow intestinal transit — no bowel dilatation
   a. Valves
   b. Reversed segments
   c. Colon interposition

4. Operations to increase mucosal surface area.
   a. Creation of neomucosa
   b. Sequential intestinal lengthening

Slow transit in patients with short bowel syndrome is uncommon and should, in all cases, prompt a search for strictures, adhesions, and blind loops causing partial obstruction. These are usually left over from the original underlying disease, such as necrotizing enterocolitis or Crohn's disease, and should be treated expeditiously. We have on rare occasions found prior unsuspected pathology such as duodenal webs and missed intestinal atresias, successful treatment of which allows a favorable outcome.

Rapid intestinal transit is a more frequent occurrence in patients with short bowel syndrome. Rapid transit may be a result of inappropriate enteral nutrition, extremely short length of bowel, or small bowel bacterial overgrowth. Once nutritional issues have been addressed, persistent rapid transit with increased stool/ostomy losses should prompt investigation to rule out potential structural causes for the rapid transit. These are manifest most often by segmental bowel dilatation. Figure 18.2 demonstrates significant small bowel dilatation on the contrast study of an 18-month old patient with short bowel syndrome and a history of episodic abdominal distension with increased stool outputs. Dilated bowel segments exhibit poor antegrade peristalsis, an observation first characterized by de Lorimier et al.[34] It is believed that such dilated segments result in significant stasis of intestinal content, leading to small bowel bacterial overgrowth and rapid transit. While the latter is consistent with clinical experience, hard evidence for bacterial overgrowth and episodic translocation in this setting is lacking. Nevertheless, it is our practice to attempt aggressive gut decontamination on an empirical basis when dealing with rapid intestinal transit in a patient with intestinal failure. The demonstration of a dilated segment of bowel in such a patient usually presages failure of medical treatment and the need for surgical intervention. It must be emphasized that the indication for surgery is the failure of medical treatment in a patient with a significantly dilated segment of small bowel; the demonstration of bowel dilatation in a patient who is advancing satisfactorily toward enteral autonomy from parenteral nutrition (PN) and is free of complications is in itself not an indication for surgical intervention.

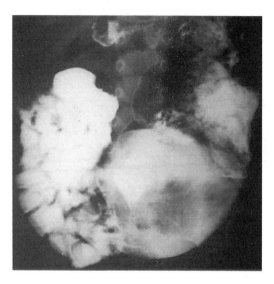

FIGURE 18.2 Contrast radiograph showing segmental small bowel dilatation.

The choice of surgical procedure to tackle the dilated bowel segment in the patient with intestinal failure often requires careful judgment. The simplest expedient of resecting the dilated segment is applicable only in the rare instance where bowel length is demonstrably a non-issue with early enteral autonomy having been achieved in a patient with adequate remnant bowel length and a very limited segment of dilated bowel. More often, the choice rests between a simpler tapering procedure or a procedure that combines tapering with some potential gain in length. De Lorimier and Harrison first described an intestinal plication technique that achieved the goal of creating a narrower, and therefore it was hoped, a more streamlined and propulsive loop of bowel, without any loss of mucosal surface area.[35] They achieved these twin objectives by simple in-folding of the dilated loop of bowel and suturing adjacent sero-muscular surfaces.[35] The principle of the intestinal plication technique is shown in Figure 18.3. Unfortunately, though the operation is effective in the short term, the plication is prone to partial or complete breakdown with recurrence of the dilatation and its attendant complications. Tapering enteroplasty as performed by most surgeons today consists of removal of a portion of the dilated bowel along the antimesenteric border, leaving behind a segment that is of normal caliber. Due care must be taken to avoid narrowing the residual bowel excessively with a resultant stricture. If there is any concern, a small enterotomy allows passage of a wide-bore tube (e.g., 24 Fr, in a neonate), with tapering of the bowel around the tube, to ensure a satisfactory remnant lumen. This is usually not necessary, and placement of stay sutures along the antimesenteric border prior to the actual tapering allows visual estimation of the lumen to be left behind, as shown in Figure 18.4. Tapering can be done simply and swiftly with repeated firings of a linear mechanical stapling device incorporating a cutting blade, with additional imbrication of the staple line along the antimesenteric border if desired.

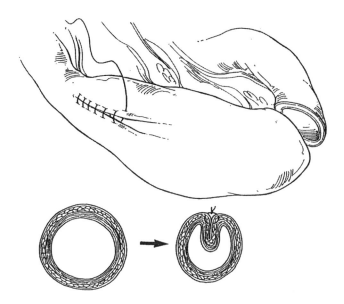

FIGURE 18.3   Intestinal plication. (From O'Neill, J.A. et al., *Pediatric Surgery, Volume 2: Short Bowel Syndrome*, Elsevier, 1998, p. 1227. With permission.)

The Longitudinal Intestinal Lengthening and Tapering (LILT/Bianchi) procedure first described by Adrian Bianchi in 1980 is based on the principle that the mesenteric blood supply of the bowel can be separated into two layers, with vessels alternately ending in opposite surfaces.[36,37] Development of an avascular window in the mesenteric border of a dilated bowel loop between the two leaves of the mesentery and careful allocation of alternate blood vessels to either side allows division of a dilated loop of bowel into two "hemi-loops," each with half the original blood supply. Anastomosis of the two hemi-loops, end-to-end in isoperistaltic fashion in a "lazy-S" configuration, completes the operation, as shown in Figure 18.5. The actual longitudinal division of the bowel may be accomplished relatively rapidly with a mechanical stapling device, dividing the hemi-loops between two double rows of staples, or the division may be carried out by hand using bipolar diathermy with fashioning of the hemi-loops by tedious hand suturing.

We have recently encountered three patients who developed hemi-loop fistulae between adjacent hemi-loops having undergone LILT elsewhere in childhood, using a stapled technique. The first of these was referred to us for isolated small bowel transplantation with recurrent life-threatening fungal infections. A dilated loop at the site of his previous LILT was found to be due to complete breakdown of the adjacent walls of the two hemi-loops, essentially forming a giant recirculating loop. At operation at our institution, the fistulae and adjacent staple lines were excised; the mesenteric borders were redefined, preserving the blood supply to the hemi-loops, and a hand-sewn LILT was redone. At over 18 months follow-up, the child has achieved full enteral autonomy off PN and is free of all infections. This case has led us to abandon the stapling technique and adopt a traditional freehand

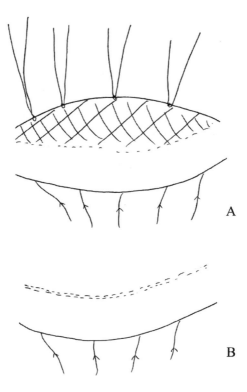

FIGURE 18.4 Tapering enteroplasty. Shaded portion of dilated loop is excised (stay-sutures on anti-mesenteric border).

technique in all cases on the basis that it may allow more precise visualization and protection of the mesenteric blood vessels without the additional dissection required to create the space needed for insertion of a stapling device. While Bianchi's follow-up paper indicated that hemi-loop fistulae occurred in two of five study animals, this complication has not been reported since, until our recent inclusion of the above case in a larger report.[38] It is unclear whether reported failures following the Bianchi LILT procedure may at least partially be due to this unrecognized complication. It is also unknown whether adoption of a freehand technique using bipolar diathermy and hand-suturing as opposed to using a stapling device will reduce the incidence of this complication. A modification of the Bianchi procedure has been proposed by Chahine and Ricketts, using a single wide tapered anastomosis, thus avoiding the need for three smaller anastomoses as originally proposed by Bianchi.[39]

The results of the Bianchi procedure are somewhat difficult to assess, and are largely in the form of individual case series. Formal studies of the physiological effects of this operation are few. In a series of carefully conducted experiments in dogs, Thompson et al. demonstrated that LILT attenuated the normal adaptive response.[40] Animals that had undergone lengthening had diminished body weight, albumin levels, and absorption as compared to animals that had undergone resection alone at 4 and 12 weeks of study.[40] Transit time was prolonged after lengthening —

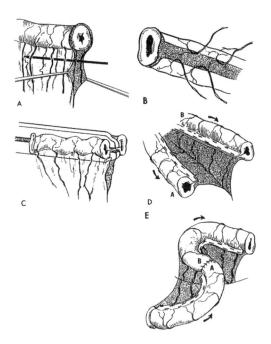

FIGURE 18.5 Bianchi (LILT) procedure. (A) Dissection between peritoneal leaves of mesentery. (B) Intervascular space on mesenteric border. (C) Bowel loops between jaws of stapling device. (D) Hemiloops resulting from stapling and division of bowel. (E) Isoperistaltic anastomosis between hemiloops. (From Bianchi, A., Intestinal loop lengthening — A technique for increasing intestinal length, *J. Pediatric Surgery*, 15, 145–151, 1980. With permission.)

these changes appeared related to hypergastrinemia and possibly to decreased enteroglucagon and increased somatostatin levels. [40] The same group reported on their early clinical experience with the procedure in six children — overall outcome was improved in five of six children, with four of the five achieving full enteral autonomy from PN and some improvement being achieved in the fifth. [41] However, the authors reported that one of the six patients died from sepsis related to an anastomotic leak and one of the five survivors had necrosis of one of the hemi-loops. [41] This early report emphasizes the potential morbidity and even mortality from the operation, related as much to the fragility of the patient population as to the procedure. In one of the few objective studies of the procedure, Weber and Powell documented reduced stool frequency (mean of 8 preoperatively to 3 per day, 6 months after), increased transit time, and normalization of D-xylose and fat absorption after Bianchi LILT procedures in five patients. [42] Four of the five patients attained full enteral autonomy from PN six months after the lengthening procedure. A follow-up report on 16 patients from the same group confirmed their early experience with objective improvements in measured aspects of bowel motility and absorption, as well as achievement of enteral autonomy from PN in 14 of the 16 patients (88%).[43]

Waag et al. reported on their experience with application of the procedure in 25 children with short bowel syndrome.[44] With a mean follow-up of 6 years, PN was discontinued in 17 of 18 survivors at a mean of 5.1 months after operation.[44] The authors emphasized the frequency of metabolic and septic complications occurring in this group of patients. The group required constant vigilance and medical and nutritional treatment in order to achieve overall acceptable outcomes in 13 of their 18 survivors. None of the 7 deaths in their series were related directly to the procedure — 3 were due to end-stage liver disease in association with PN, and 2 were due to sepsis.[44]

Spitz and coworkers from the Hospitals for Sick Children in London reported on the problems leading to failure of the procedure in three children with "very short bowel syndrome."[45] In all three cases, the authors concluded that the combination of technical problems and worsening complications of short bowel syndrome may have been reduced considerably by deferring application of the procedure to a time when the infants were bigger and normal adaptation had been completed.[45] Occurrence of hemi-loop entero-enteric fistulae appeared to be the cause of failure in the first patient in the series. We believe loss of early functional improvement following the LILT procedure must be vigorously investigated particularly to rule out anastomotic narrowing or entero-enteric fistulae between hemi-loops. These may be hitherto underrecognized complications leading to some of the "failures" following the procedure. Bianchi's own experience with the procedure in 20 children resulted in 7 of 9 survivors attaining enteral autonomy from PN at a median follow-up of 7 years.[46] In general, survivors had at least 40 cm of small bowel at the time of lengthening and had minimal or no liver disease.[46] A follow-up report (Bianchi, A.: personal communication) in over 25 children indicates that the experience is sustained, with perhaps a slightly higher percentage of patients coming off PN in the longer term.

Bianchi's own experience with autologous gut salvage supports the generally accepted view that the LILT procedure, and indeed other procedures aimed at autologous gut salvage should not be applied in patients with any degree of PN-associated liver disease other than in its earliest stages. We have recently reported on our experience with extended application of autologous gut salvage procedures in the intestinal transplant era.[38] This series included application of the Bianchi LILT procedure in four carefully selected children with advanced liver disease, all of whom had clinical evidence of portal hypertension, significant hyperbilirubinemia, and biopsy evidence of fibrosis in the liver, up to and including cirrhosis. The four were part of a series of patients with advanced liver disease who were aggressively treated for PN-associated liver disease with attempts at autologous gut salvage. Four of the ten children attained full enteral autonomy from PN, and four others had significant (> 50%) decrease in PN requirements. Of greatest interest, eight of the nine survivors in this cohort exhibited full biochemical and functional liver recovery following the procedure, as did the one patient who died from catheter-related sepsis while being close to full enteral autonomy. Twelve of the 13 children in this report were originally referred for intestinal transplantation, in isolation or combined with the liver. We now believe that the presence of even advanced degrees of liver dysfunction in very carefully selected children with short bowel syndrome may not be an absolute contraindication to attempts at autologous gut salvage. This conclusion must be tempered by the fact that patients with intestinal failure and advanced liver disease may have a very limited window of opportunity for successful combined liver-intestinal transplantation; we firmly believe that the needs of such a high-risk group of patients are best served by a multidisciplinary team with expertise and experience in all aspects of management of intestinal failure and liver disease, while having rapid access to transplantation.

A small percentage of patients who undergo the Bianchi procedure develop secondary dilatation of the lengthened segment with evidence of dysmotility in the dilated segment. Additionally, some patients have dilatation of only the second and third parts of the duodenum or very proximal jejunum. These patients are not candidates for longitudinal intestinal lengthening, in the former case because the mesentery is now reduced to a single layer and in the latter case for anatomic reasons. For this small cohort of patients, Kimura and Soper reported on a technique of Transverse Bowel Lengthening, using an isolated bowel segment.[47,48] The operation relies on developing neovascularization of the dilated segment of bowel by creating a wide myo-enteropexy, anchoring the bowel after denuding it of the sero-muscular layer on its antimesenteric aspect to the undersurface of similarly denuded liver or rectus sheath. At a second stage about six weeks later, if the dilated bowel loop shows evidence of having successfully "parasitized" itself to its neo-vascular source, the loop can be divided transversely, effectively achieving transverse intestinal lengthening and tapering. While the bowel loop so isolated appears capable of normal function, the actual situations where such novel procedures can be applied are few and far between.[24,48] Attachment of a loop of bowel to the undersurface of the abdomen does also significantly complicate abdominal reentry, which may be a factor if a patient is failing all therapies and being considered for intestinal transplantation.

The recently described STEP (Serial Transverse Enteroplasty Procedure) has generated considerable interest.[49,50] In principle, lengthening of a loop of bowel is achieved by serial transverse applications of a GIA stapler, from opposite directions, to create a zig-zag channel, as shown in Figure 18.6. The authors reported their initial observations in a group of six pigs in which bowel dilatation was first accomplished by creating a reversed jejunal segment. Bowel lengthening was accomplished and the animals were studied radiologically prior to terminal examination of the bowel at six weeks.[49] There appeared to be a significant gain in length of bowel in animals following the procedure and the zig-zag channel appears to straighten out at six weeks. All lengthened animals gained weight. In their first case report that followed soon after, the authors reported improved bowel function in a two-year-old patient who had apparent "failure" of a Bianchi procedure performed at the age of 11 months, with significant dilatation of the previously lengthened segment. Bowel length was increased again by application of the novel STEP procedure, from a total of 130 cm to 200 cm. Improvement in bowel function was paralleled by some improvement without normalization of D-xylose absorption.[50] The remarkable technical simplicity of this novel procedure in comparison to the relative complexity of the Bianchi and other lengthening procedures may explain the considerable interest it has generated including in the lay press (*New York Times*, 2003). Several groups have each performed a small number of STEP procedures. Our own experience suggests the need for caution and further study (Iyer, unpublished observations). Of

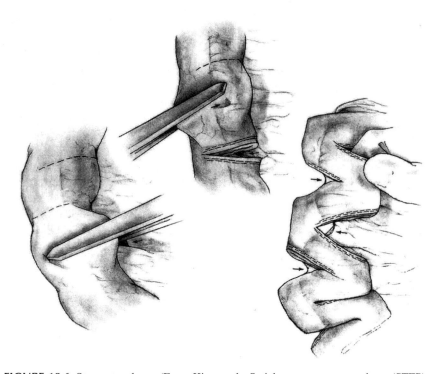

FIGURE 18.6 Step enteoplasty. (From Kim et al., Serial transverse enteroplasty (STEP): a novel bowel lengthening procedure, *J. Pediatric Surgery*, 38, 425–429, 2003. With permission.)

four patients who underwent the STEP procedure, one had some dilatation after a Bianchi procedure approximately 18 years ago; this patient, receiving approximately 50% of her caloric intake via PN experienced no benefit from the procedure, as did one other adult patient with extreme short bowel (45 cm ending in a stoma). The third patient, who had excessive stoma losses with minimally dilated bowel, underwent the STEP and appears to have reduced ostomy losses with modest improvement in PN requirements following the procedure. The fourth patient had rapid worsening of her advanced liver disease following the STEP procedure and died from the complications of end-stage liver disease. This limited early experience suggests the need for further study to better understand the choice of candidates and potential contraindications for what appears to be a technically simple operation.

The occurrence of refractory rapid intestinal transit in a patient with short bowel syndrome in the absence of bowel dilatation is particularly challenging. Nipple valves, constructed in the manner of an everted ileostomy at the site of small bowel-colonic anastomosis, have been shown to be of benefit.[24] The biggest drawbacks of the technique are the fact that the optimal length of the valve is unclear — a short valve is ineffective while too long a valve may cause complete intestinal obstruction. Further, constructing an optimal valve may require 8–10 cm of bowel in a patient who may not be able to afford the additional loss of length. Prosthetic valves address these concerns and require only 2–3 cm of bowel for their placement, but may be complicated by erosion of the valve into the bowel lumen or obstruction caused by tissue reaction or prosthetic dislodgement.[24]

The potential benefit of reversed intestinal segments in management of short bowel syndrome has been referred to earlier. Panis and coworkers reported on segmental reversal of the small bowel in eight patients at the time of restoration of intestinal continuity.[10] The mean length of remnant small bowel at the time of reversal was 46 ± 18 cm and the mean length of segment used for reversal was 12.7 ± 2.8 cm, with the reversed segment being distal small bowel in all but one patient. Complete mesenteric rotation was avoided by appropriate juxtaposition of the segments to be anastomosed. At a median follow-up of 35 months (range 2–108 months), four patients attained full enteral autonomy from PN, with significant reduction in PN requirements in the remaining patients.[10] Unpredictable bowel growth in children makes the use of reversed segments much less reliable; although reversed loops may initially slow transit, they can cause progressive intestinal obstruction as they grow with the child.

Isoperistaltic colonic interposition to slow intestinal transit has seen only limited clinical application perhaps, because of the risk of eosinophilic colitis causing refractory bleeding.[10] While the potential value of colonic salvage of undigested carbohydrates, converting them into short-chain fatty acids is recognized, it is unclear why a segment of colon taken out of colonic continuity and interposed in the small bowel should be of greater value than in its original anatomical position.

The tantalizing prospect of creating neomucosa and thus truly expanding mucosal surface area has drawn extensive research over the last decade, but clinically meaningful success remains elusive at this time.[52,53] Georgeson and coworkers have adopted a novel approach toward the same goal.[54] In eight children with refractory short bowel syndrome and no signs of intestinal adaptation, dilatation of the small bowel was accomplished by creating a nipple or artificial valve. When the bowel was deemed to be satisfactorily dilated, intestinal lengthening was carried out in a conventional Bianchi-type procedure. Seven of eight patients achieved a decrease in PN requirement with this approach.[24,54]

CONCLUSIONS AND FUTURE DIRECTION

Surgical management of intestinal failure has evolved considerably over the last four decades, paralleling advances in parenteral and enteral nutrition. Improvements in understanding of the physiology of intestinal failure and adaptation have also contributed to the improvement in outcomes. There is also a growing realization that indications for surgical intervention in this high-risk patient population are for the most part related to failure of nutritional and medical treatment or to onset of complications. A challenge for the future is to better define the position and timing of potentially risky surgical intervention aimed at autologous gut salvage, weighed against early referral for intestinal transplantation with the prospects of improved post-transplantation outcomes. Perhaps the answer will lie in intestinal transplantation programs working alongside intestinal rehabilitation programs, providing a whole range of expertise, from nutritional and medical intervention to autologous intestinal reconstruction and intestinal transplantation. Patients with intestinal failure will then have specific therapy directed to their disease state rather than having to find different centers offering one or other but not comprehensive therapy. Such comprehensive "intestinal failure/rehabilitation centers" may be the practical solution to improved outcomes for the patient with intestinal failure, while we await clinically meaningful advances in creating neomucosa and tissue-engineered bowel.

REFERENCES

1. Toloukian, R. and Walker-Smith, G., Normal intestinal length in preterm infants, *J. Pediatr. Surg.*, 18, 720, 1983.
2. Nightingale, J., Bartram, C., Lennnard-Jones, J., Length of residual bowel after partial resection: correlation between radiographic and surgical measurements, *Gastrointest. Radiol.*,16, 305, 1991.
3. Alpers, D., How adaptable is the intestine in patients with short-bowel syndrome? *Am. J. Clin. Nutr.*, 75, 787, 2002.
4. Sondheimer, J., Cadnapaphornchai, M., Sontag, M., and Zerbe, G., Predicting the duration of dependence on parenteral nutrition after neonatal intestinal resection, *J. Pediatr.*, 132, 80, 1998.
5. Messing, B., Crenn, P., Beau, P., Boutron-Rualt, M., Rambaud, J., and Matuchansky, C., Long-term survival and parenteral nutrition dependence in adult patients with the short bowel syndrome, *Gastroenterology*, 117, 1043, 1999.
6. Cywes, S., The surgical management of massive bowel resection, *J. Pediatr. Surg.*, 3, 740, 1968.
7. Budding, J. and Smith, C., Role of recirculating loops in the management of massive resection of the small intestine, *Surg. Gyn. Obst.*, 125, 243, 1967.
8. Hutcher, N. and Salzberg, A., Pre-ileal transposition of colon to prevent the development of short bowel syndrome in puppies with 90 percent small intestinal resection, *Surgery*, 70, 189, 1971.
9. Hutcher, N., Mendez-Picon, G., and Salzberg, A., Prejejunal transposition of colon to prevent the development of short bowel syndrome in puppies with 90 percent small intestine resection, *J. Pediatr. Surg.*, 8, 771, 1973.
10. Pannis, Y., Messing, B., Rivet, P., Coffin, B., Hautefeuille, P., Matuchansky, C., Rambaud, J., and Valleur, P., Segmental reversal of the small bowel as an alternative to intestinal transplantation in patients with short bowel syndrome, *Ann. Surg.*, 225, 401, 1997.
11. Wilmore, D. and Dudrick, S., Growth and development of an infant receiving all nutrients exclusively by vein, *JAMA*, 203, 860, 1968.
12. Wilmore, D. and Dudrick, S., Safe long term venous catheterization, *Arch. Surg.*, 98, 256, 1969.
13. Wilmore, D. and Dudrick, S., An in-line filter for intravenous solutions, *Arch. Surg.*, 99, 462, 1969.
14. Wilmore, D., Groff, D., Bishop, H., and Dudrick, S., Total parenteral nutrition in infants with catastrophic gastrointestinal anomalies, *J. Pediatr. Surg.*, 4, 181, 1969.
15. Dudrick, S., Wilmore, D., Vars, H., and Rhoads, J., Long-term parenteral nutrition with growth, development and positive nitrogen balance, *Surgery*, 64, 134, 1968.

16. Dudrick, S., Wilmore, D., Vars, H., and Rhoads, J., Can intravenous feeding as the sole means of nutrition support growth in the child and restore weight loss in an adult? An affirmative answer, *Ann. Surg.,* 169, 974, 1969.

17. Dudrick, S., Groff, D., and Wilmore, D., Long term venous catheterization in infants, *Surg. Gyn. Obst.,* 129, 805, 1969.

18. Hanson, W., Osborne, J., and Sharp, J., Compensation by the residual intestine after intestinal resection in the rat: I. Influence of amount of tissue removed, *Gastroenterology,* 72, 692, 1977.

19. Hanson, W., Osborne, J., and Sharp, J., Compensation by the residual intestine after intestinal resection in the rat. II. Influence of postoperative time interval, *Gastroenterology,* 72, 701, 1977.

20. Kurkchubasche, A., Rowe, M., and Smith, S., Adaptation in short bowel syndrome: reassessing old limits, *J. Pediatr. Surg.,* 28, 1069, 1993.

21. Wilmore, D., Dudrick, S., Daly, J., and Vars, H., The role of nutrition in the adaptation after massive resection, *Surg. Gyn. Obst.,* 132, 673, 1971.

22. Wilmore, D. and Dudrick, S., Effects of nutrition on intestinal adaptation following massive small bowel resection, *Surg. Forum,* 20, 398, 1969.

23. Quigley, E. and Thompson, J., The motor response to intestinal resection: motor activity in the canine small intestine following distal resection, *Gastroenterology,* 105, 791, 1993.

24. Georgeson, K., Short-Bowel Syndrome. In *Pediatric Surgery,* 5th ed., O'Neill J. Jr., Ed., Mosby-Year Book., St. Louis, MO, 1998, 1223–1232.

25. Di Abriola, G., De Angelis, P., Dall'oglio, L., and DiLorenzo, M., Strictureplasty: an alternative approach in long segment bowel stenosis Crohn's disease, *J. Pediatr. Surg.,* 38, 814, 2003.

26. Dietz, D., Fazio, V., Laureti, S., Strong, S., Hull, T., Church, J., Remzi, F., Lavery, I., and Senagore, A., Strictureplasty in diffuse Crohn's jejunoileitis: safe and durable, *Dis. Colon Rectum,* 45, 764, 2002.

27. Kosloske, A. and Jewell, P., A technique for preservation of the ileocecal valve in the neonatal short intestine, *J. Pediatr. Surg.,* 24, 369, 1989.

28. Thompson, J., Iyer, K., DiBaise, J., Young, R., Brown, C., and Langnas, A., Short bowel syndrome and Crohn's disease, *J. Gastrointest. Surg.,* 7, 1069, 2003.

29. Vaughan, W., Grosfeld, J., West, K., Schere, L., Villamizar, E., and Rescorla, F., Avoidance of stomas and delayed anastomosis for bowel necrosis: the "clip and drop-back" technique, *J. Pediatr. Surg.,* 31, 542, 1996.

30. Moore, T., Management of midgut volvulus with extensive necrosis by "patch, drain and wait," *Ped. Surg. Int.,* 6, 313, 1991.

31. Moore, T., Management of necrotizing enterocolitis by "patch, drain and wait," *Pediatr. Surg. Int.,* 4, 110, 1989.

32. Weber, T. and Lewis, E., The role of second-look laparotomy in necrotizing enterocolitis, *J. Pediatr. Surg.,* 21, 323, 1986.

33. Nguyen, B., Blatchford, G., Thompson, J., and Bragg, L., Should intestinal continuity be restored after massive intestinal resection? *Am. J. Surg.,* 158, 577, 1989.

34. de Lorimier, A., Norman, D., Goodling, C., and Preger, L., A model for the cinefluoroscopic and manometric study of chronic intestinal obstruction, *J. Pediatr. Surg.,* 8, 1973.

35. de Lorimier, A. and Harrison, M., Intestinal plication in the treatment of atresia. *J. Pediatr. Surg.,* 18, 734, 1983.

36. Bianchi, A., Intestinal lengthening: an experimental and clinical review, *J. R. Soc. Med.,* 77, 35, 1984.

37. Bianchi, A., Intestinal loop lengthening — a technique for increasing small intestinal length, *J. Pediatr. Surg.*, 15, 145, 1980.

38. Iyer, K., Horslen, S., Torres, C., Vanderhoof, J., and Langnas, A., Functional liver recovery parallels autologous gut salvage in the era of intestional transplantation, *J. Pediatr. Surg.*, 39, 340, 2004.

39. Chahine, A. and Ricketts, R., A modification of the Bianchi Intestinal lengthening procedure with a single anastomosis, *J. Pediatr. Surg.*, 33, 1292, 1998.

40. Thompson, J., Quigley, E., and Adrian, T., Effect of intestinal tapering and lengthening on intestinal structure and function, *Am. J. Surg.*, 169, 111, 1995.

41. Thompson, J., Pinch, L., Murray, J., Vanderhoof, J., and Schultz, L., Experience with intestinal lengthening for the short-bowel syndrome, *J. Pediatr. Surg.*, 26, 721, 1991.

42. Weber, T. and Powell, M., Early improvement in intestinal function after isoperistaltic bowel lengthening, *J. Pediatr. Surg.*, 31, 61, 1996.

43. Weber, T., Isoperistaltic bowel lengthening for short bowel syndrome in children, *Am. J. Surg.*, 178, 600, 1999.

44. Waag, K., Hosie, S., and Wessel, L., What do children look like after longitudinal intestinal lengthening? *Eur. J. Pediatr. Surg.*, 9, 260, 1998.

45. Huskisson, L., Brereton, R., Kiely, E., and Spitz, L., Problems with intestinal lengthening, *J. Pediatr. Surg.*, 28, 720, 1993.

46. Bianchi, A., Longitudinal intestinal lengthening and tailoring: results in 20 children, *J. R. Soc. Med.*, 90, 429, 1997.

47. Kimura, K. and Soper, R., Isolated bowel segment (Model 1): creation by myoenteropexy, *J. Pediatr. Surg.*, 25, 512, 1990.

48. Kimura, K. and Soper, R., A new bowel elongation technique for the short bowel syndrome using the isolated bowel segment Iowa models, *J. Pediatr. Surg.*, 28, 792, 1993.

49. Kim, H., Fauza, D., Garza, J., Oh, J-T., Nurko, S., and Jaksic, T., Serial transverse enteroplasty (STEP): a novel bowel lengthening procedure. *J. Pediatr. Surg.*, 38, 425, 2003.

50. Kim, H., Lee, P., Garza, J., Duggan, C., Fauza, D., and Jaksic, T., Serial transverse enteroplasty for short bowel syndrome: a case report, *J. Pediatr. Surg.*, 38, 881, 2003.

51. Glick, P., de Lorimier, A., Adzick, N., and Harrison, M., Colon interposition: an adjuvant operation for short-gut syndrome, *J. Pediatr. Surg.*, 19, 719, 1984.

52. Bianchi, A., Lendon, M., and Ward, I., Assessment of surgical techniques for neomucosal growth, *Ped. Surg. Int.*, 7, 41, 1992.

53. Saday, C. and Mir, E., A surgical model to increase the intestinal absorptive surface: intestinal lengthening and growing neomucosa in the same approach, *J. Surg. Res.*, 62, 184, 1996.

54. Georgeson, K., Halpin, D., Figueroa, R., Vincente, Y., and Hardin, W.J., Sequential intestinal lengthening procedures for refractory short bowel syndrome, *J. Pediatr. Surg.*, 29, 316, 1994.

19 Intestinal Failure and Visceral Transplantation: A New Era of Colossal Achievement

Geoffrey Bond, Guilherme Costa,
George Mazariegos, Jorge Reyes, and
Kareem Abu-Elmagd*

CONTENTS

* Support in part by research grants from the Veterans Administration and Project Grant No. DK-29961 and R01 DK 54232 from the National Institutes of Health, Bethesda, MD.

Recently, the center for Medicare and Medicaid Services (CMS) qualified intestinal, combined liver-intestinal, and multivisceral transplantation as the standard of care for patients with irreversible intestinal and parenteral nutrition (PN) failure. The decision was supported by the cumulative improvement in survival over the last decade. Prior to the current era, the worldwide experience was plagued with uncontrolled rejection, graft versus host disease (GVHD), and fatal infection. These undefeated barriers stemmed from the large gut lymphoid mass and the intramural microbial load with the absence of an effective immunosuppressive and antimicrobial therapy. With the emergence of small bowel and multivisceral transplantation in 1990, multiple factors, in addition to the clinical introduction of tacrolimus, have sustained and increased these efforts, including evolution of surgical techniques and improvement in postoperative care. The most valuable achievement, however, has been the effective control of rejection and treatment of life-threatening opportunistic infections. This chapter outlines the common current practice, surgical techniques, and postoperative management of the three different types of intestinal transplantation. In addition, new strategies to overcome some of the current immunologic and biologic challenges are defined with the aim of raising the level of such a creative surgery to be a better therapy for PN-dependent patients.

The Department of Health and Human Services (HSS) has recently considered, in response to the senior author's formal request, that intestinal, liver-intestinal and multivisceral transplantation be the standard of care for patients with irreversible intestinal and PN failure. The submitted documents clearly demonstrated the therapeutic efficacy and improved survival outcome of each of the three types of intestinal transplantation with long-term rehabilitation and cost-effectiveness comparing favorably with Medicare expectations for other abdominal and thoracic organ transplantation.[1-6]

Based on compiled data in the literature,[1,2,7] we can safely define the clinical criteria of PN failure as follows: (1) significant liver damage, (2) limited central venous access, (3) multiple line infection/sepsis, and (4) frequent episodes of severe dehydration. The manifestations of substantial hepatic injury include elevated liver function tests, enlarged spleen, low platelet counts, gastroesophageal/stomal varices, coagulopathy, and liver cirrhosis.

INDICATIONS

Irreversible intestinal failure is an essential requirement for consideration of transplantation. The diagnosis should be made after the optimal utilization of the currently available medical and surgical therapeutic modalities to enhance intestinal adaptation and long-term rehabilitation. Short gut syndrome, whether surgical or congenital, is the most common indication for intestinal transplantation. Other common indications include dysmotility and malabsorption syndromes.

In addition, intestinal or multivisceral replacement is an innovative therapy for patients with gastrointestinal neoplasm. The three different types of intestinal transplantation are illustrated in Figure 19.1, with the following indications for each procedure.

Isolated Intestine

The indications for isolated intestinal transplant include: (1) short-gut syndrome: intestinal atresia, midgut volvulus, gastroschisis, abdominal trauma, necrotizing enterocolitis, Crohn's disease, mesenteric vascular thrombosis, and surgical adhesions; (2) motility disorders: hollow visceral myopathy/neuropathy and total intestinal aganglionosis; (3) malabsorption syndromes: microvillus inclusion disease, selective autoimmune enteropathy, radiation enteritis, and inflammatory bowel disease; (4) gastrointestinal neoplasm: mesenteric desmoid tumor, diffused intestinal polyposis, Gardener's syndrome, and other large benign unresectable mesenteric masses. The coexistence of portal hypertension should be considered in patients with long-term PN therapy and/or hypercoagulable syndromes. In these patients, gastroesophageal varices and ascites are uncommon features because of reduced or absent mesenteric arterial flow with short gut syndrome. For those with documented portal hypertension, the components of the intestinal allograft are determined by the type and degree of portal hypertension, as well as the extent of liver damage.[1] Patients with isolated splenic vein thrombosis should undergo splenectomy or preferably shunt surgery along with isolated intestinal transplantation. On the contrary, those with extensive portomesenteric and splenic vein thrombosis should be considered for either combined liver-intestinal or multivisceral transplantation. Patients with modest portal hypertension presented with mild splenic enlargement, platelet count > 50,000, no gastroesophageal varices, and modest portal fibrosis without severe intrahepatic cholestasis should be cautiously considered for isolated intestinal transplantation. In such patients, the venous outflow of the intestinal graft should be drained into the recipient systemic circulation.

Combined Liver-Intestine

The en-bloc hepatointestinal transplantation is indicated for patients with irreversible failure of both organs. In most of these cases, the liver failure is commonly associated

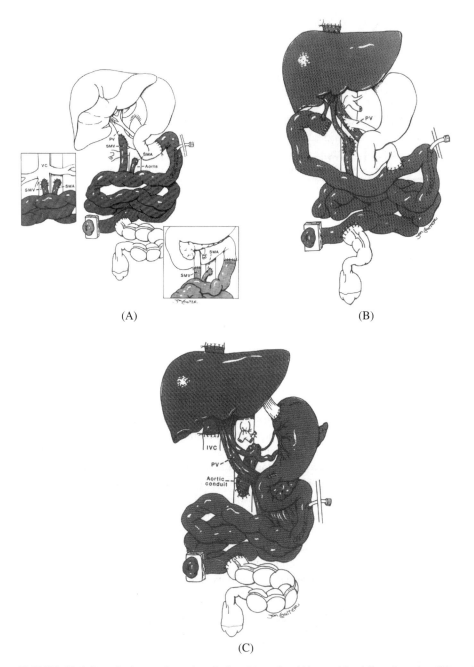

(A)

(B)

(C)

FIGURE 19.1 Intestinal transplantation: isolated intestine (A), combined liver-intestine (B), and full multivisceral (C). Note the old technique of Roux-en Y choledochojejunostomy with combined liver-intestinal transplant. (From Todo, S., Tzakis, A., Abu-Elmagd, K. et al., *Ann. Surg.* 1992; 216: 223–234. With permission.)

with the chronic use of PN. In addition, the procedure could be the only feasible therapeutic modality that can be successfully performed for liver failure patients with concomitant portomesenteric thrombosis. The coexistence of hypercoagulability without liver failure is no longer an indication for simultaneous liver replacement but with lifelong commitment for anticoagulation therapy.[8]

MULTIVISCERAL

Multivisceral transplantation whether full or modified is indicated for irreversible failure or neoplastic disorder of the abdominal visceral organs, including the small bowel. The common causes are massive gastrointestinal polyposis, mesenteric desmoid, gastrointestinal stomal tumors, hollow visceral myopathy/neuropathy, and symptomatic extensive splanchnic vascular thrombosis.

CONTRAINDICATION

Contraindications for intestinal transplant have been established based on past experience with solid organs. These include significant cardiopulmonary insufficiency, advanced malignancy, acquired immune deficiency syndrome, and existence of life threatening intra-abdominal or systemic infections.

PATIENT EVALUATION

Candidacy for intestinal and composite visceral transplants is initially guided by careful patient assessment, including the nutritional status and residual gut functional capacity. Failure of PN weaning despite optimal medical management, including rehabilitation measures, is usually a surrogate marker of poor gastrointestinal functional reserve. The primary cause of intestinal failure guides the subsequent steps of the evaluation process. Patients with enterocyte diseases should undergo thorough radiologic, endoscopic, and histologic examination of the residual gastrointestinal tract. Patients with pseudo-obstruction require gut motility studies to define the type and extent of the disease. A specific hematologic test to define the hypercoagulable syndrome is frequently needed for patients with thrombotic disorders. In addition, abdominal visceral angiography is helpful to assess the extent of thrombosis. In these and other high-risk patients, imaging of the upper and lower extremities central venous system is mandatory for the safe establishment of the required central venous accesses at the time of transplant. A full assessment of the native liver, including biochemical functions, abdominal imaging, and liver biopsy, is essential to determine the need for simultaneous hepatic replacement. The extent of the work-up needed to carefully assess the cardiopulmonary and other body organ systems is commonly guided by patient age, complexity of the medical/surgical history, and nature of the primary disease.

DONOR MANAGEMENT

A good quality and suitable size graft is essential for successful intestinal transplantation. Stable and ABO identical young cadaveric donors are preferred. Smaller size donors are ideal to compensate for the contracted recipient abdominal cavity. The current shortage in cadaveric donors stimulated the utilization of newborn, reduced sized (Figure 19.2), and ABO compatible composite visceral grafts for a few pediatric recipients at our and other transplant centers.[9] No attempts have been made by most centers to deplete the donor lymphoid tissue by antilymphocyte antibodies or to match donor and recipient Human Leukocyte Antigen (HLA). Immune-modulation of the human intestinal allograft with low-dose *ex-vivo* irradiation and donor bone marrow cell infusion has been introduced at our institution[1] after successful preclinical trials.[10, 11] The isolated intestinal grafts, if possible, should not be transplanted across a positive T cell lymphocytotoxic cross-match, and cytomegalovirus (CMV) negative patients should receive CMV negative grafts.[12] Selective gut decontamination should be attempted in all donors in addition to intravenous antibiotic prophylaxis.[13] Further donor management details are described elsewhere.[13]

SURGICAL TECHNIQUES

DONOR PROCEDURE

The embryonic origin and segmental vascular supply of the different abdominal visceral organs (Figure 19.3) is the Achilles heal for successful retrieval.[14,15] The full multivisceral specimen is envisioned as a grape cluster with a double central stem consisting of the celiac and superior mesenteric trunks. The grapes or individual organs can be divided or retained according to the surgical objectives. The three successive phases of the subdiaphragmatic organ procurement procedure are: organ dissection to be used with an intact donor circulation, in-situ cooling by aortic infusion (UW solution) with simultaneous exsanguination, and back-table preparation of the individual organs to be transplanted.

Isolation of the Intestinal Graft

The first step is total colectomy with dissection of the root of the mesentery from its avascular retroperitoneal attachments. After transection of the proximal jejunum, the main stem of the superior mesenteric artery and vein are exposed by dividing the anterior and lateral peritoneal sheath distal to the level of the ligated middle colic vessels. With the more frequent successful use of solitary pancreatic and intestinal transplantation, we recently described a procurement procedure that permits successful retrieval of both organs as well as the liver from the same donor for transplantation to different recipients (Figure 19.4).[15] The back-table vascular reconstruction of a composite intestinal-pancreatic allograft is shown in Figure 19.5.

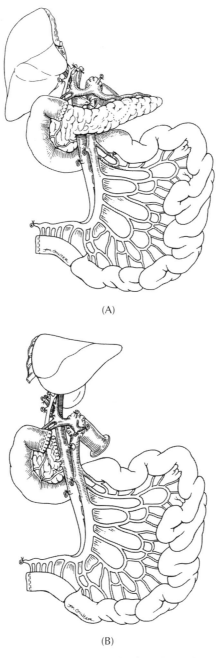

(A)

(B)

FIGURE 19.2 Combined liver-intestinal allograft with reduced liver that consists of the right lobe and medial hepatic segment (A) or the left lateral segment (B). Note that the vascular and biliary structures of the hepatic segments are maintained in continuity with the intestine. (From Bueno, J., Abu-Elmagd, K., Mazariegos, G. et al., *J. Ped. Surg.* 2000; 35(2): 291–295. With permission.)

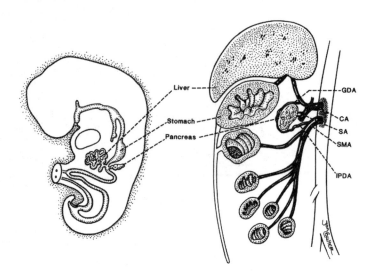

FIGURE 19.3 Embryonic origin of liver, pancreas, and alimentary canal. Note the shared axial blood supply and its segmental distribution. (From Abu-Elmagd, K., Fung, J., Bueno, J. et al., *Ann. Surg.* 2000; 232(5): 680–687. With permission.)

En-bloc Removal of the Liver and Intestine

The liver and small bowel are retrieved in continuity with their central vascular structure. The in-situ technical steps include dissection of the hepatic hilus, isolation of the intestine, exposure of the central vessels, and en-bloc removal of the cooled composite graft.[14,16] Our previously described technique (Figure 19.1B) has been recently modified with preservation of the duodenum in continuity with the donor jejunum and biliary system (Figure 19.6).[12] It is our current practice to preserve the whole pancreatic gland (Figure 19.2A). After in-situ perfusion, the composite graft is removed en bloc by fashioning a single Carrel patch around the orifice of both the celiac and superior mesenteric arteries. During the backbench procedure, the vena cava margins are freed, the duodenum stump is over-sewn with nonabsorbable sutures, and the spleen is removed. The final step is the revision and suturing of the common Carrel patch to a previously prepared segment of the donor thoracic aorta.

Multivisceral Retrieval

The procedure is an extension of the techniques used for multiple abdominal organ procurement.[17] The graft, which usually includes stomach, duodenum, pancreas, intestine, and liver, can be tailored, according to patient needs, by excluding the liver (Figure 19.7)[15] or including the kidney (Figure 19.8).[18] Accordingly, the technique used for the combined hepatic-intestinal retrieval is modified to include the stomach as part of the graft. Therefore, the different gastric vascular arcades are preserved and the organ is disconnected by transecting the abdominal esophagus. The back-table procedure includes placement of the arterial conduit as with

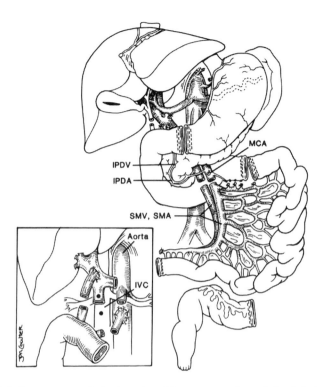

FIGURE 19.4 Procurement of the intestine. Note preservation of the inferior pancreati-coduodenal artery (IPDA) and vein (IPDV) with the pancreatic graft. Vascular conduits are anastomosed to the recipient infrarenal aorta and portal vein or inferior vena cava (inset). (From Abu-Elmagd, K., Fung, J., Bueno, J. et al., *Ann. Surg.* 2000; 232(5): 680–687. With permission.)

combined liver-intestine, over-sewing the transected gastroesophageal junction, and performing pyloroplasty. With the modified grafts, the back-table procedure involves separation of the liver by dissecting the hepatic hilus close to the superior wall of the duodenum and transecting the bile duct, as well as the common hepatic artery and portal vein. The transection of the hepatic artery is usually carried out at or below the level of the gastroduodenal artery and the portal vein is transected above its confluence.[15]

RECIPIENT OPERATION

The surgical implantation of the three generic types of the intestinal allograft starts with a liberal midline abdominal incision with unilateral or bilateral transverse extension, when needed, particularly with composite visceral transplantation.[13] The surgical procedure is often complicated by the presence of extensive abdominal adhesions, contracted abdominal cavity, and severe portal hypertension particularly in patients who require multiple abdominal visceral organ replacement.

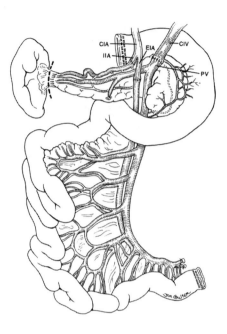

FIGURE 19.5 Back-table vascular reconstruction of the composite intestinal-pancreatic allograft. Note continuity of the pancreas, duodenum and small intestine with intact vascular pedicle. (From Abu-Elmagd, K., Fung, J., Bueno, J. et al., *Ann. Surg.* 2000; 232(5): 680–687. With permission.)

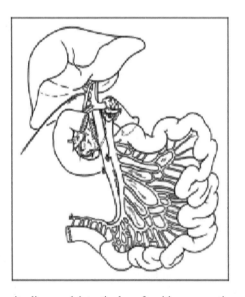

FIGURE 19.6 Composite liver and intestinal graft with preservation of the duodenum in continuity with the graft jejunum and hepatic biliary system. (From Abu-Elmagd, K., Reyes, J., Todo, S. et al., *J. Am. Coll. Surg.* 1998; 186: 512–527. With permission.)

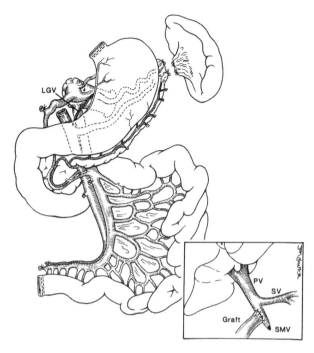

FIGURE 19.7 Modified multivisceral graft that contains stomach, duodenum, pancreas and small intestine. Note preservation of the gastroepiploic arcade and left gastric pedicle with venous drainage to the side of the recipient superior mesenteric vein stump (inset). (From Abu-Elmagd, K., Fung, J., Bueno, J. et al., *Ann. Surg.* 2000; 232(5): 680–687. With permission.)

Intestine Alone

Dissection of the residual native organs and lysis of the surgical adhesions are the first initial steps of the operation. However, the crucial part of the procedure is graft revascularization. The initial step is dissection of the recipient infrarenal aorta and a segment of the portomesenteric venous system or infrarenal inferior vena cava. The technique of graft revascularization by anastomosing the vascular conduits to the recipient vessels (Figure 19.4, inset) rather than to the graft mesenteric vessels on the back table, avoids difficult exposure and possible prolongation of the warm ischemia time.[15] Portal venous drainage of the isolated intestinal graft depends primarily on the technical feasibility of gaining access to the recipient portomesenteric axis. Because of its hemodynamic and metabolic advantages, this type of drainage should always be attempted in all patients particularly with inadequate hepatopetal portal flow, previous splenectomy, dearterialized native liver, and those with caval filters. The systemic caval drainage should be limited to patients with frozen hepatic hilus, portal vein thrombosis, significant hepatic fibrosis, and prior intestinal transplant. Continuity of the gastrointestinal tract is usually restored by conventional surgical procedures. At the end of the operation, a jejunostomy and gastrostomy tube is inserted for immediate postoperative decompression and early

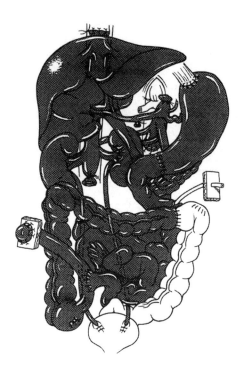

FIGURE 19.8 Full multivisceral graft with inclusion of the kidney. (From Todo, S., Tzakis, A., Abu-Elmagd, K. et al., *Transplantation* 1995; 59(2): 234–240. With permission.)

enteral feeding. The creation of a temporary vent chimney or simple loop ileostomy is always needed to provide easy access for surveillance endoscopy. Closure of the latter, which is usually 3 to 6 months after transplantation, is determined by the postoperative course and functional status of the intestinal graft.

Liver-Intestine

The principles of combined hepatic-intestinal transplantation are the same as that of liver alone. The basic surgical principal is to create a portocaval shunt during the early phase of the operation with the aim of decompressing the residual recipient splanchnic venous bed (Figure 19.9).[6,13,14] The piggyback technique with the avoidance of the venovenous bypass has been our common practice, because of the coexistence of the central venous occlusion particularly of the upper extremities in most of these patients. Arterial revascularization of both the liver and intestine is achieved by anastomosing the common arterial conduit (Figure 19.6) to the infrarenal recipient aorta. The gastrointestinal tract is reconstructed as with isolated intestinal transplantation. The recently described technique of combined hepatic-intestinal retrieval with preservation of the duodenum in continuity with the bile duct and graft jejunum (Figure 19.6) eliminates the need for biliary reconstruction and consequently reduces the operative time and avoids the potential complications of biliary reconstruction.[12]

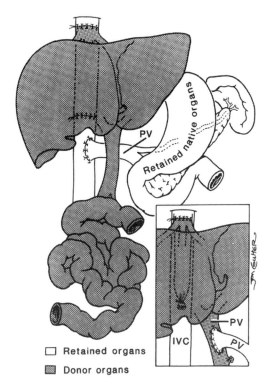

FIGURE 19.9 Drainage of the venous outflow of the retained native viscera in liver-intestinal recipients into their inferior vena cava by portocaval shunt. Note our earlier practice of disconnecting the shunt and reanastomosing the end of the recipient portal vein (PV) to the side of graft portal vein (inset). (From Starzl, T.E., Todo, S., Tzakis, A, et al., *Surg. Gynecol. Obstet.* 1991; 172(5): 335–344. With permission.)

Multivisceral

With multivisceral transplantation, the stomach, duodenum, and pancreas are transplanted en-bloc with the liver and intestine as shown in Figure 19.1C. The procedure can be modified, according to the patient need, to contain all of these organs with exclusion of the liver. This operation is quite different from the originally described cluster procedure since the latter includes only small portions of the jejunum and stomach with the pancreas and duodenum en bloc with the liver. With full multivisceral transplantation, the arterial inflow and venous outflow are reconstituted as with combined liver-intestinal transplant (Figure 19.1C). Total excision of the native upper abdominal organs eliminates the need for a portocaval shunt. With the modified (without liver) graft when the native pancreas, spleen, and duodenum is retained, the venous outflow is drained into the recipient portal circulation and the biliary system is maintained intact as illustrated in Figure 19.10A. This new technique of venous outflow reconstruction maintains the portosplenic circulation intact during graft placement and preserves the spleen that may protect the patient from the risk of post-transplant lymphoproliferative disease (PTLD).[1] In recipients who require

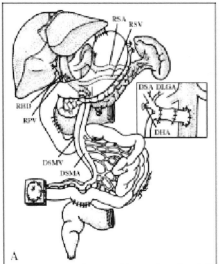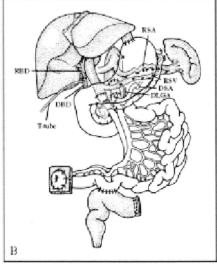

FIGURE 19.10 Transplantation of a modified multivisceral graft (unshaded organs) containing the pancreas and all of the hollow intra-abdominal viscera. (A) Native liver, spleen, pancreas, and a C-loop of duodenum have been retained and drained through a side-to-side host to graft duodenal anastomosis. (B) Native spleen is preserved with maintenance of the recipient portosplenic circulation during graft insertion. Note the duct-to-duct biliary reconstruction. (From Abu-Elmagd, K., Reyes, J., Bond, G., Mazariegos, G. et al., *Ann. Surg.*, 2001; 234(3): 404–417. With permission.)

pancreatoduodenectomy, the biliary system is reconstructed by preserving a segment of donor distal bile duct and performing a duct to duct anastomosis (Figure 19.10B). To reestablish continuity of the gastrointestinal tract, the anterior wall of the transplanted stomach is anastomosed to the recipient gastric cuff or abdominal esophagus (Figure 19.10). Distal reconstruction is preformed as previously described for the isolated intestinal graft.

POSTOPERATIVE MANAGEMENT

The standard postoperative care of the intestinal and multivisceral recipient has been fully described elsewhere.[19,20] The primary focus of this report, however, is the recent advances in the postoperative care of this unique population, with a special emphasis on graft immune-modulation and enhancement of acquired tolerance.

IMMUNOSUPPRESSION

The primary universal immunosuppressive regimen for the intestinal recipients is tacrolimus and steroids. In addition, prostaglandin E1 is infused intravenously as an adjunct during the first postoperative week. Various induction protocols have been recently adopted by different centers to reduce the observed high risk of rejection. Azathioprine, mycophenolate mofetil, and more recently sirolimus are used from the outset as a third agent in selected cases.[1] Steroids, OKT3, rATG, and Campath 1H are utilized to treat rejection episodes. Induction therapy was first used for our intestinal recipients in 1995.[1] This immunoprophylactic approach was triggered by the proven deleterious effect of rejection on survival outcome.[12,21] Cyclophosphamide was first used until the clinical emergence of the humanized IgG1 monoclonal antibody daclizumab. This antibody is directed at the subunit of the human interleukin-2 receptors. Daclizumab (Zenapax®) is used at our institution in an intravenous dose of 1–2 mg/kg body weight for a total of 5 doses.[22] The first dose is administered within a few hours before surgery and the remaining 4 doses were given at 2, 4, 6, and 8 weeks after transplantation.

GRAFT IMMUNE-MODULATION AND RECIPIENT PRECONDITIONING

Despite some improvement in survival with induction therapy, the chronic need for heavy maintenance immunosuppression continues to limit the applicability of the procedure. To overcome such an impediment, a novel immunomodulatory strategy has been recently introduced in Pittsburgh to enhance tolerogenicity and acceptance of the human intestinal allograft. A series of exquisitely controlled rat studies[10] have shown that the quantity and lineage profiles of the passenger leukocytes contained in different organ grafts strongly affect the quantity and lineage of microchimerism, graft survival, and function. In these experiments, the intestinal passenger leukocytes have shown to be less tolerogenic with a higher risk of graft versus host disease (GVHD) than the passenger leukocytes of the liver and bone marrow cells, both of which include large numbers of immature leukocytes and cells of myeloid origin. Accordingly, depletion of the mature T cells in the intestinal allograft with low-dose ex-vivo irradiation combined with donor bone marrow cell replacement should improve the survival benefits of intestinal transplantation by reducing the risk of rejection without increasing the risk of GVHD.[11] The intestinal component of the allograft is irradiated on the back table with a single dose of 750 cGy. The encouraging preliminary results of combined graft irradiation and leukocyte infusion[1] together with the recent revelation of the mechanism of graft acceptance[23,24] stimulated the recent initiation of a clinical trial of thymoglobulin preconditioning and posttransplant tacrolimus monotherapy.[25] With host pretreatment and limit use of post-transplant immunosuppression, the seminal mechanism of clonal exhaustion-deletion may be protected with the achievement of donor-specific nonreactivity and organ engraftment that may not require maintenance therapy for stability. The thymoglobulin pretreatment intravenous dose is 5–10 mg/kg which is covered with two grams of intravenous methylprednisolone. Campath 1H is given intravenously at a total dose of 30-60 mg over 2–4 hours. The total dose of either drug is usually completed before graft revascularization. Post-transplant immunosuppression is with tacrolimus only with a 12-hour trough level of 10–15 ng/ml. Rejection episodes are treated with the conventional therapy.

IMMUNOLOGIC MONITORING

Rejection of the intestine allograft is diagnosed from clinical observations, endoscopic findings, and histopathologic studies of mucosal biopsies.[13,19] Surveillance endoscopy with random mucosal biopsies, particularly of the allograft ileum, is performed at least once per week for the first three months, and every three to six months thereafter and whenever it is clinically indicated. The clinical, endoscopic, and histologic criteria adopted for the diagnosis of intestinal rejection are described elsewhere.[7,13,20,26] The zoom video endoscopy[27] and serum citrulline levels[28] have been recently utilized for the diagnosis of early rejection. The future availability of noninvasive, more sensitive, and highly specific tools to detect early rejection will undoubtedly improve the therapeutic advantages of the procedure. The early diagnosis of GVHD requires a high index of clinical suspicion and availability of a highly advanced immunohistochemical technology.[1,12] The examination of suspicious skin and gastrointestinal tract lesions allow the identification of donor leukocytes with the in-situ hybridization technique using the Y-chromosome-specific probe or the immunohistologic staining of donor-specific HLA antigens. Other GVHD target organs also should be closely observed and biopsy samples are taken when indicated. Prompt augmentation of immunosuppressive therapy including steroids is usually effective with the early diagnosis of GVHD.

NUTRITION AND GRAFT FUNCTION

The achievement of full nutritional autonomy requires flexible and complex management strategies, particularly for recipients of multivisceral grafts.[12] The conversion from parenteral to enteral alimentation is gradual and usually commences within the first two postoperative weeks. Opiates, loperamide, and kaolin-pectin mixture are used for high stomal output/diarrhea, and prokinetic agents are used to treat gastrointestinal dysmotility. Standard hepatic and pancreatic function tests are used to track the functional status of these organs. Successful complete withdrawal of PN with establishment of full gastrointestinal nutritional autonomy has been a most valuable tool in assessing intestinal graft function. Anthropometric measures, including weight, height (children), and upper-arm measurement of fat and muscle as well as serum albumin levels, are frequently utilized for longitude follow-up.

INFECTION PROPHYLAXIS

Protocols for antimicrobial prophylaxis and active treatment are similar to those used for solid organ recipients.[13] In addition, selective gut decontamination is used for 1–2 weeks postoperatively and during moderate to severe rejection episodes.[12,19] Chronic viral and protozoal prophylaxis is with gancyclovir for CMV/Epstein-Barr Virus (EBV) and bactrim for *Pneumocystis carinii*. The newly developed techniques of PP65 antigenmia test and semiquantitative polymerase chain reaction (PCR) assay of EBV in the peripheral blood has allowed early detection, preemptive treatment, and monitoring of the virus associated syndromes with better survival outcome.[1] The concept of infectious implications of rejection that have been previously demonstrated with liver transplantation is even more applicable with the intestine because a disrupted mucosal barrier quickly creates a lethal environment for the total body. The paradoxical therapeutic philosophy of treating infection relatable rejection with prompt increase in immunosuppression, in addition to systemic and local antibiotic therapy, is of utmost importance to prevent or stop bacterial translocation among intestinal transplant recipients.[12,13]

CURRENT CLINICAL STATUS

WORLDWIDE EXPERIENCE

Between April 1985 and May 2003, a total of 923 patients received 989 intestinal transplants at 61 centers.[29] Of these, 76% (n = 747) were transplanted in the U.S. with 33% (n = 247) being performed at the University of Pittsburgh Medical Center (UPMC). There has been a steady increase in the number of centers and the procedures performed per year. Of the 923 recipients, 61% were children and 54% were male. Most of the donors were cadaveric with only 32 grafts obtained from living donors, including an identical twin and a triplet. The liver was more commonly transplanted en-bloc with the intestine in the younger recipients because of the higher incidence of PN associated liver failure in children compared to the adult population. The leading causes of intestinal failure and indications for transplant were gastroschisis (21%), volvulus (17%), dysmotility (16%), necrotizing enterocolitis (12%), intestinal atresia (8%), and microvillus inclusion (6%) in children; and ischemia (23%), Crohn's disease (14%), gastrointestinal neoplasm (16%), and trauma (10%) in adults. The retransplantation rate was 8% among children and 6% for adults.

SURVIVAL

As of May 31, 2003, a total of 484 intestinal recipients were currently alive worldwide with an overall survival rate of 52%.[29] The leading causes of death were sepsis (49%), rejection (11%), technical complications (9%), lymphoma (6%), and respiratory failure (6%). With the cumulative increase in survival over the last 10 years, the one-year patient and graft survival rates for those who were transplanted after February of 1998 were 77% and 65% for isolated intestine, 60% and 59% for combined liver-small bowel, and 66% and 61% for multivisceral grafts, respectively. There was no difference in survival between the three different types of the intestinal allografts. As expected, survival rates were significantly higher in patients who were called in from home for their transplant (p = 0.0004). Another significant survival risk factor was center size, with higher survival rates at centers that performed more transplants. Of great achievement was the significant improvement in the one-year survival with the recent use of pretreatment/induction therapy, particularly with rATG or campath 1H.[29] Such a novel immunosuppressive regimen has recently been introduced by Starzl and Abu-Elmagd et al.[25]

The University of Pittsburgh decade of experience has been recently published as a single-center experience.[1] Between May 1990, and February 2000, a total of 165 transplants were given to 155 consecutive recipients. The Kaplan-Meier

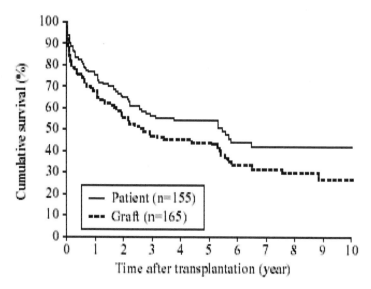

FIGURE 19.11 Kaplan-Meier patient and graft survival curves for the Pittsburgh population. (From Abu-Elmagd, K., Reyes, J., Bond, G., Mazariegos, G. et al., *Ann. Surg.*, 2001; 234(3): 404–417. With permission.)

actuarial survival rate for the total population was 75% at 1 year, 54% at 5 years, and 42% at 10 years (Figure 19.11), with achievement of full nutritional autonomy in more than 90% of the survivors.[1] Recipients of liver-intestinal grafts had the best prognosis for continued survival beyond 5 years (Figure 19.12). Both patient and graft survival improved since 1994 compared with the premoratorium experience (Figure 19.13) with 1- and 5-year patient survival rate of 78 and 63%, respectively. Although the reasons for improvement must be considered indeterminate because of the complexity of the cases and of the treatment strategies, induction therapy, bone marrow augmentation, low dose *ex vivo* allograft irradiation, and rATG pretreatment have significantly contributed to the cumulative increase in survival among the Pittsburgh recipients and subsequently the worldwide experience.[1,25] The recent analysis of our rATG/campath 1H experience showed a one- and three-year patient survival of 91% and 81% with a graft survival rate of 95% and 70%, respectively (unpublished data).

RISK FACTORS

Multivariate analysis of the Pittsburgh experience identified multiple risk factors that significantly affect patient and graft survival.[12, 21] With rejection and the need for heavy immunosuppression being the most detrimental variable, cold ischemia time, number of previous abdominal operations, operative time, development of PTLD, CMV disease, and inclusion of a large segment of colon with the graft were significant risk factors that influenced the survival outcome. Based on the 1999[2] and 2004[29] reports of the International Intestinal Transplant Registry, the worldwide survival outcome with intestinal transplantation has been influenced by five important factors:

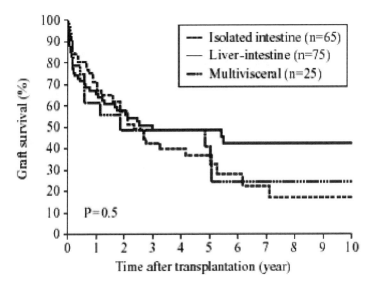

FIGURE 19.12 Kaplan-Meier survival of the three different types of the intestinal allografts. (From Abu-Elmagd, K., Reyes, J., Bond, G., Mazariegos, G. et al., *Ann. Surg.*, 2001; 234(3): 404–417. With permission.)

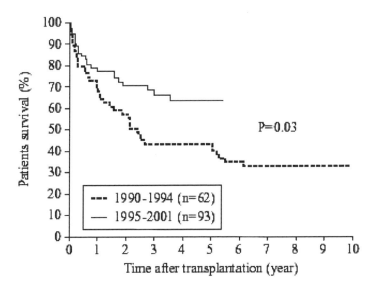

FIGURE 19.13 Patient survival before and after the 1994 moratorium at the University of Pittsburgh. (From Abu-Elmagd, K., Reyes, J., Bond, G., Mazariegos, G. et al., *Ann. Surg.*, 2001; 234(3): 404–417. With permission.)

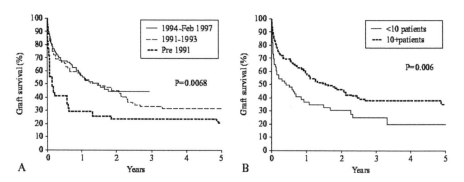

FIGURE 19.14 Graft survival by: (A) time of transplant, (B) center size. (From Grant D., *Transplantation*, 1999, 67: 1061–1064. With permission.)

era of transplantation, disease gravity (home versus hospital bound) at the time of transplant, transplant center size, pretreatment/induction therapy, and recipient's age. Graft survival has significantly improved over time (Figure 19.14A) and both patient and graft survival outcomes were significantly better at centers that have performed more than a total of 10 intestinal transplants (Figure 19.14B).

REJECTION

Despite the use of new adjunct immunosuppressive agents with different cellular and molecular targets, including cyclophosphamide, mycophenolate mofetil, daclizumab, and sirolimus, the overall incidence of intestinal rejection or the ease of management has not dramatically improved.[1] Therefore, we recently introduced the conceptual and clinical application of recipient pretreatment with antilymphocyte depleting agents such as rATG and campath 1H.[25] Although it is too early to make a definitive conclusion, the pretreatment protocol is associated with significant reduction in the need for maintenance immunosuppression. Early acute rejection has been documented at a significantly higher rate among the isolated intestinal grafts compared with intestine contained in a composite graft.[1,2,12] Although the cumulative risk by the end of the first postoperative year was similar among both types of the intestinal graft,[12] the cumulative risk of graft loss due to acute/chronic rejection was significantly greater among the isolated compared to the composite grafts that contained liver (Figure 19.15). It remains to be seen if the degree of long-term destructive immunity among the intestinal allografts will be significantly affected by the HLA mismatch, systemic venous drainage (isolated intestine), and positive lymphocytotoxic cross-match.[1,10] Chronic rejection has been reported at an overall rate of 7% to 10%.[1,2,12] The cumulative risk is significantly greater among the isolated intestinal grafts compared with the composite grafts that contained liver with a 5-year rate of 31% versus 7%.[1] In addition to the type of the allograft, the frequency and severity of acute rejection, recipient age (adults), and race (black) are significant risk factors for development of chronic rejection.[30]

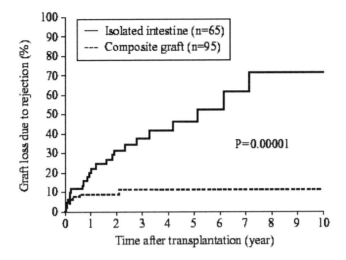

FIGURE 19.15 Cumulative risk of graft loss from rejection in the intestine-only and composite visceral grafts that contained liver. (From Abu-Elmagd, K., Reyes, J., Bond, G., Mazariegos, G. et al., *Ann. Surg.*, 2001; 234(3): 404–417. With permission.)

Graft vs. Host Disease

Unexpectedly, the incidence of GVHD has been relatively low despite the large lymphoid mass being contained in the transplanted intestine with a documented incidence of 5%.[1] With similar risk among recipients of all three types of intestinal allografts, the disease is self-limited in most cases with augmentation of immunosuppression.

Success of Weaning

Out of a total of 89 bowel transplants that were performed at the University of Pittsburgh between July 2001 and December 2003, and were given to rATG-pretreated recipients with post-transplant tacrolimus monotherapy, 57 (64%) cases underwent attempts of weaning. The criteria of weaning were: 1) postoperative follow-up more than 90 days, 2) rejection-free interval of more than 60 days, and 3) baseline biopsy free of rejection on tacrolimus monotherapy. The weaning process consisted of dose-spacing of tacrolimus to every other day or longer intervals. Of the 57 weaned recipients, 31 (54%) experienced rejection that was successfully treated with steroids (n = 15), OKT3 (n = 11), and campath 1H (n = 4). With a median weaning follow-up of 13 months (range: 2.4–25.4), 19 (33%) recipients are currently on spaced doses of tacrolimus monotherapy: every other day (n = 7), three times per week (n = 9), and twice per week (n = 3). In addition, another 17 (20%) recipients are on a single daily dose of tacrolimus. The type of allograft, bone marrow infusion, and bowel irradiation did not significantly affect the success of weaning.

Long-Term Rehabilitation

The long-term rehabilitation with all three kinds of the intestinal transplant procedure is similar to that achieved with other types of thoraco-abdominal organ transplant.[1,12] Out of a total of 406 worldwide survivors who passed the sixth postoperative months, 85% maintained fully functioning grafts with complete enteric nutritional autonomy. Interestingly enough, 80% of these recipients achieved a modified Karnofsky performance score of 90–100%.[2,29] These therapeutic indices are even higher at centers with vast experience.[1]

COST-EFFECTIVENESS

With combined liver-intestinal and full multivisceral transplantation being a life-saving procedure, the cost-effectiveness of only the isolated intestinal and modified (without liver) multivisceral transplants can be examined because of the availability of PN as an alternative therapeutic modality. Based on Medicare data, the average cost of PN in 1992 was more than $150,000 per patient per year, not including the cost of frequent hospitalization, medical equipment, and nursing care.[6] With the current average cost of the intestine only transplant, the procedure becomes cost-effective by the second year after surgery.[31]

CURRENT CONTROVERSIES

The recent evolution of combined liver, intestinal, and multivisceral transplantation has questioned the therapeutic role of isolated liver replacement in children with PN induced liver failure. This controversial issue is fueled by the previously reported unsatisfactory outcomes with sole liver transplant[32] and the current high mortality among children waiting for composite visceral grafts.[33] A satisfactory short-term outcome, however, has been recently achieved with isolated liver transplant in a highly select group of children who have shown evidence of increasing enteral feeding tolerance and have sufficient length of small bowel that complete enteral adaptation can be reasonably expected.[34] Even with such careful selection, some of these isolated liver allografts may not escape the long-term deleterious effects of PN. The recently defined syndrome of hollow visceral neuropathy and/or myopathy is not an uncommon indication for intestinal transplantation among both the pediatric and adult population. The frequent involvement of the stomach at the time of referral and the well-known progressive nature of the disease dictate, in our opinion, the need for modified (without liver) or full multivisceral replacement.[1] Others have advocated a less extensive operation by limiting the visceral replacement to the small intestine only with surgical drainage of the native stomach to the proximal jejunum of the transplanted bowel.

FUTURE PROSPECTS

With the recent improvement in patient and graft survival after intestinal transplantation, the procedure should be considered as a definitive therapy and before the development of PN induced liver failure. Early referral for isolated intestinal transplant will undoubtedly eliminate the need for combined organ replacement and save a significant number of cadaveric donor livers that could be used to rescue other patients with isolated liver failure. In addition, further improvement in the survival advantage and cost-effectiveness of the procedure is greatly anticipated as clearly demonstrated in the most recent analysis of the Intestinal Transplant Registry database. The current results of our preconditioning protocol with the minimal need for maintenance immunosuppression is expected to raise the level of intestinal transplantation to be the standard of care for most patients with chronic intestinal failure. The clinical availability of a reliable serum or tissue marker will undoubtedly ease the management of these patients with increase in the therapeutic indices of the operation. The temporary and permanent effects of enteric ischemia-reperfusion injury, central gut denervation, and lymphatic disruption are important nonimmunologic factors that may contribute to suboptimal recovery of the complex metabolic and neuroenteric functions of the intestinal allografts. Better understanding of the mechanisms and sequelae of these injuries may increase the practicality of the procedure by opening the way for further refinement in the current methods of organ preservation, graft implantation, and recipient management.

ACKNOWLEDGMENTS

The author would like to thank Eileen V. Misencik for preparing the manuscript and the staff of the Intestinal Rehabilitation and Transplant Center at the University of Pittsburgh Medical Center for their hard work and collaborative efforts.

REFERENCES

1. Abu-Elmagd, K. et al., Clinical intestinal transplantation: a decade of experience at a single center, *Ann. Surg.,* 234, 404, 2001.
2. Grant, D., Intestinal transplantation: 1997 report of the international registry, Intestinal Transplant Registry, *Transplantation,* 67, 1061, 1999.
3. Reyes, J. et al., Current status of intestinal transplantation in children, *J. Pediatr. Surg.,* 33, 243, 1998.
4. Grant, D., Current results of intestinal transplantation, The International Intestinal Registry, *Lancet,* 347, 1701, 1996.
5. Abu-Elmagd, K., Bond, G., Reyes, J., and Fung, J., Intestinal transplantation: a coming of age, *Adv. in Surg.,* 36, 65, 2002.
6. Todo, S. et al., Intestinal transplantation in composite visceral grafts or alone, *Ann. Surg.,* 216, 223, 1992.
7. Howard, L. and Hassan, N., Home parenteral nutrition: 25 years later, *Clin. Nutr.,* 27, 481, 1998.
8. Giraldo, M. et al., Intestinal transplantation for patients with short gut syndrome and hypercoagulable states, *Transplant Proc.,* 32, 1223, 2000.
9. Bueno, J. et al., Composite liver-small bowel allografts with preservation of donor duodenum and hepatic biliary system in children, *J. Pediatr. Surg.,* 35, 291, 2000.

10. Murase, N. et al., Variable chimerism, graft-*versus*-host disease, and tolerance after different kinds of cell and whole organ transplantation from Lewis to Brown Norway rats, *Transplantation,* 60, 158, 1995.

11. Murase, N. et al., Immunomodulation for intestinal transplantation by allograft irradiation, adjunct donor bone marrow infusion, or both, *Transplantation,* 70, 1632, 2000.

12. Abu-Elmagd, K. et al., Clinical intestinal transplantation: new perspectives and immunologic considerations, *J. Am. Coll. Surg.,* 186, 512, 1998.

13. Abu-Elmagd, K. et al., Three years clinical experience with intestinal transplantation, *J. Am. Coll. Surg.,* 179, 385, 1994.

14. Starzl, T.E. et al., The many faces of multivisceral transplantation, *Surg. Gynecol. Obstet.,* 172, 335, 1991.

15. Abu-Elmagd, K. et al., Logistics and technique for procurement of intestinal, pancreatic, and hepatic grafts from the same donor, *Ann. Surg.,* 232, 680, 2000.

16. Casavilla, A. et al., Logistics and technique for combined hepatic-intestinal retrieval, *Ann. Surg.,* 216, 605, 1992.

17. Starzl, T.E., Miller, C., Bronznik, B., and Makowka, L., An improved technique for multiple organ harvesting, *Surg. Gynecol. Obstet.,* 165, 343, 1987.

18. Todo, S. et al., Abdominal multivisceral transplantation, *Transplantation,* 59, 234, 1995.

19. Abu-Elmagd, K. et al., Management of intestinal transplantation in humans, *Transplant Proc.,* 24, 1243, 1992.

20. Reyes, J. et al., Nutritional management of intestinal transplant recipients, *Transplant Proc.,* 25, 1200, 1993.

21. Todo, S. et al., Outcome analysis of 71 clinical intestinal transplantations, *Ann. Surg.,* 222, 270, 1995.

22. Abu-Elmagd, K. et al., The efficacy of daclizumab for intestinal transplantation: preliminary report, *Transplant Proc.,* 32, 1195, 2000.

23. Starzl, T.E. et al., M. Cell migration, chimerism, and graft acceptance, *Lancet,* 339, 1579, 1992.

24. Starzl, T.E. and Zinkernagel, R., Antigen localization and migration in immunity and tolerance, *New Engl. J. Med.,* 339, 1905, 1998.

25. Starzl, T.E. et al., Tolerogenic immunosuppression for organ transplantation, *Lancet,* 361, 1502, 2003.

26. Lee, R.G., Nakamura, K., and Tsamandas, A.C., Pathology of human intestinal transplantation, *Gastroenterology,* 110, 2009, 1996.

27. Kato, T. et al., Improved rejection surveillance in intestinal transplant recipients with frequent use of zoom video endoscopy, *Transplant Proc.,* 32, 1200, 2000.

28. Pappas, P.A. et al., Serum citrulline and rejection in small bowel transplantation: a preliminary report, *Transplantation,* 72, 1212, 2001.

29. Grant, D. et al., 2003 Report of the Intestine Transplant Registry. A new era has dawned, submitted *New Engl. J Med.,* 2004.

30. Parizhskaya, M. et al., Chronic rejection of small bowel grafts: a pediatric and adult study of risk factors and morphologic progression, *Ped. Dev, Path.,* 6, 240, 2003.

31. Abu-Elmagd, K.M. et al., Evolution of clinical intestinal transplantation: improved outcome and cost effectiveness, *Transplant Proc.,* 31, 582, 1999.

32. Lawrence, J.P. et al., Isolated liver transplantation for liver failure in patients with short bowel syndrome, *J. Pediatr. Surg.,* 29, 751, 1994.

33. Bueno, J. et al., Factors impacting the survival of children with intestinal failure referred for intestinal transplantation, *J. Pediatr. Surg.*, 34, 27, 1999.
34. Horslen, S.P. et al., Isolated liver transplantation in infants with total parenteral nutrition-associated end-stage liver disease, *Transplant Proc.*, 32, 1241, 2000.

20 Medication Delivery in Intestinal Failure

Rex A. Speerhas, Andrew Bragalone, and Susan Wagner

CONTENTS

In the patient with intestinal failure resulting in short bowel syndrome (SBS), many of the factors that affect bioavailability of oral medications may be compromised. Studies have shown that the absorption of orally administered medications was proportional to the length of the remaining small bowel.[1] The choice of medication delivery system (tablet, solution, cream, suppository, injection, etc.) for any drug can make the difference between successful treatment and treatment failure (inability to produce the desired drug effect). Treatment of short-term clinical disease (e.g., urinary tract infections) and long-term disease (e.g., hypertension) can be altered if the bioavailability of a medication is compromised. This chapter will explain the varying delivery systems, giving the clinician the rationale for making the appropriate choice for medication delivery for the patient with malabsorption.

PHARMACOKINETICS

The pharmacokinetics of any medication is related to its rate of absorption, distribution and elimination (metabolism and excretion) within the body (Table 20.1).

TABLE 20.1
Factors that Effect the Pharmacokinetics and Bioavailability of Drugs

- Residual intestinal length and absorptive surface area
- Mucosal integrity of the bowel
- Intestinal motility
- Expected site of release of the drug from its dosage form
- Rate of release of the drug from its dosage form
- Drug solubility
- Physiologic requirements of drug dissolution
- Binding and localizing in tissues
- Distribution to the site of action
- Drug biotransformation
- Drug excretion

The drug must be absorbed into the circulation and distributed to the site of action in order to produce its pharmacological effect. The bioavailability of a medication is the measurement of the rate and amount of systemic absorption of the active drug moiety.

Selection of the most appropriate medication delivery system, therefore, depends on the physical and chemical properties of the drug, the dose of the drug, the route of administration, the desired therapeutic effect, the physiologic release of the drug from the delivery system, the concentration of the drug at the absorption site, and the pharmacokinetics of the drug (Figure 20.1).

The bioavailability of the medication depends on the following processes: disintegration or dissaggregation of the delivery system, dissolution of the drug, diffusion of the drug molecules to the absorbing surface, and absorption of the drug across cell membranes into the systemic circulation. The rate-limiting step in the bioavailability of a medication is the slowest step in this series. For tablets and capsules, the dissolution rate of the drug is the rate-limiting step. For controlled-release systems, the release of the medication from the dosage form is the rate-limiting step.

MEDICATION DELIVERY SYSTEMS

The delivery system that is used when a medication is manufactured directly affects the time and rate of medication absorption. The process of absorption is the entry of substances from the lumen of the gastrointestinal (GI) tract into the body. Medications may be absorbed by passive diffusion from all parts of the GI tract. The delivery system used to administer the medication can have a significant effect on the site of absorption.

Medications administered orally have contact with the oral cavity, the esophagus, the stomach, and the small and large intestine. Any remains of the medication and its delivery system that are not absorbed eventually exit the body through the anus.

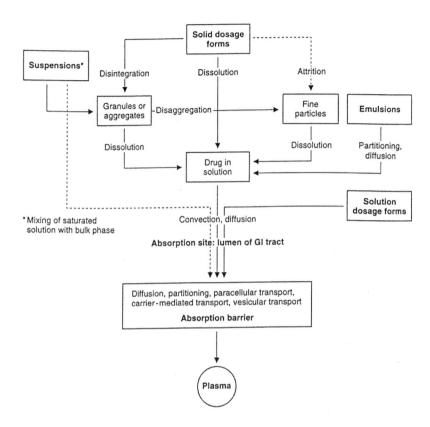

FIGURE 20.1 Schematic representation of the processes involved in drug release from oral dosage forms.

The most prominent site for medication absorption is the small intestine. In most cases, if absorption is not complete by the time the medication leaves the small intestine, the drug's effect may be erratic or incomplete.

Factors influencing absorption include drug solubility, physiologic requirements for dissolution, the absorptive surface area, mucosal integrity, intestinal motility, and timing of medication release from the delivery system. The patient with SBS may be compromised in one or more of these factors and therefore is likely to have medication absorption altered.

BUCCAL/SUBLINGUAL DRUG ADMINISTRATION

An alternative route of drug administration for patients who have impaired GI function is the oral cavity. Buccal and sublingual administration offers the same advantages as oral agents while avoiding a few of their disadvantages. A soft, compressed tablet is placed in the side of the cheek and the gums (buccal) or under the tongue (sublingual) and the drug is absorbed through the oral mucosa, bypassing the GI tract.

The oral mucosa has a thin epithelium but a large blood supply, a favorable environment for drug absorption. Placing medications under the tongue or in the side of the cheek prolongs the drug's residence time and allows for a more complete absorption process. Drugs administered provide an immediate systemic effect because first pass metabolism by the liver is avoided. Medications that have been formulated for absorption in the oral cavity include morphine, fentanyl lozenges, nitroglycerin, and Remeron Soltabs. Rapid disintegration and acceptable taste are required for this delivery system to be appropriate. Sucrose is commonly found in these medications to add sweetness and increase palatability.

TABLETS AND CAPSULES

Administration of drugs orally is the preferred route of medication delivery for both the clinician and patient due to convenience, cost, and stability. Absorption of drugs using this route is multifactorial; pH changes along the GI tract, intestinal length, surface area and mucosal integrity, intestinal transit time, delayed gastric emptying, presence of bile and digestive enzymes, and blood supply can all influence the bioavailability of a drug. A drug administered orally will pass through many parts of the alimentary canal, including the mouth, esophagus, stomach, and the small and large bowel. Each part can expose a drug to different pH levels, secretions and enzymes, and time of contact. In normal healthy patients, the total transit time from mouth to rectum for food or drug is 0.4 to 5 days. Transit through the small intestine typically ranges from 3 to 4 hours. For most drugs, absorption occurs in the upper portion of the small intestine, primarily due to the presence of a large surface area. Patients with intestinal failure have multiple GI physiological differences that can impair the absorption and bioavailability of orally administered drugs.

Two common solid dosage forms given orally are tablets and capsules. Each has its own unique formulation and undergoes different processes in the GI tract to release the drug. Drug dissolution is the rate-limiting step in absorption for both dosage forms.

Tablets contain both active drug and excipients, compressed under high pressure to form a uniform solid mass. Excipients are used as filler material and to aid in the dissolution process. Common excipients that enhance drug dissolution include disintegrants and surfactants. Disintegrants aid in breaking up the solid tablet form rapidly, exposing a larger surface area to the dissolving fluids so the drug dissolution process can begin. Surfactants improve the contact between solid drug particles and GI fluids, allowing for an increased drug dissolution rate and bioavailability.

Capsules are composed of hard or soft gelatin shells that contain the drug and fillers for volume. The gelatin shells absorb water from the GI fluids, swell, and dissolve in the GI tract. The drug is released rapidly and bioavailability is usually good. Hard gelatin capsules generally contain a powder blend of drug and fillers, whereas soft shells can contain powered blends, drug solutions, or suspensions.

Once the active drug is released from its respective dosage form, bioavailability is affected by drug dissolution in the GI fluids, diffusion of the drug to the intestinal epithelium, and finally absorption of the drug across the epithelium and entrance into the systemic circulation. The upper portion of the small intestine, the duodenum, is the primary site of drug absorption. However, the drug must travel through the stomach first, where it is exposed to acid pH's ranging from as low as 1.5 to as high as 6. While there are a limited number of drugs whose bioavailability is enhanced by acidic pH levels (i.e., itraconazole, ketoconazole), most are unstable and degrade into inactive products, causing a decrease in bioavailability. The presence of food in the stomach can greatly affect the bioavailability of those drugs degraded and inactivated by low pH levels. Food (especially any high in fat content) causes a delay in gastric emptying time. This increases the amount of time a drug is exposed to the pH of the stomach, which can lead to increased degradation of active drug and lowered bioavailability.

Optimal bioavailability occurs in the fasted patient who takes the drug with a large amount of water, which aids in solubility and dissolution. Impaired peristalsis due to drugs (e.g., anticholinergics), disease state, or surgery also leads to increased gastric emptying time, causing a delay in onset of drug action. The gastric cells do release enzymes such as gastrin and pepsin, as well as substances such as intrinsic factor. Prolonged exposure to these substances may aid in the digestion and absorption of certain drugs. These substances mix with the drug before the gastric contents are emptied into the duodenum, where absorption can occur.

The duodenum has multiple features that make it the ideal location for drug absorption. Bile and pancreatic enzymes such as trypsin, carboxypeptidase, and lipase are secreted into the small intestine and form a diverse medium in which otherwise insoluble drugs can dissolve. These substances aid in digestion, hydrolysis, and cleavage of complex molecules. Impairment of these digestive secretions can significantly impact a drug's bioavailability.

The small intestine has a rich vascular supply that consists of a network of capillaries, which produces a concentration gradient that moves dissolved drug from the intestine to the general circulation. Drug absorption in this area is complex and involves one or more of the following processes: passive diffusion, carrier-mediated transport, vesicular transport, and pore transport. Drugs diffusing via passive transport freely cross the concentration gradient that requires no further energy sources. A drug possessing more lipophilic characteristics will traverse the lipoid cellular membranes and have improved bioavailability. Carrier-mediated transport requires that the drug form a complex with an intrinsic substance and travel across the membrane bound to this carrier. Only a limited number of such carriers exist, so the saturation level of drug to carrier limits the absorptive process. If all carriers are occupied by drug, then no further absorption will occur until more carrier sites become available. Vesicular transport involves the engulfment of drug particles by the cell, as in phagocytosis (large molecules) or pinocytosis (relatively small particles and solutes). It is through this vesicle that drug is transported across the intestinal epithelium. Pore transport is the transfer of drug through channels in the cell membrane, through which only small molecules such as urea and water may pass.

Once absorption is complete, the drug enters the systemic circulation, where it is subjected to the first-pass metabolism effects of the liver. Bioavailability of all oral agents will always be less than 100% due to the liver metabolism. If a drug is prone to enterohepatic recycling, the bioavailability will be further lessened.

In the patient with SBS, drug absorption that requires active transportation across the cell membranes can be limited. A shortened bowel decreases the number of pores, channels, and carriers available to transport drug into the systemic circulation.

Decreased intestinal transit time can lead to incomplete absorption of the drug at the site of its administration, thereby decreasing overall drug bioavailability. Presence of food and irregular contractions of the bowel can move intestinal contents toward the lower small intestine and colon, taking undissolved drug with it. Increasing dosages beyond recommended guidelines may be necessary to overcome physiologic complications in the intestinal failure patient.

In patients who have impaired swallowing or who have a feeding tube in place, some tablets can be crushed or capsules can be broken prior to administration. These medications should be formulated for immediate release. An immediate release drug that is crushed should be absorbed to the same extent and produce the same effects as if it were delivered as an intact tablet or capsule.

Enteric coated or controlled release drugs should never be crushed. Certain medications such as Prilosec® must be mixed with water before being put down a feeding tube. Depakote Sprinkle® capsule contents should be mixed with applesauce prior to administration to improve the taste in the patient with impaired swallowing.

SOLUTIONS AND SUSPENSIONS

A solution is a homogenous mixture of one or more substances dispersed in a dissolving medium. The bioavailability of a medication in a solution is enhanced before administration since the initial process of dissolution has already taken place. The rate-limiting step for a medication delivered in solution is the absorption process. A medication dissolved in an aqueous solution is in its most bioavailable form. Solutions may, therefore, be a very effective delivery system for the intestinal failure patient.

Solutions can be aqueous, hydroalcoholic (e.g., elixirs, tinctures), or viscous (e.g., emulsions, syrups). Medications that are not completely soluble in water may have solubility enhanced by alcohol and are prepared as elixirs or tinctures. Emulsions are solutions of oil dispersed and stabilized in an aqueous medium. They are unique for fat-soluble medications. Syrups are viscous sugar-dense media and decrease gastric emptying time, which may increase or decrease absorption and these effects must be closely monitored.

Solution delivery systems have the advantage of providing increased flexibility of medication administration. They may be formulated for use by injection, rectally, orally, as an ophthalmic, or topically. They are very useful for patients who cannot or refuse to take tablets and capsules. Solutions also allow for ease in adjusting dosages of medications.

Solutions have disadvantages as well. Many chemicals are less stable when in solution. Some drugs do not dissolve in liquids that are acceptable for pharmaceutical use. Chemicals with objectionable taste may not be well tolerated in liquid delivery systems. Solutions and their containers are more difficult to handle, package, transport, and store.

Medications in solution require measurement by the patient or caregiver that is often less accurate than a solid dosage form. Solutions that are hyperosmolar (i.e., syrups) may induce an osmotic diarrhea in the short bowel patient.

Suspensions are dispersions of small solid particles of a drug in a liquid medium in which the drug is not soluble. The bioavailability of medications from suspensions may be similar to solutions because the finely divided drug particles are dispersed and provide a large surface area for rapid dissolution.

Suspensions have most of the same advantages and disadvantages over solid delivery systems as solutions. Additional disadvantages, however, include necessary suspending agents that may prolong gastric emptying time, slow drug absorption, and decreased absorption rate. Another disadvantage is the need to shake most of these systems prior to dose measurement. If not shaken, the medication will not be evenly distributed and dosing errors will result.

CONTROLLED RELEASE DRUG PRODUCTS

The goal of any medication delivery system is to reach a therapeutic level of drug at an intended site of action and to maintain that level long enough to produce an effect. This goal is often achieved orally by administering medication in multiple doses given at a specified frequency. The dosing interval is based largely on the pharmacokinetics of the drug. However, there are some potential problems with the multiple dosing approach. It may result in large peaks and troughs in the drug blood levels of the drug. This may mean that the drug is not within the therapeutic range for a sufficient amount of time. Another problem inherent in multiple-dose therapy is patient compliance. Inability to adhere to a complex dosing regimen may result in therapeutic failure. In recent years, pharmaceutical companies have searched for ways to meet the goal of achieving therapeutic levels while avoiding these problems. As a result, many drugs have been reformulated as controlled-release products.

Extended-release products are formulated to allow the drug to be released over an extended period of time following ingestion. These dosage forms are intended to provide at least a twofold reduction in dosing frequency as compared to the immediate-release dosage form. They have been referred to as "repeat-action," "prolonged-action," or "sustained release."

Delayed-release products are designed to release the drug in discreet amounts over an extended period of time. They may also be designed to release a quantity of drug immediately and the remaining drug at a later time. These drug products may be coated or encapsulated to allow them to pass through the acidic secretions of the stomach, avoiding gastric irritation or drug inactivation. The most common example of a delayed release product is an enteric-coated tablet (such as Ecotrin®).

Controlled release is a combination of processes involving dissolution, permeation, and diffusion. Oral-controlled release mechanisms can be segregated into the following systems:

Diffusion systems — The release of drug is determined by its diffusion through a water-insoluble polymer. This polymer is usually expelled unchanged in the feces after the entire drug has been leached out.

Dissolution systems — Hindering the dissolution rate of drugs that are highly water-soluble controls the release. This is achieved by coating the drug with a varying thickness of slowly soluble polymers, a process known as microencapsulation.

Osmotic systems — These systems consist of an outside semipermeable layer with a core-containing drug. A small opening in the outside layer allows water into the product, which forces drug out. Controlling the flow rate of water into the system controls the outflow of drug.

Ideally, the rate of drug release from any controlled release product would be constant, similar to an intravenous infusion. Once at a steady state, the rate of drug release would equal that of drug elimination.

The half-life ($t^1/_2$) of the drug must be taken into consideration when formulating controlled release products. Generally a drug with a $t^1/_2$ greater than 8 hours is not a good choice for formulating into a controlled-release product as it would not provide any benefit over a conventional dosage form. Conversely, to achieve a long duration of activity for a drug with a very short $t^1/_2$ would require an amount of drug that might make the final product impractical for a patient to swallow.

There are numerous advantages to use of controlled-release products. First is the ability to achieve sustained therapeutic levels of a drug. Decreasing fluctuations in drug levels may improve control of the condition being treated. This in turn should result in a prolonged and more consistent response to the drug therapy. Second, controlled release products can improve patient compliance to the drug therapy regimen by decreasing the number of daily doses taken. Third, it is possible that a single controlled-release product may be economically advantageous to patients in that decreasing the number of doses may reduce their prescription costs.

Controlled-release products also have disadvantages. Removal of the drug from the systemic circulation may be more difficult in cases of overdose or adverse effect. The absorption of the drug may be incomplete or erratic due to patient specific GI tract problems. Finally, controlled-release products could fail, resulting in release of more of the drug than desired or release of the drug at a greater rate than anticipated. Given these limitations, controlled-release delivery systems may not be the best choice for use in patients with SBS.

SUPPOSITORIES AND ENEMAS

Rectal administration of drugs, if the intestinal failure patient has an intact colon and rectum, can be used as an alternative route for drug delivery, although it is usually not the first choice of most clinicians. This route can be used to produce local or systemic effects, depending on the type of drug used. Anti-inflammatory agents, vasoconstrictors, and astringents are mainly used for local effect. When placed in an appropriate, stable delivery system, nearly all drugs can be administered rectally to provide a systemic effect. However, due to slow and unpredictable absorption from the rectum, it is challenging to determine the correct dose of any medication to provide the desired effect.

The rectum forms the last 15–20 cm of the colon. The internal epithelial layer inside is one cell thick and produces approximately 3 ml of fluid each day over the entire surface area of the rectum. Considering that drug absorption occurs via passive diffusion in this section of the GI tract, the volume of fluid and residence time are the two most important factors that influence absorption from this route. The rectum receives its blood supply from the upper, middle, and lower hemorrhoidal veins. Drug molecules that enter the middle or lower hemorrhoidal veins will be emptied into the systemic circulation, thereby bypassing the liver and first-pass metabolism and increasing overall bioavailability. Drug that is absorbed into the upper hemorrhoidal veins will be metabolized by the liver first before entering the general circulation, causing bioavailability to be less than 100%. Therefore, it is most favorable to administer drugs to the lower rectum to increase bioavailability.

The colon contains a diverse microflora, including aerobic and anaerobic bacteria that are necessary to modify certain drugs (e.g., sulfasalazine, balsalazide, digoxin, levodopa) before they can be absorbed. The intestinal failure patient, who is predisposed to bacterial overgrowth and complications resulting in diarrhea, may be placed on antibiotics that alter this bacterial population. This may lead to decreased bioavailability for these select drugs.

The most common way to administer a drug rectally is in suppository form. Suppository bases are one of two types: water-soluble or glycerin-based. In order for the drug to be released from the suppository, the base must melt at body temperature on the mucus membranes inside the rectum or be able to dissolve in the small amount of rectal fluid available to allow drug dissolution and absorption to occur. The drug itself must have some degree of lipid solubility in addition to water solubility in order to be absorbed across the mucus lining of the rectum. The release of a drug from the suppository and its subsequent absorption can be a slow process, given the small amount of fluid in the rectum that can be utilized for drug dissolution and the affinity of the drug for the fluid. Drugs with limited solubility will take longer to dissolve in the surrounding fluids, and the rate of absorption will be retarded.

In addition to suppository base and drug characteristics, there are other factors that can affect drug dissolution and absorption from the rectum. Any condition that causes an increase in rectal fluid volume (e.g., diarrhea, enema administration) can alter drug absorption. The composition of the rectal fluid, primarily its viscosity and surface tension, can affect drug dissolution and absorption. Increased colonic motility and presence of fecal matter can cause premature expulsion of the suppository from the rectum, thereby decreasing overall absorption of the drug due to a shortened residence time. The suppository can move further up the rectum from where it was originally placed, thereby altering the site of drug absorption and possibly exposing the drug to the metabolic processes of the liver instead of being drawn into the general circulation.

Enemas and microenemas have an increased drug absorption and bioavailability because the drug is already in solution. Enemas, therefore, bypass the drug dissolution step. Absorption occurs at a faster rate than suppositories and is more complete. Despite the absorptive advantages of the enema solution, administration is more difficult and can be painful for the patient.

TOPICAL SYSTEMICS

Numerous medications are available in topical dosage forms. Creams and ointments and patches are generally considered as locally acting products with no appreciable systemic absorption. New modes of drug delivery (patches) have been developed that allow improved systemic absorption of a drug when applied topically. These products are limited in number and scope but may be useful in treatment of patients with SBS.

For a medication to be absorbed systemically through the skin, it must be able to permeate the various tissue layers of the skin. In addition, the drug must be nonirritating and nonsensitizing to the skin. Even with acceptable permeation, the amount of drug that will reach the systemic circulation is probably going to be limited. Topical administration of drugs in infants results in greater absorption than in older children and adults. This is due to a greater skin surface area to body size ratio as well as greater skin hydration and a thinner stratum corneum. The early 1980s saw the development of the adhesive patch transdermal drug delivery system. These patches were designed with several types of reservoir systems to resolve the contact time problem. The drugs to be formulated into transdermal products are usually of high concentration to ensure that the product can be physically contained in the small patch. Example transdermal products are nicotine, clonidine, estrogen, and fentanyl patches. In addition, the patch serves to keep the skin hydrated, which increases permeation and drug absorption. The limitations of the transdermal systems are skin reactions to the adhesives used and the small number of drugs that are candidates for transdermal delivery.

For patients who are intolerant or allergic to intravenous fat emulsion, a topical safflower oil lotion can be prepared to prevent essential fatty acid deficiency. This lotion is specially compounded by a pharmacy and is applied daily by the patient.[8]

Alternative products are being developed. For certain ionic drug products, percutaneous absorption is facilitated by application of an electrical current. This is known as iontophoresis. However, the number of drugs that can be administered in this way is limited and skin irritation can be a problem. Drugs can also be delivered using mechanically modulated systems such as sonophoresis, where drugs are moved through the skin using ultrasound. Again, the number of products that can be used in this way is limited.

INHALANTS

Originally, inhalation therapy was restricted to the aerosolized administration of drugs by difficult-to-use equipment. This changed after the development of the metered-dose-inhaler (MDI). The MDI is now the primary drug delivery system for treatment of chronic respiratory disorders such as asthma and emphysema. Drugs administered in this way have the advantage of being convenient and easy for the patient to use. If properly used, the drug is delivered locally to the lung in a lower dose than required orally. This has the potential to decrease systemic side effects of medications such as beta-agonists and steroids that are frequently used to treat respiratory problems.

Inhalation therapy is also being increasingly used to deliver drugs into the systemic circulation. Examples of newer aerosol therapies include drug delivery through the nasal mucosa of calcitonin for treatment of osteoporosis, sumatriptan for treatment of migraine headaches, and nitroglycerin spray through the oral mucosa for treatment of angina.

INJECTIONS

Parenteral delivery of medication is a common practice, especially for hospitalized patients. The advantages to this route are that the drug will have a much more immediate effect on the patient, especially if given intravenously. Drugs administered parenterally are 100% bioavailable, that is, the rate and extent of absorption are maximized. This route is effective for drugs that may not be orally active or are inactivated in the gastrointestinal tract. For the unconscious or nauseated patient, administration of medications by injection may be the only option. Depending on the site of administration, drugs given by injection may also be used for local effects such as injected anesthetics for dental procedures. There are disadvantages to administration by injection. The primary disadvantage is that the effect of the drug is not easily reversible once the injection is complete. Administration of drug by injection requires more time and preparation skills than a drug given orally. Giving a drug by this route requires training in aseptic procedures to prevent contamination, which may induce sepsis. Parenteral administration may be more painful for the patient either in gaining intravenous access or during intramuscular or subcutaneous administration of the drug. Drugs given parentally must also be manufactured to much more rigorous standards of sterility and physiological compatibility. As a result, parenteral products are more expensive than oral or topical medications.

There are several routes available for parenteral therapy. The desired effect, the volume of drug to be delivered or the characteristics of the drug itself determine which route is selected. **Intradermal** injections are given into the superficial layer of the skin. The limitation to this route is that only small volumes (approximately 0.1 ml) can be comfortably given or blisters may form. This is the route used for diagnostic tests or for some vaccines. Absorption by this route is slow. **Subcutaneous** injections (e.g., enoxaparin, insulin) are given in the loose tissue beneath the skin. As with intradermal injections, the volume of drug that can be given is limited but the onset of action is more rapid. Patients with low body fat percentages may find subcutaneous injections uncomfortable. **Intramuscular** injections (e.g., iron dextran, octreotide, vitamin B12) are given into a muscle mass, usually the large muscle of the upper arm or thigh. The volume of drug that can be comfortably given to the patient intramuscularly is less than 5 ml. Absorption is faster than intradermal or subcutaneous injection, except when the medication is formulated as a depot, such as Sandostatin LAR®. Depot injections slowly release drug over a long period of time. Depot injections are ideal in patients with chronic concurrent conditions such as diarrhea. Intramuscular injections should be considered when the subcutaneous route is problematic, such as when a large dose volume is required or the patient is experiencing pain and irritation at the subcutaneous site. This route may not be ideal for patients with low muscle mass. **Intravenous** injections (e.g., Protonix®,

Phenergan®) are administered directly into the vein. Once injected, the drug is distributed to the entire body immediately. The volume of drug that can be given intravenously is much greater than the other routes. Depending on the drug characteristics and/or the desired effect, the drug may be given as intermittently or as a continuous infusion. Injections of drug can also be **intraspinal**, **intrathecal**, or **intrasynovial** although these routes are less frequent and are for highly specific therapies.

CONCLUSION

Many medication delivery systems have been developed by the pharmaceutical industry. Each has advantages that promote effective delivery of medications so that maximum benefit is obtained, but not all pharmaceuticals are available in all delivery systems. In the patient with an uncompromised gastrointestinal tract, the choice of delivery system may not be a complicated one. However, in the patient with intestinal failure resulting in SBS, the choice of delivery system may determine the success or failure of therapy. The clinician must be familiar with all available delivery systems and be able to make a selection that will maximize drug therapy for the intestinal failure patient.

REFERENCES

1. Menardi, G. and Guggenbichler, J.P., Bioavailability of oral antibiotics in children with short-bowel syndrome, *J. Ped. Surg.*, 1984, 84–86.
2. Block, L.H. and Collins, C.C., Biopharmaceutics and Drug Delivery Systems, in *Comprehensive Pharmacy Review,* Shargel, L., Mutnick, A.H., Sourney, P.F., and Swanson, L.N., Eds., Lippincott Williams & Wilkins, Baltimore, MD, 2001, pp. 78–87.
3. Shargel, L. and Yu, A., Physiologic Factors Related to Drug Absorption, in *Applied Biopharmaceutics & Pharmacokinetics,* Shargel, L. and Yu, A., Eds., Appleton & Lange, 1999, chap. 5.
4. Shargel, L., Bioavailability and Bioequivalence, in *Comprehensive Pharmacy Review,* Shargel, L., Mutnick, A.H., Sourney, P.F., and Swanson, L.N., Eds., Lippincott Williams & Wilkins, Baltimore, MD, 2001, 131.
5. Aulton, M.E., Ed, *Pharmaceutics & The Science of Dosage Form Design*, Churchill Livingston, New York, 1988, pp. 304–340 and 412–422.
6. Block, L.H., Medicated Topical Drugs in *Remington: The Science and Practice of Pharmacy*, Limmer, D., Ed, Lippincott Williams & Wilkens, Baltimore, MD, 2000, chap. 44.
7. Lee, T.W. and Robinson, J.R., Controlled Release Drug-Delivery Systems in *Remington: The Science and Practice of Pharmacy*, Limmer, D., Ed., Lippincott Williams & Wilkens, Baltimore, MD, 2000, chap. 47.
8. Miller, D.G. et al., Cutaneous application of safflower oil in preventing essential fatty acid deficiency in patients on home parenteral nutrition, *Am. J. Clin. Nutr.*, 1987, 419–423.

21 Survival and Quality of Life on Home Parenteral and Enteral Nutrition

Lyn Howard

CONTENTS

In the past 30 years, long-term home parenteral and enteral nutrition (HPEN) have become widely available therapies in medically advanced countries for persons with severe intestinal dysfunction. The dysfunction can result from a critical loss of absorbing surface or an inability to convey food to and through the intestinal tract. Figure 21.1 shows the type of diseases where these therapies are typically used.[1]

0-8493-1803-3/05/$0.00+$1.50
© 2005 by CRC Press LLC

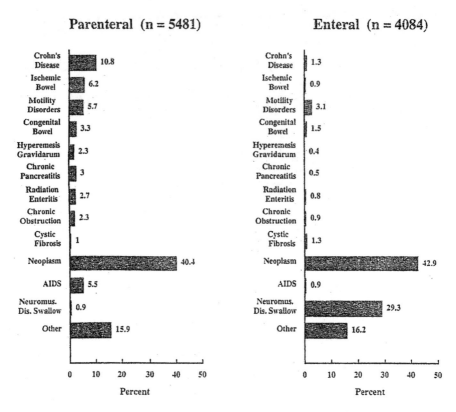

FIGURE 21.1 The distribution of diagnoses in new patients receiving HPN and HEN reported to the North American HPEN (NAHPEN) Registry from 1985 to 1992. The values shown were percents of the total for each therapy category.

Home parenteral nutrition (HPN) was first attempted in the early 1970s in chronic short bowel patients.[2–9] In these individuals low complication rates and good rehabilitation were reported, and this success led to a willingness to offer HPN to patients with relatively short-term needs, such as pregnant women with hyperemesis gravidarum or cancer patients with metastatic disease and bowel obstruction.[10]

Home tube enteral nutrition (HEN) is a long-established therapy for obstructive dysphagia from cancer or functional dysphagia from vascular or neurologic disorders. More recently, HEN has been extended to patients with intestinal absorption deficits who can stay compensated with round-the-clock use of their limited gastrointestinal tract.[11]

Because these therapies are intrusive and expensive, assessing their impact on survival and quality of life are important. Although these two aspects of clinical outcome are related, they are not synonymous and need to be separately evaluated. Perhaps because HPN is more expensive than HEN, there are more studies evaluating HPN outcome than HEN outcome.

FACTORS INFLUENCING SURVIVAL ON HPEN

PRIMARY DIAGNOSIS

The underlying disease has the strongest and most predictable influence on HPEN survival.[1,10–12] This has led to an international agreement to describe HPEN clinical outcome as a profile for a particular disease such as Crohn's or a diagnostic group such as cancer.

Death, if it occurs, is principally due to the primary disease or some other medical illness; it rarely occurs from an HPEN complication, particularly with short-term use. HPN cancer patients have a mean survival of 4 months.[10,12–14] The majority die from progression of their malignancy and a few die from another medical disease; only 1% die from an HPN complication.[15] In more chronic conditions, such as Crohn's disease, survival on HPN can extend for many decades.[16] Over a long period of time an HPN user accrues a 10–15% chance of dying from a therapy complication both in the U.S.[10] and Europe.[12,17]

Table 21.1 summarizes the 12-month outcome for 11 disorders managed with HPN and 3 disorders managed with HEN. It shows the duration on HPEN is less than a year for most patients. This is true in part because cancer is the leading diagnosis for HPN and HEN patients on both sides of the Atlantic.[11,12,18,19] However, the majority of patients with nonmalignant disorders (Crohn's, ischemic bowel disease, etc.) also use HPEN for less than a year. Most of these patients resume full oral nutrition; very few die. In the U.S. only 25% of HPN Crohn's patients and 48% of ischemic bowel patients continue on HPN therapy beyond a year.[10] In Europe only 44% of Crohn's patients and 68% of ischemic bowel patients continue on HPN beyond six months.[12] This means no more than 15–20% of patients who start HPN become really long-term users. In the U.S. this translates into 6000–8000 persons chronically dependent on HPN.

For HEN therapy the largest diagnostic categories are cancer and neuromuscular disorders of swallowing (Table 21.2). In the North American Home Parenteral and Enteral Registry, only 6% of HEN cancer patients continue HEN beyond a year; 59% die and 30% resume full oral nutrition. With neuromuscular disorders, at one year 25% continue HEN, 48% die, and 19% resume full oral nutrition. In the small category of HEN patients with impaired intestinal absorption, at one year 82% are alive, 45% resume full oral nutrition, and 28% continue HEN.[11]

AGE

The influence of age on HPEN outcome is not easy to study because the underlying disease process tends to be different in the very young and the very old. In adult HPN patients with nonmalignant chronic intestinal failure studied in France and Belgium,[17] 2-year survival in patients under 40 years was 95%, in the 40-60-year-old group it was 80%, and in the over-60-year-old group it was 68%. This increased mortality with age greatly exceeds the expected death rate in the general population. It implies older persons withstand a major insult less readily than younger persons,

TABLE 21.1
Summary of Outcome on HPEN

Diagnosis/ Therapy	No. of Patients	Age (year [a] [SDI])	Survival on Therapy (% [observed deaths/ expected deaths])	Therapy Status at 1 year (% [SEM])[b]			Rehabilitation Status in First Year (% [SEM])[c]			Complication[d] (per patient yr)	
				Full oral nutrition	Continued on HPEN Therapy	Died	Complete	Partial	Minimal	HPEN	Non-HPEN
HPN											
Crohn's disease	562	36	96	70	25	2	60	38	2	0.9	1.1
Ischemic bowel disease	331	49	87	27	48	19	53	41	6	1.4	1.1
Motility disorder	299	45	87	31	44	21	49	39	12	1.3	1.1
Congenital bowel defect	172	5	94	42	47	9	63	27	11	2.1	1.0
Hyperemesis Gravidarum	112	28	100	100	0	0	83	16	1	1.5	3.5
Chronic pancreatitis	156	42	90	82	10	5	60	38	2	1.2	2.5
Radiation enteritis	145	58	87	28	49	22	42	49	9	0.8	1.1
Chronic adhesive obstructions	120	53	83	47	34	13	23	68	10	1.7	1.4
Cystic fibrosis	51	17	50	38	13	36	24	66	16	0.8	3.7
Cancer	2122	44	20	26	8	63	29	57	14	1.1	3.3
AIDS	280	33	10	13	6	73	8	63	29	1.6	3.3

HEN											
Neurological disorders of swallowing	1134	65	55	19	25	48	5	24	71	0.3	0.9
Cancer	1644	61	30	30	6	59	21	59	21	0.4	2.7
Impaired small bowel absorption	329	36	99	45	28	17	43	42	15	0.4	2.7

N/A, not applicable because the group was too small

[a] Survival rates on therapy are values at 1 year calculated by the life table method. This will differ from the percentage listed as died under therapy status because all patients with known end points are considered in this latter measure. The ratio of observed vs. expected deaths is equivalent to a standard mortality ratio.

[b] Not shown are those patients who were readmitted to the hospital or who had changed the type of therapy by 12 months.

[c] Rehabilitation is designated complete, partial, or minimal relative to the patient's ability to sustain normal age-related activity.

[d] Complications refer only to those complications that resulted in rehospitalization.

Data from North American Home Parenteral and Enteral Nutrition Patient Registry, Annual Reports 1985–1992, Albany, NY: Oley Foundation, 1987–1994.

TABLE 21.2
Clinical Diagnosis of Patients Receiving Long-Term Enteral Feeding

	NA HPEN Patient Registry[a] (%)	VAH PEG Study[b] (%)	East Anglian UK Study[c] (%)	Spanish HEN Registry[d] (%)
Cancer	42	32	14	33.3
Head and neck	15	16		
Esophageal	8	5	13	
Gastric	5	—	—	
Other GI tumors	5	—	1	
Leukemia, lymphoma	2	—	—	
Other tumors	7	11	—	
Neuromuscular disorder	29	48	54	41.2
Cerebrovascular disease	—	19	9	
Other neurologic disorders	—	29	45	
Small bowel malabsorption	8	—	4	
Nutritional depletion, other causes[e]	21	21	15	
Total No. Patients Studied	3931	7369	191	2986

[a] North American Home Parenteral and Enteral Nutrition Patient Registry, Annual Reports 1985–1992, Albany, NY: Oley Foundation, 1987–1994.
[b] Veterans Administration Hospital percutaneous endoscopic gastrostomy study 1990–1992[51]
[c] East Anglia UK prospective home enteral tube feeding study, November 1992 to November 1993[20]
[d] Spanish National Registry for the year 2000.[19]
[e] A heterogeneous group of metabolic, cardiorespiratory, and congenital disorders.

perhaps because they already carry a greater disease burden. Figure 21.2 shows the separate survival rates for pediatric, middle-aged, and geriatric patients in North America receiving HPN for Crohn's disease, ischemic bowel, or motility disorders.[10] These three diagnostic groups were selected because these disorders affect all age groups, yet have high survival rates on HPN therapy and above average rehabilitation. The comparison showed that like the European data, younger individuals survive better than older subjects. They also have a greater likelihood of resuming full oral nutrition and experience more complete rehabilitation. The one aspect where younger individuals fare worse is a 50% greater likelihood of hospital readmission for sepsis. The conclusion from this study was that while younger patients had a better outcome, the clinical outcome was reasonably good in all age groups, so age per se should not disqualify anyone from HPN therapy. Children and geriatric subjects generally require extensive family support, so initiating HPN must be manageable and acceptable to family caregivers. Long-term institutional care is rarely an option.

There is one study on the influence of age on HEN outcome.[1] Table 21.3 summarizes clinical outcome in neuromuscular disorders of swallowing in all ages and then separates out the very young and very old. The geriatric patients (65 years and over) have remarkably poor outcome, with 46% survival at 12 months and 86%

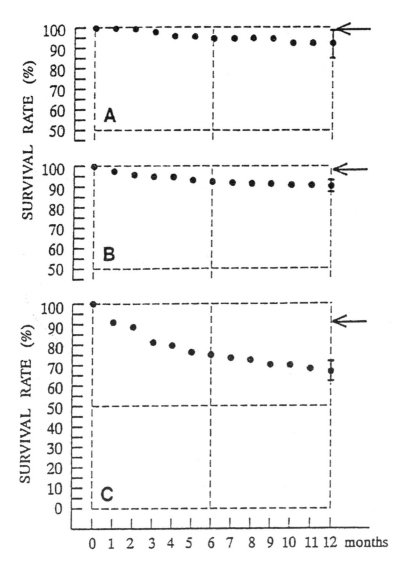

FIGURE 21.2 Survival rates on HPN for (A) pediatric (age range, 0–18 years), (B) middle-aged (age range, 35–55 years), and (C) geriatric (age range, 65 years or older) patients with Crohn's disease, ischemic bowel, and motility disorders showing the 95% confidence interval for patients surviving 12 months and indicating expected mortality rates (*arrows*) for the age and sex-matched individuals in the general U.S. population.[1]

experiencing minimal rehabilitation. Patients 25 years and under have an 89% survival rate, with 54% experiencing complete or partial rehabilitation. HEN therapy complications resulting in hospitalizations were infrequent in both young and old patients, occurring once every three years. Part of the reason for age having such a major HEN impact is that the causes of the neuromuscular dysphagia were quite different in the two age groups. The East Anglian study of home enteral tube feeding

TABLE 21.3
Neuromuscular Disorders of Swallowing: HEN
Clinical Outcome Measured by Age Group

	All Ages	Under 25	65 and Over
Number of patients	1134	146	787
Female:Male	587:547	60:86	436:351
Average (S.D.) age in years	65 (26)	6 (6)	79 (8)
Survival on HEN[a]			
% at 12 mo	54	89	46
Expected survival (%)	95	99	93
Rehabilitation status			
% at 12 mo			
Complete	4	15	2
Partial	20	39	12
Minimal	6	46	86
HEN therapy status			
% at 12 mo			
Resume oral intake	19	23	17
Continue HEN	27	59	21
Died	46	14	53
Complication rates			
Rehospitalizations/patient year			
HEN related	0.29	0.27	0.34
Non-HEN related	0.91	0.95	0.94

SD = standard deviation

[a] Survival rates on therapy are values at 1 year calculated by the life-table method.

provided the most detailed breakdown of diagnosis in relation to age[20] (in Table 21.2 also). In this study older subjects commonly had cerebrovascular disease, multiple sclerosis, motor neuron disease, and head injury, diagnoses that frequently lead to progressive deterioration. Younger subjects had chiefly cerebral palsy, which is a relatively stable clinical condition.

LENGTH AND TYPE OF REMAINING BOWEL

This issue chiefly relates to HPN survival; however, partial adaptation can enable a short bowel patient to graduate to HEN. It is not known if this switch improves survival but it may, since it reduces therapy complications requiring hospitalization from 1 to 0.4 per year.

Studies in France have shown that survival is significantly influenced by the length of the remaining small bowel and this is closely linked to the probability of achieving HPN independence.[22] In 2 years 80% of patients with 100–150 cms of small bowel become HPN independent and survival probability is close to 100%. In contrast, patients with less than 50 cm of small bowel, at 2 years, have a 90% chance of being still HPN dependent and a survival probability of 75%. These investigators have also shown that a short bowel patient with an end jejunostomy has a significantly higher risk of death than patients with similar small bowel length but an incontinuity colon. Studies from Denmark have demonstrated the important role of the colon in the adaptation process, capturing calories, nitrogen, fluid, and electrolytes.[22] The presence of the ileocecal valve and cecum improves the chance of getting off HPN.[23]

Chronic bowel obstruction increases mortality in HPN patients. The French group found obstruction increased the risk of death 2.6 times (95% confidance interval 1.1–5.8).[17] This may in part be due to a higher risk of sepsis. In the North American HPEN Registry, patients with chronic adhesive obstruction were hospitalized for sepsis 0.87 times per year, compared to Crohn's patients who were hospitalized for sepsis 0.46 times per year.[1]

EXPERIENCE OF THE SUPERVISING PHYSICIAN

There are preliminary data from both North America and France that experience of the supervising clinician influences survival of patients on HPN. Table 21.4 shows that Crohn's patients managed in large centers in North America have a significantly lower mortality risk than Crohn's patients managed in smaller community hospitals.[23] Messing et al. found that HPN patients started before 1984 had a risk of death that was 5.6 (95% confidence interval 2.4–21) times higher than patients started after 1987. Since the managing physician team were relatively stable during this entire period, they believe the improvement in mortality reflects a learning curve for physicians managing these complex patients.[17]

TABLE 21.4
Mortality Rate of Crohn's Disease Patients in Teaching Programs vs. Nonteaching Programs

	Teaching Programs	Nonteaching Programs
Number of patients	328	79
Average HPN duration (years)	1	0.8
Deaths	17	7
Average mortality rate/year[a]	5.2%	12.5%
North American Home PEN Registry[1]		

[a] $p < .025$.
HPN, home parenteral nutrition

Factors That Influence Complications but Not Yet Demonstrated to Influence Survival

A small study of patients dependent on opiates and benzodiazepines to control pain and anxiety found that in a 12-month period, compared to nondrug-dependent patients, addicted patients had significantly more septic events and other complications. [24]

A study of peer support found HPN patients and their families who join a national organization that brings them together and provides education have significantly fewer episodes of sepsis.[25]

FACTORS INFLUENCING QUALITY OF LIFE ON HPEN

Measurement of Quality of Life (QoL)

The essential features of a QoL instrument are validity, reliability, responsiveness, appropriateness, and practicality.[26] In HPEN evaluation most studies have used two popular methods, the short-form 36-profile (SF-36) questionnaire,[27] which documents the burden of illness in several key spheres, and the Euro QoL index,[28] which yields a single figure on a QoL scale. A Euro QoL assessment is brief and easily administered and is becoming a standard measurement in Europe in the clinical setting.[29] These instruments are well standardized for patients with chronic disorders, but they are not specific for HPEN patients and are what Patrick and Deyo refer to as generic QoL methods.[30] Smith et al. have sought to develop more HPN specific QoL instruments.[25,31,32]

In all these QoL studies the patient or a close family member is answering the questionnaire, and since the perception of health status and suffering are subjective life values, the patient and family assessment, especially over time, gives the most valuable information.[29]

Other approaches to measurement of health status are the assessment of rehabilitation by the managing clinicians.[1] This has been used in large multicenter studies involving several thousands of patients, where collecting the patients viewpoint directly was not feasible. These scales use a simple 1--3[1] or 1--4[33-35] scoring system. As shown in Table 21.1, the North American Home Parenteral and Enteral Nutrition Registry designated rehabilitation as complete when the individual resumes full age-related activity, as partial when only part-time resumption is possible, and as minimal when the person is barely ambulatory or bedridden.[1]

There are also economic instruments such as a cost-effective analysis, which compares the QoL and cost of two different treatments for the same disease. In the future this may be appropriate in intestinal failure patients for comparing HPN to small bowel transplant (SBT). Another economic approach is a cost utility analysis. In this method, survival is weighted by increases in QoL achieved and expressed as quality-adjusted life year (QALY). These economic measures, which take into account both the cost of treatment and its measured benefit, are important in deciding health-care priorities.

QoL for HPN Patients with Nonmalignant Chronic Intestinal Failure

On the SF 36 and Euro QoL questionnaires, HPN patients with benign disease have scores in the 60–70s compared to a general population score of 100.[36-40] A British study shown in Table 21.5 evaluated family life, social life, and sex life for patients on HPN and compared it to the patients assessment of these same parameters before they became ill and after they become ill but before they started HPN. As the table shows, satisfaction was in the high range before the illness, was very poor during the illness, and significantly improved after HPN was established, although it did not return to the original pre-illness score.[40]

In the first several months on HPN, the patient's emotional status is commonly influenced by the clinical circumstances that led to his or her need for therapy. A Crohn's patient who has gone through many small bowel resections, incurring more and more diarrhea and loss of energy, often welcomes HPN for its promise of restored strength and physical independence. On the other hand, an individual who suddenly suffers a mesenteric infarct requiring massive bowel resection wakes from the anaesthetic to find themselves abruptly dependent on HPN, and such an individual often suffers significant depression, making it difficult to engage them in the learning of the self-infusion technique. This difference in response evens out after a year, when

---

TABLE 21.5
Quality of Life Before and After HPN

	Very Poor %	Poor %	Satisfactory %	Good %	Very Good %
Family Life					
Before illness (n = 88)	0	6	6	25	63
After illness (before HPN (n = 78)	14	24	15	24	22
Now (on HPN (n = 87)	3	10	17	33	36
Social life/activities					
Before illness (n = 86)	8	3	5	21	63
After illness (before HPN (n = 76)	49	26	12	5	8
Now (on HPN (n = 84)	17	32	23	18	11
Sex life					
Before illness (n = 69)	6	6	11	22	55
After illness (before HPN (n = 63)	32	40	17	6	5
Now (on HPN (n = 68)	17	10	28	9	18
Overall					
Now (on HPN) (n = 94)	4	26	45	18	7

* The quality of family life, social life, and sex life while on HPN was significantly worse than before illness ($p < 0.001$) but significantly better than after the illness (before HPN) ($p < 0.001$) chi squared statistic).[40]

confidence in life and self-autonomy are generally restored. The early QoL scores of these two types of patients are very different but by a year they are similar.[36,37]

Detsky et al.[36] found that QoL scores improved slowly over time, peaking at 4–5 years. Malone studied 12 long-term HPN patients with an average duration of 7 years on HPN, and again 3 years later, and found their health status and QoL remained stable.[44] Richards et al.[39] found younger individuals (< 45 years) had better SF 36 than older individuals (> 55) and that narcotic addiction significantly lowered QoL, probably, as mentioned earlier, because it increased septic events and hospitalizations.

Smith et al. have studied several aspects of life for HPN patients and their families using more HPN specific questionnaires. She found a high QoL was experienced by patients with strong self-esteem and a good family relationship. These aspects seemed critical to weathering the loss of employment, loss of income, and decreased social interaction that commonly occurs with HPN.[31] Smith et al. also demonstrated that affiliation with a national organization promoting HPN education and peer support (the Oley Foundation, Albany, NY; http://www.oley.org) led to higher QoL and lower depression scores than experienced by nonaffiliated controls matched for diagnosis, duration on HPN, age, and sex.[25] As mentioned earlier the affiliated patients also had fewer episodes of sepsis. In a third study, Smith et al. showed that videotaped interactive education sessions could also reduce depression in HPN patients and lower the frequency of septic events.[32]

As summarized in Table 21.1, rehabilitation status is either complete or partial for most patients with nonmalignant chronic intestinal failure. Crohn's disease patients, for example, have a 98% complete or partial rehabilitation after one year on therapy; in fact, this disorder tends to be the gold standard for good HPN outcome. Some benign disorders, radiation enteritis, chronic adhesive disorders, and cystic fibrosis have less complete rehabilitation, perhaps reflecting episodes of bowel obstruction and extra intestinal complications.[17]

Economic evaluations of HPN in nonmalignant short bowel patients have shown home management to be more cost effective than prolonged hospitalizations. Studies in Canada[36] and Great Britain[39] found HPN costs 30–60% less than hospital parenteral nutrition and provides a better quality of life. HPN costs show less savings in the first year compared to subsequent years, so the cost benefit may chiefly be with long-term users. Reddy and Malone assessed the cost per year for 30 HPN patients between 1991 and 1996. The annual cost per patient per year was $55,193 ± $30,596 (mean ± SD) for the infusion and outpatient monitoring and 0 to $140,220 for rehospitalization.[42]

QoL for HPN patients with Nonmalignant Chronic Intestinal Failure Compared to Other Patients with Chronic Illness

HPN QoL has been compared with the renal transplant recipient QoL and found to be lower.[38] In two small studies from the University of Pittsburgh, QoL was the same in stable HPN patients and stable post small bowel transplant (SBT) patients. However, HPN patients suffering from severe HPN complications and awaiting SBT had more anxiety and more depression and consequently a significantly lower QoL.[43,44]

Jeppesen et al. examined the Danish HPN population between 1991 and 1995 to see how many of their 129 patients might have benefited from SBT. They found only a small percentage were in reality potential candidates. A small number of their patients died from HPN-related deaths mainly caused by liver failure. Such patients they felt could benefit from the SBT option in the future.[45] These same investigators compared QoL in HPN patients to short bowel patients not dependent on HPN and found the HPN-dependent individuals had a lower QoL. This was not explained by any difference between the two groups in regard to the presence stomas. The authors felt the difference reflected difficulty with dependence on complex technolgy.[46]

QoL for HPN Patients with Cancer

The use of HPN in cancer patients varies quite widely depending on the cultural ethical and economic orientation of the country. In the U.S., most European countries, and Japan,[12,13,47] cancer is the underlying diagnosis for 40–60% of HPN patients. In France the percentage drops to 18% and in Great Britain to 5%.[18,33,34]

It is widely agreed that randomization of bowel-obstructed cancer patients to HPN versus simple hydration would not be an ethically acceptable study. The concern is twofold, first burdening terminal patients (surviving three months or less) with the complexity and risks of HPN and, second, not nutritionally supporting patients able to survive for an extended period of time. The central dilemma is predicting who will survive a short time and who is capable of surviving a long time. The average cancer patient survives four months[1] but as shown in Table 21.1, 20% survive one year. Some of these patients may have had a curable disease.

A multicenter study from Italy of 75 noncurable cancer patients found that HPN preserved nutritional status and Karnofsky performance in patients who survived > 3 months. QoL was judged to have improved on HPN in only 9% who survived < 3 months but in 68% who survived > 3 months. Karnofsky performance status > 50 at the start was strongly predictive of longer survival. These investigators concluded HPN should be avoided when the cancer is noncurable and the Karnofsky status is < 50.[48] A second multicenter study in Italy compared length of survival and QoL in 69 HPN noncurable cancer patients. The median survival was 4 months (range 1–14). About one third of patients survived over 7 months. QoL remained stable until 2–3 months before death. Cancer-related symptoms of weakness, pain, edema, and dyspnoea, if present at the onset, persisted in most patients (96%) on HPN. Nutritional indices remained stable until death. The investigators concluded HPN sustained QoL if the patient survived longer than 3 months. They recommended a Karnofsky score of > 50 at the onset, as a predictor of long-term survival, plus a valid medical indication and the patient's and family's interest in HPN be the criteria for initiating HPN in noncurable cancer patients.[49]

A Japanese study evaluated the reaction of families and home nurses to HPN in cancer patients. Families felt very stressed in giving this care to the patient; nurses felt the undertaking was worthwhile and wanted HPN if they had terminal cancer.

These results suggest families feel more burden than professionals realize and emphasizes the importance of taking into account the family's wishes as well as those of the terminal patient, and not forcing the medical staff's opinion on the family.[50] This observation is important in the U.S., because sending a patient home is cost saving but clearly may be traumatic to the family. This issue suggests a meeting with the family, before HPN is presented as an option to the patient, is a wise step.

QoL for HEN Patients with Cancer

The North American Home Parenteral and Enteral Registry describes outcome in 1644 HEN cancer patients (Table 21.1), 50% of whom are dead in 4 months.[11] However, 30% return to full oral nutrition, suggesting that for many of these patients, HEN was therapy for a potentially curable tumor. Twenty-nine percent of cancer patients experience minimal rehabilitation but most experienced at least partial rehabilitation. Rehospitalization occurred on average 3 times in the first year, chiefly for complications related to the cancer and only 0.4 times for an HEN complication. This HEN complication rate is 1/3 of the HPN cancer rate.

A number of other studies found similar outcome. In the large retrospective Veterans Administration study the survival rate in 1157 head and neck cancer patients was 30% at 1 year.[51]

There are no detailed QoL studies in HEN cancer patients. Most clinicians involved in long-term HEN apply the same standards used for HPN cancer patients.[52] However, the decision to withhold tube feeding from a person who is terminally ill has not been totally resolved. An important study evaluated the role of nutrition and hydration in 32 patients predicted to have a life expectancy of 3 months or less. All 32 patients did in fact die in that time period. These dying patients rarely experienced hunger or thirst, and there was no evidence that food and fluid, beyond that requested by the patient, contributed to the patients comfort.[53] However, these patients were able to take food and water by mouth, and this is not true of many dysphagic patients with upper airway-GI cancers. In the U.K., bowel-obstructed patients with advanced malignant disease are not usually treated with any from of artificial nutrition support.[54] In the U.S., intravenous hydration or an endoscopic, radiological, or surgical gastrostomy is provided in most cases.

QoL for HEN Patients with Neuromuscular Disorders of Swallowing

This is the other large category of HEN disorders. As mentioned earlier most of the older patients have experienced a cerebrovascular accident, multiple sclerosis, motor neuron disease, or head trauma, and most of the younger subjects have cerebral palsy.[20] In the North American Home Parenteral and Enteral Patient Registry 12% of these patients were 25 years or less, 19% were 26–64 years, and 69% were 65 years or older. The age distribution was similar in the VA study, where 68% were 65 years or older.[51] As noted earlier, because age and primary diagnosis are closely related, the clinical outcome is very different in the young and old, even though both groups tend to have chronic tube dependence (Table 21.3).

Because dysphagia due to neuromuscular disease is a classic indication for tube enteral nutrition and because outcome data paints a rather dismal rehabilitation picture, especially for older patients, QoL studies are urgently needed to determine when tube feeding makes sense and when it does not. Wolfsen et al. have raised a similar issue; in 191 patients who had a PEG placed for long-term enteral nutrition, all died within a year, and 21% temporally resumed oral nutrition.[55] Moran and Frost described outcome in 41 PEG patients, 75% of whom had a neuromuscular disease of swallowing. A third of their patients were dead in 3 months, but a third resumed oral nutrition, and they felt gastrostomy feedings may have speeded recovery of speech and swallowing in cerebrovascular accidents.[56]

QoL studies are not easy to do in many stroke patients, but clearly there is a critical need for QoL evaluation from the patients' and families' viewpoint. Also, clinical pointers are needed to distinguish between those stroke patients likely to die quickly and those likely to experience substantial rehabilitation. Once initiated, tube feeding is difficult to withdraw, especially where it involves a gastrostomy.

QoL for HEN Patients with Small Bowel Malabsorption

As shown in Table 21.3, a total of 85% of these patients experience complete or partial rehabilitation and 82% survive one year on therapy.[11] One year after starting therapy 45% resumed full oral nutrition. Malone[41] included 4 long-term short bowel enteral patients in her 3-year longitudinal study of 17 HPEN patients. There were no significant differences between SF-36 scores of parenteral or enteral patients. The scores were 50%–70% of those from the general population. The patients limitations were related mostly to impaired physical health and lack of vitality. The scores were stable over the 3-year study period.

Patients with short bowel syndrome who make the switch from parenteral to enteral nutrition often experience initial difficulty with nausea, cramping, and diarrhea and need strong medical and psychosocial support. They also need careful monitoring of their hydration, fat-soluble vitamins, and divalent cation status. In many respects managing a short bowel patient enterally is more challenging than managing them parenterally. Most patients eventually recognize the switch as desirable, getting away from the sepsis risk of HPN.

QoL for HEN Patients with Other Disorders

HEN has been shown to have clinical benefit in cystic fibrosis, HIV disease, and chronic renal failure. However, formal QoL studies have not been done in these disorders.

Another group urgently needing QoL studies are children on HEN and the viewpoint of their parents. Intestinal failure children are usually managed with a combination of parenteral and enteral nutrition support. This often implies two pumps, creating significant mobility problems for these children. Creative parents have addressed some of these issues with a harness to prevent tubes being pulled out in active children[57] and clothes designed to keep children's hands away from their tubes or catheters.[58]

OUTSTANDING ISSUES IN REGARD TO HPEN SURVIVAL AND QOL

While many factors that influence HPEN outcome are relatively immutable (primary disease, length and type of remaining bowel, age), other factors can be changed to the positive benefit of the patient, notably the experience of the supervising clinician and the degree of patient and family involvement with an effective education and peer support organization.

Unfortunately, the training of physicians in nutrition support is limited so only a few centers have large, experienced programs. This suggests a yearly or twice yearly consultation at a major center may be appropriate even if most of the care is delivered locally.[59]

Quality of life studies are urgently needed, especially in home enteral patients. It should be emphasized that home enteral patients outnumber home parenteral patients 5 to 1.[10]

HPN and SBT are sometimes presented as competing therapies. This will not be true until it is shown that SBT long-term survival and QoL are equal to HPN outcome. SBT outcome is steadily improving[60] and eventually may be a feasible alternative to long-term HPN. In the interim it is important that managing clinicians agree when referral to a surgeon for autologous gastrointestinal reconstruction or transplant is appropriate. Table 21.6 summarizes current thinking on this medical-surgical cross management.

Although most nursing homes will accept patients on tube feeds or simple intravenous hydration, very few accept patients on parenteral nutrition. This means if terminal HPN patients need institutional care they may be placed a long distance

---

TABLE 21.6
Medical — Surgical Management of Intestinal Failure Patients

- The patient may require a combination of HPN, intravenous hydration, and HEN. With bowel adaption the patient progresses to greater enteral dependence and eventually may come off artificial nutrition.
- Presence of strictures, dilated bowel with poor motility, out-of-continuity bowel, or clinical evidence of bacterial overgrowth indicates need to consider autologous gastrointestinal reconstruction (AGIR).
- Less than 25 cm of proximal small bowel in a child and 50 cm in an adult, especially if no in-continuity colon, is predictive of poor HPN outcome and warrants early evaluation and joint follow-up by a surgical intestinal failure team (AGIR/SBT).
- Development of HPN-related liver failure requires urgent evaluation by a surgical intestinal failure team, since average survival from onset of jaundice is 10 months and waiting time for SBT is at least 6 months.

away from their families or end up for prolonged periods of time back in the hospital. These are rarely good solutions. For this reason, respite care for stressed families needs to be available and the issue of when to terminate parenteral nutrition should be discussed with the patient, and a living will completed, at the outset of therapy. This gives the patient and family primary control in this undertaking. Both HPN and HEN are considered active treatments, not simple supportive care, since they both carry potential for discomfort and serious complications. While this patient-centered approach to terminal care is well established, it is not common to address these issues at the early phase of a complex undertaking, which may in fact continue for years or even decades. For HPEN patients, this up-front discussion is wise.

REFERENCES

1. North American Home Parenteral and Enteral Nutrition Patient Registry, Annual Reports 1985–1992, Albany, NY: Oley Foundation, 1987–1994.
2. Shils, M.E. et al., Long term parenteral nutrition through external arteriovenous shunt, *N. Engl. J. Med.* 283: 341–344, 1970.
3. Shils, M.E., Home TPN Registry annual reports, 1978 to 1983: New York Academy of Medicine, New York.
4. Jeejeebhoy, K.N. et al., Total parenteral nutrition at home for 23 months, without complications and with good rehabilitation, *Gastroenterol.* 65: 811–820, 1973.
5. Broviac, J.N. and Scribner, B.H., Prolonged parenteral nutrition in the home, *Surg. Gynecol. Obstet.* 139: 24–28, 1974.
6. Jeejeebhoy, K.N. et al., Total parenteral nutrition at home: Studies in patients surviving 4 months to 5 years, *Gastroenterol.* 71: 943–953, 1976.
7. Fleming, C.R., McGill, D.B., and Berkener, S., Home parenteral nutrition as primary therapy in patients with extensive Crohn's disease of the bowel and malnutrition, *Gastroenterol.* 73: 1077–1081, 1977.
8. Heizer, W.D. and Orringer, E.P., Parenteral nutrition at home for 5 years via arteriovenous fistulae, *Gastroenterol.* 72: 527–532, 1977.
9. Ladefoged, K. and Jarum, S., Long term parenteral nutrition, *Br. Med. J.* 2: 262–266, 1978.
10. Howard, L. et al., Current use and clinical outcome of home parenteral and enteral nutrition therapies in the United States, *Gastroenterol.* 109: 355–365, 1995.
11. Howard, L., Patton, L., and Scheib-Dahl, R., Home enteral feeding: Outcome in long-term enteral feeding. In *Gastrointestinal Endoscopy Clinics of North America*, Shike, M., Ed., W.B. Saunders, Philadelphia, PA, 1998, chap. 11.
12. Van Gossum, A. et al., Home parenteral nutrition in adults: A European multicenter survey in 1977, *Clin. Nutr.,* 18: 135–140, 1999.
13. Howard, L., Home parenteral and enteral nutrition in cancer patients, *Cancer* 72: 3531–3541, 1993.
14. Cozzaglio, L. et al., Outcome of cancer patients receiving home parenteral nutrition, *J. Parenter. Enteral Nutr.* 21: 339–342, 1997.
15. Howard, L. and Michalek, A.V., Home parenteral nutrition, *Ann. Rev. Nutr.* 4:69–99, 1984.
16. Editorial: Oley Foundation President celebrates 20 years on total parenteral nutrition (TPN). In *Lifeline Letter*, Oley Foundation, Albany, NY, 1995.

17. Messing B. et al., Prognosis of patients with nonmalignant chronic intestinal failure receiving long term parenteral nutrition, *Gastroenterol.* 108: 1005–1010, 1995.

18. Howard, L., Home parenteral nutrition: a transatlantic view, *Clin. Nutr.* 18: 131–133, 1999.

19. Planas, M. et al., Enteral nutrition at home. National Register for the year 2000, *Nutr. Hosp.* 18: 34–38, 2003.

20. Parker, T., Neale, G., and Elia, M., Home enteral tube feeding in East Anglia, *Eur. J. Clin. Nutr.* 50: 47–53, 1996.

21. Messing, B. et al., Long term survival and parenteral nutrition dependence in adult patients with short bowel syndrome, *Gastroenterol.* 117: 1043–1050, 1999.

22. Jeppesen, B.P. and Mortensen P.B., Significance of a preserved colon for parenteral energy requirements in patients receiving home parenteral nutrition, *Scand. J. Gastroenterol.* 33: 1175–1179, 1998.

23. Howard, L. and Hassan, N., Home parenteral nutrition — 25 years later. In *Gastroenterology Clinics of North America*, Fleming, C.R., Ed., W.B. Saunders, Philadelphia, PA, 1990, 481–512.

24. Richards, D.M. et al., Opiate and sedative dependence predicts a poor outcome for patients receiving home parenteral nutrition, *J. Parenter. Enteral Nutr.* 21: 336–368, 1997.

25. Smith, C.E. et al., Home parenteral nutrition: Does affiliation with a national support and education organization improve patient outcome? *J. Parenter. Enteral Nutr.* 26: 159–163, 2002.

26. Velanovich, V., The quality of quality of life studies in general surgical journals, *J. Am. Coll. Surg.,* 193: 288–296, 2001.

27. Ware, J., SF 36 Health Survey, Manual and Interpretation Guide, Medical Outcomes Trust, Boston, MA, 1993.

28. EuroQoL Group: EuroQoL — a new facility for the measurement of health related quality of life, *Health Policy* 16: 199–208, 1990.

29. Richards, D.M. and Carlson, G.L., Quality of life assessment and cost effectiveness, Nightingale J.M.D., Ed., Greenwich Medical Media Limited, London, 2001, 447–457.

30. Patrick, D.L. and Deyo, R.A., Generic and disease specific measures in assessing health status and quality of life, *Med. Care* 27 suppl., 217–232, 1989.

31. Smith, C.E., Quality of life in long term TPN patients and their family caregivers, *J. Parenter. Enteral Nutr.* 17: 501–506, 1993.

32. Smith, C.E. et al., Clinical trail of interactive and videotaped educational interventions reduced infection, reactive depression and rehospitalizations for sepsis in patients on home parenteral nutrition, *J. Parenter. Enteral Nutr. Abstr.* 27(2), 137–145, 2003.

33. Messing, B. et al., Home parenteral nutrition in adults: a multicenter survey in Europe, *Clin. Nutr.* 8: 3–9, 1989.

34. O'Hanrahan, T. and Irving, M.H., The role of HPN in the management of intestinal failure; report of 400 cases, *Clin. Nutr.* 11: 331–336, 1992.

35. Pironi, L. et al., Home parenteral nutrition for the management of chronic intestinal failure, a 34 patient-year experience, Ital. J. *Gastroenterol.* 25: 411–418, 1993.

36. Detsky, A.S. et al., Quality of life of patients on long term TPN at home, *J. Gen. Intern. Med.* 1: 26–33, 1986.

37. Galandiuk, S. et al., A century of HPN for Crohn's disease, *Am. J. Surg.* 159: 540–545, 1990.

38. Herfindal, E.T. et al., Survey of home nutritional support patients, *J. Parenter. Enteral Nutr.* 13: 255–261, 1989.

39. Richards, D.M. and Irving, M.H., Assessing the quality of life of patients with intestinal failure on home parenteral nutrition, *Gut* 40: 218–222, 1997.
40. Elia, M. et al., Report of the British Artificial Nutrition Survey–August 1999. British Association of Parenteral and Enteral Nutrition, Maidenhead Berks, U.K.
41. Malone, M., Longitudinal assessment of outcome, health status and changes in life-style associated with long term home parenteral and enteral nutrition, *J. Parenter. Enteral Nutr.* 26: 164–168, 2002.
42. Reddy, P. and Malone, M., Cost and outcome analysis of home parentreal and enteral nutrition, *J. Parenter. Enteral Nutr.* 22: 302–310, 1998.
43. DiMartini, A. et al., Quality of life after intestinal transplantation and among home parenteral nutrition patients, *J. Parenter. Enteral Nutr.* 22: 357–362, 1999.
44. Rovera, G.M. et al., Quality of life of patients after intestinal transplantation, *Transplantation* 66: 1141–1145, 1998.
45. Jeppesen, P.B., Staun, M., and Mortensen, P.B., Adult patients receiving home parenteral nutrition in Denmark from 1991 to 1996 who will benefit from intestinal transplatation, *Scand. J. Gastroenterol.,* 33: 839–846, 1998.
46. Jeppesen, P.B., Langholz, E., and Mortensen, P.B., Quality of life in patients receiving home parenteral nutrition, *Gut* 44: 844–852, 1999.
47. Okada, A. and Takagi, Y., Home parenteral nutrition — the Japanese experience, *Abstr. ESPEN*, Budapest, Hungary, 1993.
48. Cozzaglio, L. et al., Outcome of cancer patients receiving home parenteral nutrition, *J. Parenter. Enteral Nutr.* 21: 339–342, 1997.
49. Bozzetti, F. et al., Quality of life and length of survival in advanced cancer patients on home parenteral nutrition, *Clin. Nutr.,* 21: 2812–88, 2002.
50. Fukui, A. et al., Comparison of the families of terminal stage cancer patients who underwent HPN and the nurses who cared for these patients and their thoughts on home care, *Gato Kagaku* suppl., 3: 687–689, 2000 (in Japanese).
51. Rabineck, L., Wray, N.P., and Petersen, N.J., Long term outcomes of patients receiving percutaneous endoscopic gastrostomy tubes, *J. Gen. Intern. Med.* 11: 287–293, 1996.
52. Schneider, S. et al., Standard options and recommendations for home parenteral or enteral nutrition in adult cancer patients, *Bull. Cancer* 6: 605–618, 2001.
53. McCann, R.M., Hall, W.J., and Groth-Junker, A., Comfort care for terminally ill patients, *JAMA* 272: 1263–1266, 1994.
54. Bains, M., Oliver, D.J., and Carter, R.I., Medical management of intestinal obstruction in patietns with advanced malignant disease, *Lancet* 2: 990–993, 1985.
55. Wolfsen, H.C. et al., Long term survival in patients undergoing percutaneous endoscopic gastrostomy and jejunostomy, *Am. J. Gastroenterol.* 85: 1120–1122, 1990.
56. Moran, B.J. and Frost, R.A., Percutaneous endoscopic gastrostomy outcome in 41 patients, indications and clinical outcome, *J. R. Sco. Med.* 85: 320–321, 1992.
57. Harness, A.P., Paraworks Enterprise Ltd. 179 W. 17th Ave. Vancouver, BC, Canada V5Y 1Z7 (http://paraworks@telus.net).
58. Eddie's Catheter Protective Vest, 7605 Ventura Ave., Yucca Valley, CA 92284.
59. Howard, L. and Ashley, C., Management of complications in patients receiving home parenteral nutrition, *Gastroenterology,* 124: 1651–1661, 2003.
60. Sudan, D. et al., Isolated intestinal transplantation for intestinal failure, *Am. J. Gastroenterol.* 95: 1506–1515, 2000.

22 Specialized Nutrition: The Patient Perspective

Elizabeth V. Tucker and Darlene G. Kelly

CONTENTS

This chapter is a dialogue between Elizabeth (Liz) Tucker, an experienced home parenteral nutrition (HPN) consumer, and Darlene G. Kelly, a gastroenterologist and medical director of a large HPN program. Although it refers specifically to HPN, most of the issues are also relevant to the home enteral nutrition (HEN) consumer. Occasionally we mention HPEN, which refers collectively to home parenteral and enteral nutrition, or the HPNer, another name for HPN consumer.

0-8493-1803-3/05/$0.00+$1.50
© 2005 by CRC Press LLC

INTRODUCTION TO HOME HPN BEFORE THE FACT

EVT: My introduction to HPN happened approximately five years before parenteral nutrition became a part of my life. A young woman who also had Crohn's disease, a gastroenterologist, a colon and rectal surgeon, and I were on a Public Broadcasting System (PBS) program about Crohn's. The young woman didn't look particularly healthy and most of the things she had to say about being on HPN were fairly negative. My thoughts were that I was very glad I wasn't on the therapy and hoped that I would never need it.

Three years later, after yet another surgery, my doctor brought up the subject of HPN. I was having a great deal of difficulty keeping my weight up and he thought the time had come to be evaluated. As anyone with a chronic illness can tell you, keeping a sense of control is very important. After learning about HPN, it became the experience that would represent Crohn's disease finally winning the battle to live a "normal" life. I said absolutely and positively "NO."

During the next two years I tried everything I could think of to keep my weight up. I ate at least 4,000 calories a day and drank high-caloric fluids to try to quench my insatiable thirst, but I still ended up going into the hospital for rehydration and nutrition supplementation more and more frequently. Rehydration solutions were not yet being used for people with short bowel and no one told me that all the high-caloric, high-osmolar drinks (mostly sodas) I was drinking were only making the problem worse. When the hospitalizations for rehydration and nutrition began happening every two to three weeks, I finally said "uncle" and let my doctor know I was willing to be evaluated. I was mentally and physically ready for a change.

My feeling is that the process would be much different if I hadn't known what TPN was ahead of time, made the decision myself and not had it suddenly made while I was hospitalized for something else, i.e., surgery, disease. Enteral nutrition was never brought up as an option, because I had already lost too much small bowel surface (thus severe malabsorption) so it was felt that enteral feedings would not do any good.

DGK: My introduction to home HPN as a clinician came a few years after Liz started her HPN. I was newly appointed to the medical staff, and it became apparent that a large portion of my time would involve managing our HPN program. The science of PN was introduced during my residency, but the patient or consumer's point of view was something I had to learn through experience. Much of what I now know came from individual contact, such as my interactions with Elizabeth (a.k.a. Liz) and others over the past 13 years. Additionally, my interaction with the Oley Foundation (to be discussed later in this chapter) has been a tremendous learning activity. The art of HPN is clearly something that must be acquired by the clinician. This can be greatly facilitated by developing the attitude that you will learn from your patients who have a much better vantage point than you, the clinician, do!

HOW THE CLINICAL DECISION IS MADE AND PRESENTED

EVT: After my 12th or 13th surgery I let my gastroenterologist request that the HPN team come and talk to me about going on the therapy. They also did a number of tests to determine whether PN was really necessary — they said it was. I still wasn't convinced, so they let me go home and try again.

After two weeks of recuperation I flew to San Francisco and spent a week in the Big Sur. I sunned by the pool, drove to Carmel, hiked through Point Lobos, and rested a great deal. However, by the time I got back to Minnesota, it was apparent even to me that I was very weak and dehydrated. The only sensible thing to do was call the TPN physician and say "okay, you were right" — so I did.

The next day I was back in the hospital being nourished and rehydrated. A day or two after that I had my first Hickman catheter placed. Fortunately the surgeon who placed it had a good sense of female priorities. I enjoy wearing low-cut tops and the placement allowed me to continue to wear the things I like. I also have an ileostomy and the catheter wasn't too long. I would be grateful for his expertise when I got home.

DGK: The story of each consumer's start on home nutrition support is different. For some it will be a matter of going from a normal diet and good health to a catastrophic event that makes HEN or HPN an absolute necessity. For others it will have been a progressive course that eventually has led to weight loss and chronic dehydration. When severe malabsorption has been clearly demonstrated and use of less expensive and risky alternatives to HEN and HPN are no longer possible, the steps toward considering these therapies should be begun. Whatever the story it is important that the patient be integral to the decision that specialized nutrition is required. A clear explanation of what HPN/HEN is, what care becomes necessary, how this will change the person's life, what possibilities are for doing "normal" activities, what the risks of the therapy are, and how the medical system will need to be involved is necessary.

INTRODUCTION OF THE HPN TEAM

EVT: While I had already met the HPN doctor, nurse coordinator, pharmacist, dietitian, and social worker, the most important member of the team after I got my catheter was the nurse who did the training. She was great. After I had the catheter placed, she came in and said we started my training that very day. She went through the process of hooking up that evening and unhooking the next morning; then she said it was my turn. After all the emphasis on sterility, I was really scared, but with her encouragement I did just fine. By the next evening I was doing it on my own.

Every day the TPN doctor and his entourage would come to see me. Little did I know at the time how important they would be as my years on HPN have rolled by — all 18 years.

DGK: Our HPN team consists of multiple health-care professionals who work closely together to ensure safety of the HPN consumer. The center of the team is the consumer him- or herself. Others involved in this team are the medical director(s) of the team, nurse coordinator, pharmacist, nurse educator, social worker, dietitian, surgeon or interventional radiologist who places the central venous access, primary care provider, and the home care company clinicians and reimbursement specialist. Each has a unique and critical part in the consumer's success and future[1].

TRAINING

EVT: While I do know consumers who are trained either as outpatients or at home, I believe I was fortunate to be trained while still in the hospital. I was given a very large notebook covering all aspects of HPN from catheter placement to how to work the pump, as well as sterile dressing changes, procedures for hooking up, unhooking, infection, and other potential problems. Next, a nurse/trainer showed and explained the procedure to me several times. Only then was I expected to do the various procedures myself.

DGK: In our program, nearly all new patients complete training while they are still hospitalized, or in some cases parts of training may be done in the outpatient setting. In order to do this, it is important that the primary physician is "tuned in" to the needs for this type of nutrition support and initiates the process while there is still a need for hospitalization. In some programs, all of the training is done in the home by the home care company. Both of these approaches were discussed in a recent paper[2,3]. There are no comparative studies examining the outcomes of these types of training approaches.

While the patient is training, the infusion duration is decreased in a stepwise manner, usually to 12 hours, while labs are monitored closely, especially in the very malnourished who are at risk for refeeding syndrome. This also allows us to be assured that fluid balance is achieved.

Each patient is provided with an extensive manual that provides background, step-by-step instructions, troubleshooting instructions, and most importantly, phone numbers for questions and concerns. The patient is encouraged to make phone calls to ask questions rather than wondering what is going on or worrying about it.

INSURANCE ISSUES

EVT: Insurance issues can tend to be the last thing HPENers think about once they have been accepted onto their therapy, but, in my opinion, it is one of the more important issues and should be dealt with on an ongoing basis.

Enteral nutrition does not have the overwhelming cost on a daily basis that HPN can generate, but keeping track of those hospital and home care generated costs is still important. The lifetime maximum insurance coverage can still be a problem, if there are numerous hospitalizations. While enteral nutrition is much less expensive therapy, it is often much more difficult to get insurance companies or HMOs to reimburse for it compared to HPN. One of the reasons that I have been given for this is that insurance companies consider enteral nutrition as just nutrition or food, a replacement for normal diet, but HPN is considered a life-support system. Several people I know on enteral seemed to have less difficulty if the use of a "J" tube or a "G" tube was required, as opposed to a nasogastric tube. What concerns me about this approach is whether there are people placed on HPN because of insurance issues, when HEN is what they really need.

With HPN daily costs, antibiotic costs for infection, any nursing costs or hospitalizations, a lifetime maximum can be consumed quickly. Some companies will raise their maximum if they are self-insured and have a valuable employee, but that doesn't happen often. Some states have high-risk pools that can take up the slack if a person has gone through their lifetime maximum, but not all plans are the same. Many states do not have plans at all and the states that do have a wide variance in cost, what they cover and their lifetime maximums.

Every HPEN consumer should do his or her best to make sure bills are accurate, overpayments do not occur, and to be knowledgeable about the options should another insurance plan be required. You can never be too informed!

DGK: I once attended a panel discussion of several consumers of HPN and HEN. I was very disappointed to hear these people laughing about how they just threw their bills into the wastebasket. It is important to discuss financial issues with the patient at the outset. This may help the person to realize that he or she has a responsibility to keep close tabs on charges and on the lifetime insurance allotment. In Liz's case her awareness of this proved to be critical to resolve issues related to incorrect billing that could have resulted in reaching her lifetime maximum years before this should have occurred.

GOING HOME: TRANSITION FROM THE PATIENT ROLE TO THE CONSUMER ROLE

EVT: I remember most of what occurred the day I went home from the hospital as though it were yesterday. A friend picked me up at the hospital and drove me home. I had brought my new pole-mounted pump and pole with me. Two home care nurses were waiting for me with several very large boxes and a small refrigerator. The boxes contained PN and all the ancillary supplies I would need. We talked about the role of the home care company; providing my PN and supplies on a two-week schedule, when I wanted my deliveries and I signed some papers.

After they left I took everything upstairs to my bedroom, put the pump and pole next to my bed, then sat and just looked around the room: the refrigerator in my bedroom, the large box of supplies, and the pump and pole next to my bed. I remember thinking that it had looked so much different in the hospital room and that it didn't look as though it belonged here in my bedroom. I had a nice, long cry, all the time wondering how I was going to manage this alone and why me anyway. Once I was through with my good cry, I put my mind to ways I could make it work. I put the refrigerator in a large closet in my spare bedroom. Added shelves in that closet and arranged all the ancillary supplies so they were readily available. Next I brought a drop front desk and put it into my bedroom, cleaned it out and put the things I would use every day in it. That left the pump and pole by my bed, and I knew I would just have to get used to that. I did.

DGK: Having a nurse from an experienced nursing agency at the home when the consumer first arrives can alleviate many of the initial anxieties. This also allows the individual to have professional input into laying out convenient and safe areas for cares to be done.

One of the lessons I learned from Liz is that when she is in the hospital she is a patient, but when she is not, she is a consumer. I feel that Liz's comments about having her supplies out of sight were a very healthy way for her to react to her new therapy. This probably has played a major role in her ability to be a consumer in the home setting, not a patient! Some people want their home to look like a hospital, and this makes it difficult for them to step out of the sick role rather than to be an individual who just happens to be on HPN or HEN.

INTEGRATION OF HPN INTO EVERYDAY LIFE

EVT: Part of the process I went through when I came home from the hospital was the first part of integrating it into my life. I have known other HPN consumers who leave their ancillary supplies in boxes in their living room and rummage through them when they need something. I couldn't do that. I wanted very much to resume my normal life and while HPN was a part of that, I wasn't going to let it be my entire life. Being organized and able to shut the closet door or desk front when I wasn't on HPN was psychologically important to me.

After that I made adjustments as they came along: learning to get the pump, pole, and me down the stairs to let my dog out, waking up in the night to go to the bathroom and remembering to take the pump and pole with me, clearing air-in-line alarms without really waking up, gaining my strength, and going back to work.

DGK: For individuals such as Liz, adjusting the PN to fit into his or her life is very important. I often tell the patient in the hospital that he or she should "run the PN," the PN should not "run his or her life." I feel this is a healthy attitude that is associated with better outcome for the consumer, as well as the consumer's family. However, it is not uncommon for consumers of HPN to make the therapy the center of their lives. The clinician should be alert to this and try to discourage this approach. Unfortunately, for some consumers that use their health issues for secondary gain, HPN can exacerbate this problem. This often results in unhealthy family interactions.

I also emphasize to the patient that he or she can adjust the timing of the HPN infusion to the activities of the day. It is not unusual for patients to have been told that they absolutely have to run the PN from 7 p.m. to 7 a.m. Anything we can do to make this therapy fit into the consumer's life will be helpful in encouraging compliance.

ROUTINE COMMUNICATION WITH HPN TEAM

EVT: Shortly after I came home from the hospital, I called the manager of my home care provider and made an appointment to go through the company. It was an excellent experience. I met the person who would be calling me for my orders, saw how the PN was mixed and met the people who mixed it. I got to know the people in the warehouse, the driver who would bring it out to me, and became friends with the nursing manager and company manager.

The benefits I got from doing this were enormous. I got to meet and see the people and the process. It made it more understandable and clear. They got to put a face and personality with a name. I believe that enhanced our ability to work together for the mutual benefit of both.

My interaction with members of the medical team has been even more important. Working with the physician, the nurse coordinator would call me to check on how things were going, as well as to schedule blood work. The blood tests were initially every week, every two weeks, every month, and finally, when I was very stable, every three months. The pharmacist helps me when I have questions about drugs or components in my PN and, with the team, determines the exact formula of the PN.

These people are the first ones I call if I have any problems or questions. Am I running a high fever or does it spike after I start infusing my PN? Am I feeling a little out of sorts even if I am taking extra fluids? Any unusual occurrence can be brought to them for their expertise. If they haven't heard from me for a while, I can count on them calling to check up on me!

DGK: We often ask the home care company's nurse to visit the patient while he or she is still in the hospital. This allows the person to have a link to the company before going home and, I believe, makes the transition to home an easier one.

COMPLICATIONS

EVT: I was very fortunate to have only one complication in the first 3 1/2 years. Because of my Crohn's, I had become anemic. The doctor decided I should have an iron dextran infusion. The home care company sent out a bag and I was to infuse it using gravity. While it was running in I inadvertently fell asleep. When the telephone rang, I jumped out of bed to get it, forgetting that I was hooked up, and pulled the catheter out 4 or 5 inches. I called a friend who is a nurse, and she told me to get to an emergency room *immediately.* Once there I had a chest x-ray and lay in a room waiting to see a doctor. Both he and the nurse touched the catheter and the skin around it without putting on sterile gloves or scrubbing the hands thoroughly. I hadn't learned yet that I had to speak up and not let them do it. The catheter hadn't pulled out of the major vein so they sent me home. Over several hours it actually contracted back into my chest. The miracle was that I didn't get an infection. The lesson I learned was that all medical personnel were not familiar with catheters and I needed to take charge in situations like that one.

My first catheter infection evolved very slowly. I felt a little out of sorts, had a cough, and was running a fever. I actually didn't think much about it until my fever was 102 (my normal is 95), I was having chills and sweats consistently, and I could hardly move out of bed.

I have had sepsis several times, tract infections, and even a mechanical malfunction that Dr. Kelly wrote up for *JPEN*.[4] While reading about complications is helpful, experience seems to be my best teacher. I become dehydrated very easily and have had to add extra hydration as part of my daily routine on numerous occasions.

DGK: It is essential that time be spent teaching the new HPN consumer about complications at the beginning. Not only does the individual need to know what they are and the possible consequences, but also the steps to be taken to intervene are a critical part of the initial education.

We also find that trying to readmit patients on TPN to a specific area of the hospital allows us to train the nursing staff in the exact techniques that our consumers have been taught. This avoids inevitable conflicts between patients and their caregivers. I certainly agree with Liz's comments about learning to advocate for herself. Frequently an impressed nurse tells me that a consumer has been very vocal about his or her catheter care. Often the nurse is made aware that this catheter is not just another IV line, but the consumer's lifeline!

WHAT THE OLEY FOUNDATION CAN DO
FOR THE CONSUMER

EVT: I was introduced to the Oley Foundation in 1989 by several corporate members of the home care company that took care of me. I had started a business helping people cope with chronic illness and providing stress management in the workplace. They felt I would learn a great deal from Oley and that I had talents Oley could benefit from, as well. I flew to Albany, NY, and then drove to Saratoga Springs for the meeting. I was so impressed with the information I got from the speakers and the connections I made with other HPN and enteral consumers. I met another HPN consumer from my area, which meant we could support each other. I was hooked!

The executive director and other members of the office maintain a web site, listen and try to direct callers with problems to a solution, work with medical professionals to provide information, and, in their extra time, try to solicit funds to keep this unique organization going. With this very small but dedicated staff, Oley provides a yearly conference for consumers, their families, and medical professionals. It is held in a different part of the country every year so more people have access to it without having to travel far. There is a bi-monthly newsletter, the *LifeLine Letter*, which has wonderful articles and provides a list of three consumers with explanations of their expertise (parent of a child on HPN, consumer on enteral, HPNer with experience in insurance, etc.). These people can be reached using a toll free number (800) 776-OLEY (6539) so there is no expense to the caller. The Oley Foundation has a web site (http://www.oley.org) with extensive information, including past *LifeLine Letter*s.

Every region of the country has a group of regional coordinators — consumers or parents of consumers — to set up small area meetings, to help those with questions, or to just be a sympathetic listener.

DGK: The Oley Foundation is an organization started in 1985 to support consumers and their families, to provide information on home parenteral and enteral nutrition, to analyze data regarding outcomes of these therapies, and to encourage networking among consumers and clinicians. In my opinion every consumer of either home TPN or tube feeds who is expected to require these therapies for more than a few months should be made aware of the Oley Foundation. Those who are able to attend the annual consumers' and clinicians' conference almost universally come away with new friendships (someone who understands their therapy and its challenges and is a willing listener), new information based on current scientific data that apply to their situation, and often reassurance that they are not alone. For those who cannot attend the Oley conference, the organization maintains a video library of many of the presentations from the meeting.

A recent publication[5] studied outcomes of HPNers who were members of the Oley Foundation compared to others who were not. This actually identified a lower incidence of infections and of depression among those who were active in the Oley Foundation.

PSYCHOSOCIAL ISSUES

EVT: From my perspective, while the physical aspects of taking care of a catheter or J-tube, etc. and being on HPEN are obviously very important, the psychosocial issues and how they are handled are equally important.

Grief and grieving, while a normal part of life, can be a challenge for a person on HPEN. Why? Because while everyone experiences losses in their life and deals with grief, those of us dealing with a chronic illness and complicated medical therapy can experience many more losses which still must be dealt with. Failure to get my Crohn's under control can mean pain, physical challenges, and the side effects of medications. Surgery can mean the additional loss of physical parts of me. Being on HPN means adjustments to my lifestyle. All of these things can have an impact on my ability to work.

Dealing effectively with the grieving process that occurs with these ongoing losses can have a tremendous impact on my quality of life. While we tend to think of grieving as a linier process — denial, anger, sadness, then acceptance — my own experience has shown me that it is really a spiral. In that spiral you can go through any of the emotions once, twice or even more times. Hopefully, they become less intense as I deal with them. What I don't want to do is get stuck in the denial, anger, or sadness and not move on. I have met and known any number of parents who seem to be stuck in the anger stage because this very unfair thing has happened to their child and changed their life as well. For several HPENers I know it is either the anger or sadness stages that they can't seem to get through — why me, my life will never be "normal," resentment of those not on the therapy. Not dealing effectively can lead to my next point, isolation versus interaction.

I am, fortunately, a very social person but there have still been any number of opportunities for me to pull into myself and lessen or stop my interactions with others. Keeping myself engaged in the world, particularly by doing volunteer work and helping others, is very important to me. Because I have a chronic illness and am on HPN, the opportunity to focus too much on *me* is always an option. Interaction with others by doing volunteer work allows me to see that there are many people in the world with problems and to feel good about helping someone else. I highly recommend it.

My last thought in this area has to do with the positives and negatives of having a pet. Actually, I have three — a cocker spaniel and two rescued cats. The positives are many. They give me tons of unconditional love. They are totally accepting of me just as I am — HPN and all. They give me a reason to get up in the morning and to interact with the world — I have to feed them and take the dog for walks, which also gets me moving. Those are just a few of the reasons I feel my pets are so beneficial for me. The only negative I can think of is that I must be that much more careful about sterility when I am changing my dressing, getting my PN ready, or storing my supplies. This is a small price to pay for the positives.

TRAVELING

EVT: My lifestyle before I went on HPN included a great deal of travel because of my husband's job. The fact that being on HPN could curtail that never even occurred to me. Several months after I started my therapy I wanted to attend a conference in Montreal, Canada. I just called up my home care company and asked what we needed to do to make this happen. This was the first of many trips I have made out of the U.S. During the 11 years that I did stress management and coping skills for companies and families dealing with chronic illness, I traveled all over the U.S. and Western Europe. For the first several years those trips were made I had to have my home care company send a pump and pole to my various destinations. It was in the days before ambulatory pumps. My first trip to Europe, with an ambulatory system, was for a National Health System Conference in Cardiff, Wales. Since that time I have been to Switzerland, Austria, the Netherlands, Italy, Germany, and the island of Grand Bahama. The secret to a successful trip for someone on HPEN is *plan, plan, plan* and then *plan some more*.

I always take a letter from my doctor in English and the language of the country I will be visiting which tells why I am on HPN and need the medical supplies I have brought with me. I always try to find the name of a medical professional or facility in the country that can give me the specialized care I might need. I work with my home care company to find out if there are any restrictions on bringing medical supplies into the country and whether I can ship anything beforehand. Check with the airlines to see whether you are going to have to pay extra for the additional baggage and weight. When they realize these are medical supplies, they may waive the fees. I also let them know that I am on a medical therapy during the flight but that I won't need any assistance.

Travel is an essential part of my life and I am always amazed when I meet people on HPEN who don't know they can go almost anywhere they want to, if they just *plan, plan, plan*. People I know on HPEN have taken cruises, gone to China, as well as Eastern European countries. While there may be places I wouldn't want to visit for sanitation reasons, I always feel the sky is the limit as far as travel is concerned.

DGK: The consumers in our HPN program have traveled throughout the world, even Singapore and Brazil. Those who have planned ahead and researched the rules of the destination country have had very few problems. I have encouraged them to fill out an abbreviated medical history form that can be obtained from the Oley Foundation web site. This provides information to a potential treating physician should treatment abroad be necessary. I also encourage the consumer to travel with the clinician's phone number readily available. A recent issue of the *LifeLine Letter* includes advice to the traveler.[6]

I do encourage those who wish to travel, as I feel this is an important part of maintaining normal life activities.

CHOICES AND ATTITUDE

EVT: You may have already gotten the impression that I believe I am the one responsible for my quality of life whether on HPEN or not. That is absolutely correct! I believe that when I wake up every morning I make a choice about whether I am going to have the best day possible or a miserable one. Then I do everything I can to make good things happen. That's not to say that I don't have bad days. I do. I may have a bowel obstruction and have to stay in bed or go to the emergency room. I may have sepsis. My Crohn's may be out of remission and I am in the bathroom 30 to 40 times during the day. I just take those days about 30 seconds at a time and still be as positive as I can be about each moment. When the problem is over I let the pain or difficulty go, forget about it and don't carry it around with me. I enjoy the good that is in every day. It may be a beautiful flower or the warmth of the sun. It could be a call from a friend or family member. It might be the wonderful feeling I get from doing something for someone else. It might be the love I feel from my pets as they stay close to me. I can always find something.

I am also a great lover of clichés. They help explain my attitude in just a few words and can remind me when I am having a bad day that there is always something good in my life. Here they are:

I will bend but I won't break.

A moving target is harder to hit, so I just keep moving.

I may not have always have control over *what* happens to me, but I do have control over what I do with it.

Do unto others, as I would have them do onto me.

CHILDREN ON HPEN

EVT: As I mentioned earlier, I have met and seen grow into wonderful young adults a number of babies, toddlers, and children on HPEN. They are amazing! This is their life and you rarely see self-pity or anger. They are much better at adjusting than most adults. One of the secrets of healthy kids on HPEN, from my perspective, is the parents. If the parents treat them as individuals and, as much as possible, as normal kids, they seem to blossom. If the parents are overprotective and neurotic about the child's illness or therapy, it seems to transfer to the child.

DGK: Children on HPEN present a challenge to the parents and to the siblings, as well. The process of growing up and transferring responsibility for care from the parent to the child can be a difficult time for everyone. This is one of many situations where the Oley Foundation can be particularly helpful. Many parent members of Oley have successfully accomplished this transition and can be a great resource for those about to enter this time in the child's life. Other issues that the child encounters include leaving the protective setting of "home" and entering college or the working world. Each of these steps is a new experience for the HPENer and his or her parents. Issues related to employment can be problematic, sometimes causing the interviewee who discusses his or her HPEN to be rejected for the job. Often a social worker or career counselor can be quite helpful with advice to the HPENer.

OTHER ISSUES

EVT: As you can probably tell, I look at life from a positive perspective. Does that mean that I have never experience any problems? Of course not. I have actively worked to find solutions when problems occur, and I don't carry them around with me when they are over. This section is a good opportunity to discuss some of the common problems that consumers on HPEN experience.

OSTOMIES

EVT: I, and many others on HPN, have an ostomy. The more bowel you have had surgically removed, the more the stomal output volume and liquidity seem to increase. Every time you go out of the house you have to know where the nearest bathroom will be. If you are on a road trip you have to be able to stop at a moment's notice or the bus, train, or airplane has to have a bathroom. Many of us restrict what we eat and the amount of liquid we consume in an effort to have some control over how often we need to use the restroom facility. One piece of information that has been very helpful to me, and I didn't learn it until a few years ago, is that osmolality of oral fluids can have a tremendous impact on my ostomy output. Even when my body is telling me to drink, drink, drink, putting any fluid such as soda pop and even water will just make my diarrhea worse and I will become more dehydrated and thirstier.

DGK: In the case of marked thirst the use of oral rehydration solution offers an opportunity to drink a fluid that improves absorption and minimizes the thirst. An important approach to minimizing stomal output is to limit high-osmolality fluids and to sip oral rehydration solution during waking hours.

EVT: I can't tell you how many times I have had my ostomy appliance tear or separate from my body and I had a catastrophe on my hands. It is another one of those opportunities where some aggravation and frustration are in order, but a positive attitude seems to make the cleanup go faster. Waking up at night in a large pool of feces can be particularly aggravating. As far as I know there is no perfect solution that can keep these things from happening, so you just have to adjust.

Body image is another important issue to be faced, particularly if you are single.[7] I dated and was fortunate that the men I had a relationship with never had a problem with all my accoutrements (ostomy, central catheter, etc.). For the consumer, it may mean avoiding close relationships because of assumptions that a partner would not be able to cope. On the other hand, these issues in fact, do negatively influence some relationships.

IMPACT ON FAMILIES

DGK: Because relationships are very individual, the way that families cope with this therapy are very individual. On one end of the spectrum is the overprotective spouse or adult child who causes the consumer to be overly dependent. In the other extreme, the consumer may avoid integrating the other family members into the experience and makes decisions independent of everyone else, causing family members to feel very shut out of the process. Those consumers and families who are able to find the "middle of the road" and work together seem to do better in the long run.

DEPRESSION

EVT and DGK: Depression can also be a huge problem for those on HPEN. If the disease process is not under control, and you feel ill day after day, it is hard not to become depressed. If it only occurs for a few days or a week or so and then things get better and the consumer feels better, that is one thing. What is much more difficult is when it stays with you and every day is depressing. It is important that clinicians dealing with your care be watchful for such symptoms. Often, however, it is necessary for the consumer or a family member to speak up and discuss symptoms of depression. With the useful drugs available for depression and anxiety, there is no need for a person to suffer.

Some individuals who are on HPN and many on HEN are unable to eat normal foods. This can result in a major psychological problem. Not only does the HPENer have to adjust to actually doing these therapies, but he or she also suffers loss of a significant part of normal daily life. This can result in a grieving reaction because of this loss.

THE LONG-TERM OUTLOOK ON HPEN

EVT and DGK: While there will probably always be problems associated with being on HPEN, there seems to be more and more attention being given by medical professionals to making these therapies safer. Just since I have been on PN they have changed some of the compounds they use to lessen exposure to aluminum. We have ambulatory pump systems that allow one to go almost anywhere. More and more attention is being given to fighting PN-related bone disease and liver disease. When other options fail we now have liver and small bowel transplant. An HPN consumer has recently published her experience as a transplant recipient.[8]

While we wouldn't wish these therapies on anyone, we are very grateful that they exist and are improving almost every day.

REFERENCES

1. Hammond, K.A., Szeszycki, E., and Pfister, D., Transitioning to home and other alternate sites. In Gottschlich, M.M. et al., Eds, *The Science and Practice of Nutrition Support*, American Society for Parenteral and Enteral Nutrition, 2001, 701–729.
2. Crocker, K.S., Ricciardi, C., and DiLeso, M., Initiating total parenteral nutrition at home, *Nutr. Clin. Pract.*, 14: 124–129, 1999.
3. Fish, J.A., Steiger, E., and Seidner, D., Initiating total parenteral nutrition in the hospital, *Nutr. Clin. Pract.*, 14: 129–130, 1999.
4. Burnes, J.U. and Kelly, D.G., Spontaneous separation and migration of a metal splice segment of a repaired Hickman catheter: A potentially dangerous complication of home parenteral nutrition (HPN), *JPEN,* 17: 287–288, 1993.
5. Smith, C.E. et al., Home parenteral nutrition: does affiliation with a national support and education organization improve patient outcome? *JPEN*, 26: 159–163, 2002.
6. Anonymous, Tips for traveling with home PEN, *LifeLine Letter*, http://www.c4isr.com/oley/lifeline/travtips.html.
7. Kron, A., Exploring sexual matters, *LifeLine Letter*, August, 2002.
8. Kindle, R., Life with Fred: 12 years of home parenteral nutrition, *Nutr. Clin. Pract.,* 18: 325–237, 2003.

23 Establishment of an Intestinal Rehabilitation Program

Laura E. Matarese and Ezra Steiger

CONTENTS

Intestinal failure occurs when intestinal mass falls below a critical value to allow for an adequate degree of digestion and absorption of nutrients and fluid. The principle cause of intestinal failure is short bowel syndrome, usually secondary to surgery for Crohn's disease or mesenteric ischemia or extensive mucosal disease of the small intestine. Patients with intestinal failure often present with chronic diarrhea, dehydration, electrolyte abnormalities, and significant malnutrition. Improvement and maintenance of normal nutritional, fluid, and electrolyte status may be achieved with home enteral nutrition (HEN), home intravenous fluids (HIVF), or home parenteral nutrition (HPN). Survival rates for patients with gastrointestinal (GI) disorders on HEN and HPN are good, ranging from 87–96% at one year to 70–90% at three years.[1]

Within the last decade there has been a great deal of interest in augmenting bowel adaptation and transplantation of the small intestine to allow for reduction or elimination of nonvolitional feedings. Treatment of intestinal failure encompasses a wide range of therapeutic options. The Intestinal Rehabilitation Program (IRP) at the Cleveland Clinic Foundation was established in 2001 with the goal of organizing a comprehensive range of interrelated services for the care of patients with severe intestinal failure. The program serves as an entry point that provides multiple services, including diagnostic evaluation, nutritional rehabilitation, medical management, surgical intervention, and referral for small bowel transplantation. Patients

0-8493-1803-3/05/$0.00+$1.50

have access to different therapies at different times during their illness. For example, a patient may start on HPN and, through diet modification, medication, and intestinal surgery, eventually be rehabilitated and transitioned off HPN. There are a multitude of GI and surgical specialists involved in the care of these patients who are coordinated through the IRP. This allows access to complete, interrelated, and easily accessible therapies to help the patient maximize intestinal absorption and digestion. Thus, there is improved continuity of care as the IRP works with many disciplines in a focused effort to improve digestion and absorption.

Although long-term parenteral nutrition has been safely used for over three decades,[2] intestinal transplantation[3] and intestinal rehabilitation[4] each for over a decade, the concept of offering patients a comprehensive evaluation of the potential benefits of all three therapies in one center is a relatively recent one.[5] This chapter will review the process of establishing an IRP with the goal of offering these interrelated therapies to ultimately provide the best therapy for the patient with severe intestinal failure.

INTESTINAL FAILURE: DEFINITION

It is important to clearly define intestinal failure so that the most appropriate patients can be referred and treated in the center. Intestinal failure occurs when there is reduced intestinal absorption so that macro- and micronutrient, fluid, and electrolyte supplements are needed to maintain health and/or growth. The presenting features include chronic diarrhea, dehydration, electrolyte abnormalities, and malnutrition. The principal cause of intestinal failure is short bowel syndrome (SBS), usually secondary to surgery for injury or disease of the small intestine (Chapter 2). Specific examples include small bowel volvulus, desmoid tumors, mesenteric vascular thrombosis, and major resections for inflammatory bowel disease. Resection of the stomach or colon does not constitute or result in short bowel syndrome, but loss of either can result in further complications for the patient who has had a resection of the small intestine and significant compromise of absorptive capacity. Intestinal failure may also result from disease of the small intestine interfering with normal absorption such as Crohn's disease, radiation enteritis, and scleroderma. Malnutrition and/or dehydration result if no treatment is given or if compensatory mechanisms do not occur.

Intestinal failure has also been classified on the basis of severity and underlying diagnosis.[6] It is the bowel length, anatomical configuration, and functional capacity that form the basis of the decision-making process for the IRP. This, in turn, will determine the treatment plan. In *severe* intestinal failure, parenteral nutrition or intravenous fluids are required because nutritional status cannot be maintained through the GI tract. In *moderate* intestinal failure, enteral feeding by tube is used for the administration of macro- and micronutrients or fluid and electrolytes (e.g., rehydration solutions). In cases of *mild* intestinal failure, dietary modification, oral supplements and/or oral rehydration solutions are used. These patients can be difficult to manage since many of them are bordering on moderate intestinal failure and need aggressive treatment and monitoring. A patient may progress from severe intestinal failure to mild or moderate due to compensatory mechanisms often stimulated by diet, medication, and growth factors. This is the goal of intestinal rehabilitation: to transition patients to a more normal lifestyle. In many instances, a patient may be nourished by more than one technique simultaneously. This is often the case as patients are transitioned from one therapy to another.

Intestinal failure can also be classified as acute or chronic. Acute intestinal failure generally has a surgical etiology (e.g., enterocutaneous fistula, obstruction, or volvulus) and may be reversible by spontaneous healing (fistula closure, resolution of ileus) or future surgery. There are occasions where SBS is purposely created, as in diverting jejunostomies, in order to promote healing in a more distal area of the GI tract (gastrointestinal anastomoses or repaired enterotomies). Acute intestinal failure can also result from medical treatment (e.g., enteritis from chemotherapy, radiation, or antibiotic therapy) and in most cases is expected to resolve. These patients are not considered candidates for intestinal rehabilitation therapy but may enter the IRP for evaluation and are triaged to HPN.

Chronic intestinal failure can be due to surgical resections performed to treat Crohn's disease or mesenteric ischemia that may be due to a thromboembolic event or volvulus. It can also occur with small bowel dysfunction, examples of which include pseudo-obstruction, Crohn's disease, radiation enteritis, and refractory Celiac disease. These are the patients who are most likely to benefit from IRP. Of the patients with chronic intestinal failure, SBS is the most common diagnosis.

ADMINISTRATIVE ASPECTS

Prior to initiation of a new program it is important to perform a demand analysis in order to determine the number of patients that will most likely benefit as well as the economic feasibility of embarking on an endeavor such as this. If the institution does not have the volume of patients or the professional expertise to support such a program, it would be best to refer these patients to an institution that does specialize in intestinal failure. Potential patients can be drawn from both internal and external sources. The initial potential patient pool will be most likely be derived from the current HPN patient population. Some of the HPN patients will be on for a short period of time, generally 3–6 months, until further surgery can be performed. Others are clearly long-term HPN patients who may benefit from intestinal rehabilitation or transplantation. Patients referred to the Departments of Gastroenterology, Colorectal Surgery, and General Surgery for GI dysfunction and intestinal failure are difficult management problems and the greatest source of referrals to the IRP. The strong support of the chairmen of the departments of Gastroenterology, Colorectal Surgery, and General Surgery is necessary to help establish an IRP program as well as the Nutrition Support and HPN teams. The marketing strategy must include both internal and external efforts. Once an estimate of the number of patients is determined, an annual volume of outpatient visits can be established. Services would include initial evaluation, treatment, and long-term follow-up care. Potential follow-up services are likely to include some or all of the following: outpatient lab testing conducted at regular intervals; home infusion therapy (HEN, HIVF, HPN); and outpatient/home oral supplementation, rehydration, and dietary modification. For optimal patient benefit, an IRP should be established in an institution with expertise in enteral and parenteral nutrition in the hospital and home, restorative surgery, strong diagnostic gastroenterology skills, and small bowel transplantation capabilities.

The next step is to develop the proposal and business plan that clearly outlines the objectives of the project, specific aims, an assessment of any competing programs, marketing strategy, outcome measures, and the budget. The goals of the program need to be specific enough to provide direction yet broad enough to reflect the vision for the program (Table 23.1).

The success of the program will have to be demonstrated in order to ensure continued survival and growth of the program. Outcomes can be measured by several variables. This may include patient-centered outcomes, such as improved nutritional status or discontinuation of HPN, as well as referral to other services and revenues generated (Table 23.2).

TABLE 23.1
Specific Objectives for an Intestinal Rehabilitation Program

- To provide a comprehensive range of services for patients diagnosed with intestinal failure including evaluation, nutritional rehabilitation, medical management, restorative surgery, and transplantation
- To restore nutritional status through the safest, most physiologic techniques compatible with the patient's lifestyle and wishes
- To improve continuity of patient care across the continuum of care
- To develop and implement protocols for gut adaptation and nutritional rehabilitation
- To provide clinical nutrition services and dietary education for patients
- To expand basic and clinical research efforts
- To establish the institution as a center of excellence for intestinal rehabilitation and nutrition therapy
- To establish educational opportunities for physicians and other members of the health-care team

---

TABLE 23.2
Outcome Parameters

- Enhanced absorption
- Improvement in nutritional status
- Decrease in HPN days or discontinuation of HPN therapy
- Decrease in IV fluid requirements
- Reduction in hospitalization for dehydration or malnutrition
- Referrals from IRP to Department of General or Colorectal Surgery
- Referrals from IRP to Department of Gastroenterology
- Referrals from IRP for Home Parenteral Nutrition/Home Enteral Nutrition
- Referrals from IRP to transplant center
- Referrals from Departments of Colorectal Surgery, Gastroenterology, or General Surgery to IRP
- Revenues from funded research
- Actual revenue generated

The first phase of the implementation of the program generally includes the determination of organizational structure and physical location. The logistics concerning how the program is to be organized, staffed, or funded or where the program will be physically located will depend on the individual institution and largely on the interest of the personnel involved. At the Cleveland Clinic Foundation, the Departments of Colorectal Surgery, Gastroenterology, and General Surgery have shared the responsibilities of providing funding and space since most of the IRP patients are referred from each of these departments. This particular model builds on strengths already present at this institution. This has enhanced the continuity of care for these patients. The program is located in the Digestive Diseases Center along with the Departments of Gastroenterology and Colorectal Surgery. Space had to be allocated to include exam rooms, office space for personnel, and space for patient education. In most institutions this will most likely mean reallocation or sharing of existing space.

The second phase of our program entails establishing the diagnostic, nutritional, and medical components as well as a mechanism for referral for restorative surgery or transplantation. In order to do this, effective multidisciplinary programs that address clinical practice, education and future research will have to be developed (Table 23.3). It will also be important to develop clinical pathways that outline care of these complex patients. The use of clinical pathways has arisen as a result of the movement in health care toward standardizing care and outcomes-oriented approaches to treatment. With the shift from empiricism to evidence-based strategies, methods, pathways, and algorithms are justified with evidence from the scientific literature.[7]

TABLE 23.3
Multidisciplinary Aspects of Intestinal Failure Programs

- Clinical practice
  - Standardized diagnostic medical evaluation
  - Development of assessment and monitoring tools
  - Development of protocols to replete fluid, electrolytes, vitamins, essential fatty acids, and trace elements as well as where to purchase the oral/enteral products
  - Development of optimal dietary modification
  - Development of care pathways and protocols
  - Development of template for discharge, clinic notes, etc.
  - Development of database for patient care and tracking outcomes
  - Development of inpatient program
  - Facilitate development of a pediatric program
- Education
  - Development of lesson plans and patient education tools using printed materials, CD-ROM, videos aimed at educating the patient/family about diet, changing behavior, and self-monitoring at home
  - Advanced training for physicians and other health care professionals interested in intestinal rehabilitation
- Research
  - Development of research protocols

The decision to establish an ambulatory or an inpatient program will depend on the needs and resources of the institution. In general an ambulatory program is less expensive to initiate but requires that the patient be relatively stable. There may be less control over the oral intake of the patient, and compliance to the treatment program will be imperative. However, providing an ambulatory program ensures continuity of care across the continuum of care. It allows patients to resume a more normal lifestyle.

Whether the program is set up as an ambulatory or inpatient program, the clinicians involved in the IRP will interact with staff in the hospital and the home care setting. For patients who are hospitalized, the IRP expertise can be utilized to determine the best form of therapy or to evaluate a perspective patient. This allows for early implementation of IRP therapies. For patients who are already at home on HPN, HIVF, or HEN consultation with IRP may enable some patients to decrease or discontinue these therapies.

DATA MANAGEMENT

A major part of the establishment of our IRP was the development of a database to store large volumes of complex data. Many variations of normal GI tract anatomy and function occur and need to be documented. Patients seen in IRP are often on combined therapies, including diet, medication, trophic substances, intravenous fluids, long-term enteral nutrition, and/or long-term parenteral nutrition. Some may require surgical intervention, including restorative surgery or small bowel or multivisceral transplantation. Appropriate management requires the collection of patient data, calculation of multiple formulae, and continued tracking of the patient's progress. In order to manage the volume and complexity of the data required to care for these patients, a sophisticated database was developed.

Our specific system was developed on Microsoft SQL Server 2000, with Microsoft Access as a client interface. The system tracks demographic information, gastrointestinal anatomy, and surgical and diagnostic procedures (Figure 23.1 through Figure 23.13). It also tracks fluid and nutrient intake from multiple sources, including oral intake, enteral nutrition, intravenous fluids, and parenteral nutrition. These can be analyzed along with the output studies. The database can also track nutritional status including anthropometry, laboratory data, bioelectrical impedance, and a nutritional diagnosis. Calculations performed by the computer include ideal body weight, height, frame size, body mass index, mid-upper arm muscle circumference, percentiles for anthropometric measurements, basal energy expenditure, total energy expenditure, protein requirements, and fluid requirements. All patient data are then stored for general patient care or future research purposes. The system tracks the reason for referral into the program and the disposition of the patient at discharge from the program. The system was designed to enhance patient care but not to replace the electronic chart. Data entry can be accomplished directly into the system or by use of data sheets that can be scanned directly into the system. The structure and organization of the sheets are changed to facilitate data entry as our needs changed. Additional tools and capabilities are added when the need is apparent. Development of an IRP database facilitates the daily clinical management of these

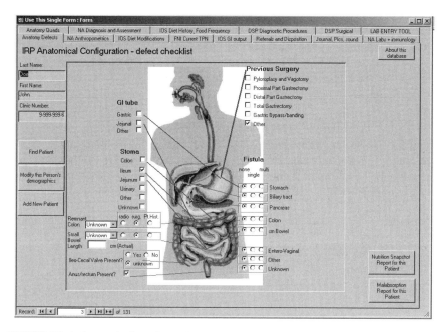

FIGURE 23.1 Anatomical configuration in IRP database

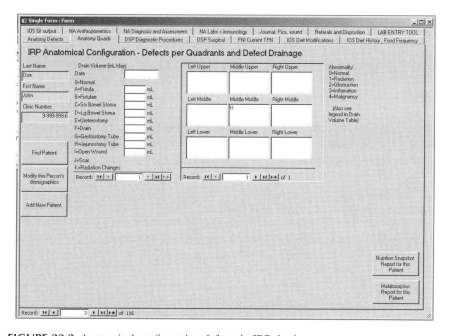

FIGURE 23.2 Anatomical configuration defects in IRP database

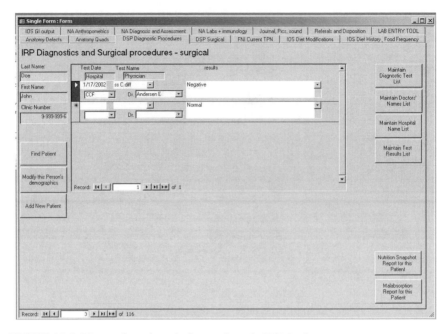

FIGURE 23.3 Diagnostic and surgical procedures in IRP database

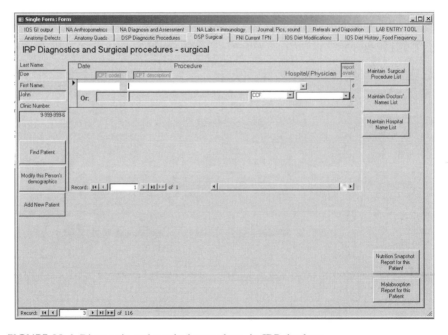

FIGURE 23.4 Diagnostic and surgical procedures in IRP database

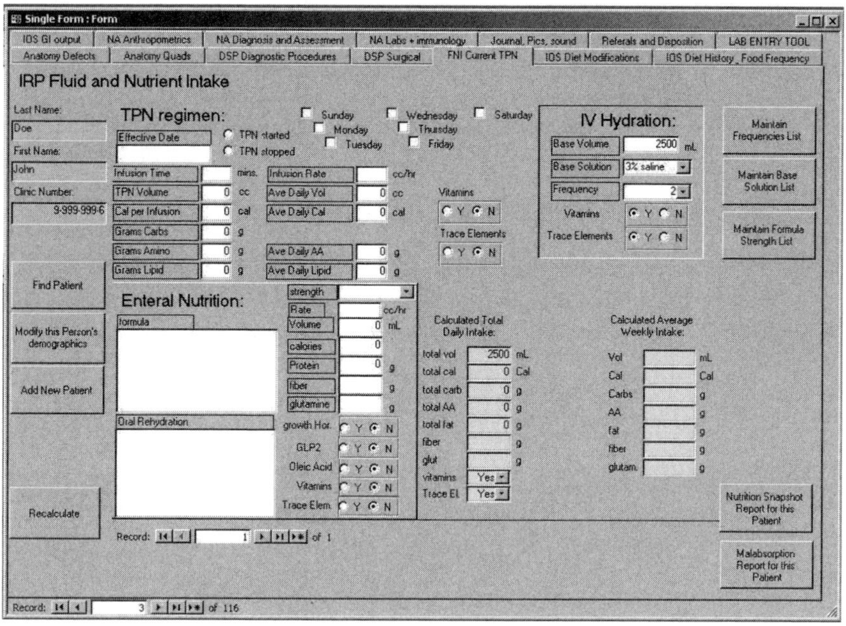

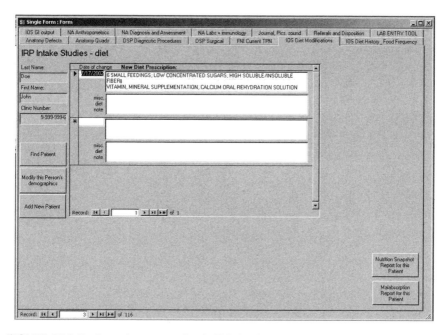

FIGURE 23.5 Fluid and nutrient intake in IRP database

FIGURE 23.6 Intake and output studies in IRP database

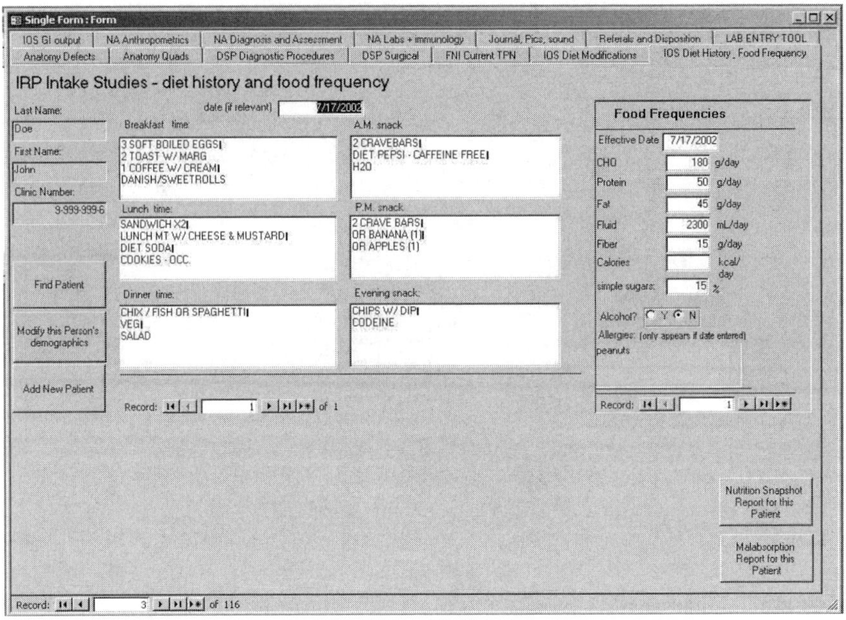

FIGURE 23.7 Input/output studies: diet history and food frequency in IRP database

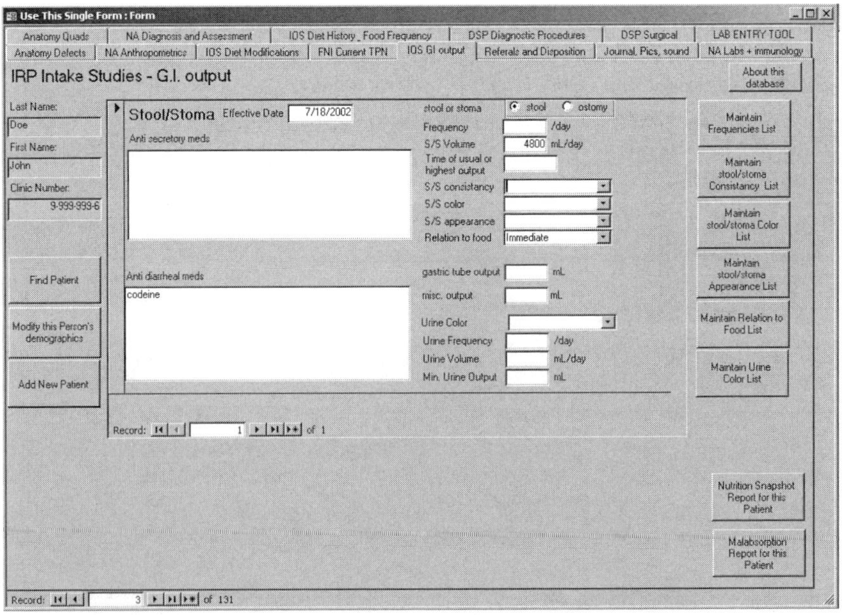

FIGURE 23.8 Input/output studies — GI output in IRP database

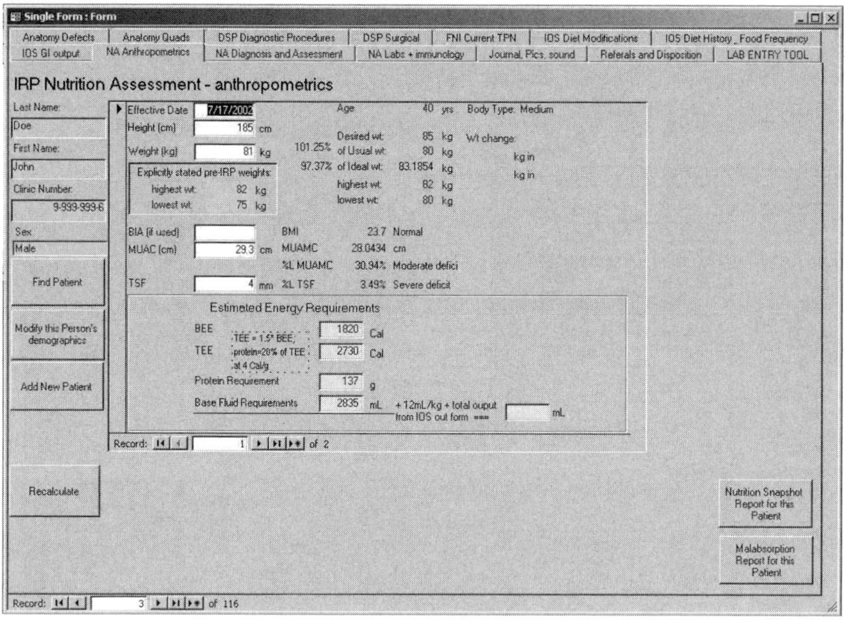

IRP Nutrition Assessment - anthropometrics

FIGURE 23.9 Nutrition assessment: anthropometry in IRP database

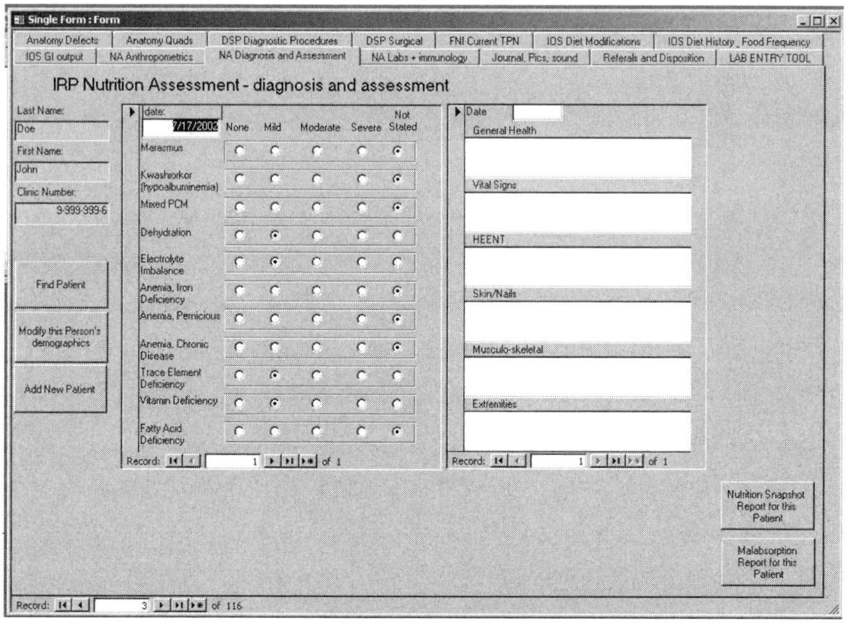

IRP Nutrition Assessment - diagnosis and assessment

FIGURE 23.10 Nutrition assessment — diagnosis and assessment in IRP database

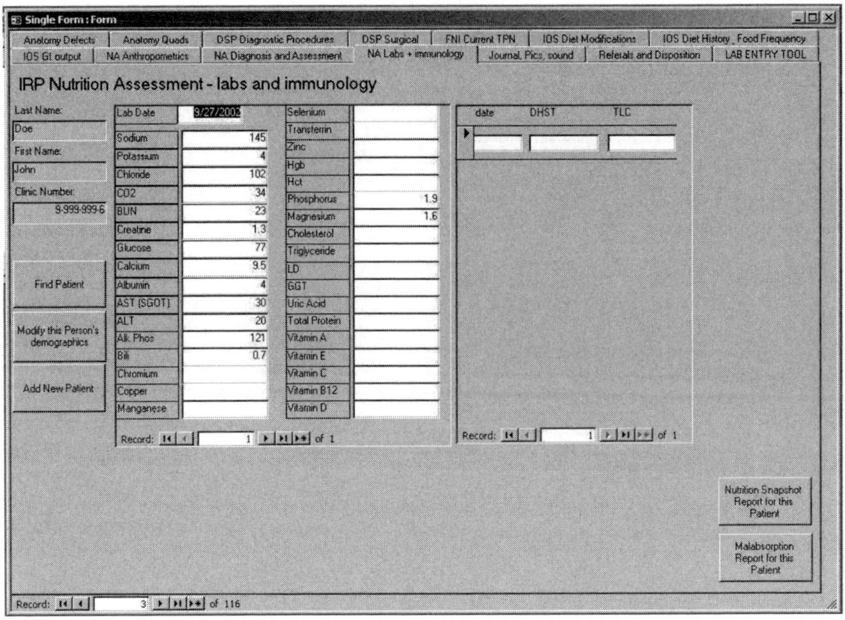

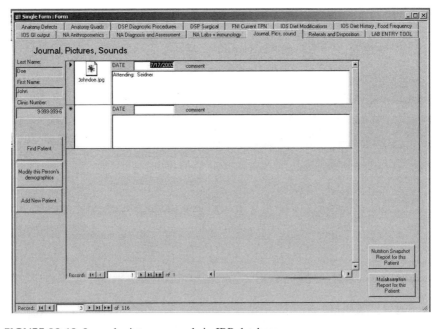

FIGURE 23.11 Nutrition assessment labs and immunology in IRP database

FIGURE 23.12 Journal, pictures, sounds in IRP database

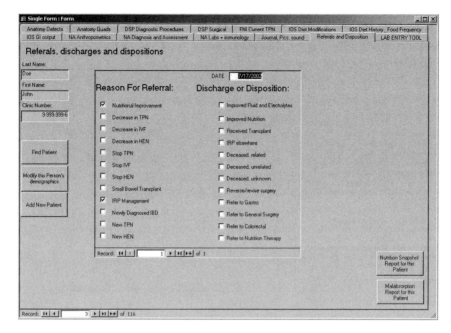

FIGURE 23.13 Referrals, discharges, dispositions in IRP database

complex patients and allows for future analysis of a large volume of multifaceted data. In addition, it allows the evaluation of the growth and outcomes of the program.

PATIENT CARE

The primary goal of the IRP is to restore nutritional status through the safest, most physiologic technique compatible with the patient's lifestyle and wishes. There are three complementary therapies involved in the management of these complex patients: (1) intestinal rehabilitation to enhance adaptation, (2) long-term enteral and parenteral nutrition and intravenous fluid replacement, and (3) surgical intervention including reconstructive surgery, intestinal, and multivisceral transplantation.

A careful and detailed nutrition assessment is a vital part of the IRP care plan (Figure 23.14).[7] The nutrition assessment defines the degree and type of malnutrition using various parameters, including medical, nutrition and medication histories, physical examination, anthropometric measures, immune status as defined by delayed hypersensitivity skin tests, and laboratory data (Chapter 6). Evaluation of nutritional status consists of two components: nutrition and metabolic assessment. Nutrition assessment measures body compartments and their alterations as caused by undernutrition. Metabolic assessment includes the evaluation of altered metabolism as it relates to the loss of lean body mass or other body compartments, and of the metabolic response to nutrition intervention.

The first priority of patient evaluation is determination of the GI anatomy, length of bowel, and presence or extent of mucosal disease. This can be very difficult, time-consuming, and complicated. Many of these patients have had multiple surgical

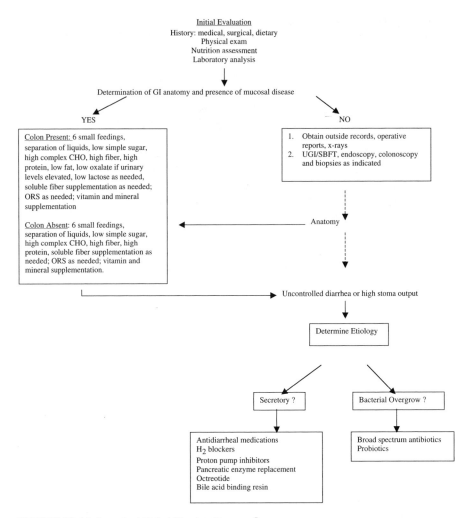

FIGURE 23.14 Intestinal Rehabilitation Program[7]

procedures in many different institutions. But this point is crucial in determining the appropriate therapy for the patient. The severity of the metabolic consequences and the ability to undergo intestinal adaptation depends on several factors. These include: 1) the extent and site of intestinal resection, 2) the presence or absence of the ileocecal valve, 3) the presence of disease in the remnant bowel, stomach, pancreas and liver, and 4) the degree of adaptation of the remaining bowel.[8] Once the anatomy and functional capacity of the gastrointestinal tract has been determined, a decision can be made as to the most effective therapy.[7]

Whenever possible, intestinal rehabilitation should be considered before long-term parenteral nutrition following bowel resection. The cornerstone of therapy for intestinal rehabilitation is dietary modification that is used to maximize fluid and nutrient absorption and minimize fecal output (Chapter 9). Medications to slow down gastrointestinal transit time or enhance absorption are used to augment dietary interventions (Chapters 10 through 12 and 20). The dietary modifications can represent significant changes in the patient's lifestyle. In order to help them implement and comply with these modifications in diet, we developed a 120-page instruction manual. The manual includes eight different dietary plans that modify the diet based on the patient's GI anatomy and mucosal disease. In order to improve compliance, ensure nutrient adequacy, and minimize monotony, a sample one-week menu pattern for each different diet was developed. The manual also includes general information on nutrition, inflammatory bowel disease, and the structure and function of the GI tract. We also included information on food safety and sanitation as well as budgeting tips. The manual covers a variety of GI-related topics such as minimizing stool and ostomy output, avoiding obstructions, and maximizing absorption. It also serves as a reference for the patients as it includes an extensive glossary of medical terms and a list of other resources available by phone, fax, post, and the Internet.

In some patients, particularly those with small bowel enterostomies or a limited length of colon, oral rehydration solutions that utilize the active co-transport system of sodium and glucose, are used to maintain hydration and decrease the dependence on intravenous fluids.[9] The method and type of fluid and electrolyte supplementation is individualized for the patients (Chapter 4). This may be accomplished by mouth with oral rehydration solutions and mineral supplementation or with intravenous fluids. Rehydration solutions can be provided via enteral feeding tubes (e.g., PEG) nocturnally to provide additional fluid replacement. At times both methods may be used until the patient can be transitioned to total oral rehydration and supplementation. Care must be taken to replace the fluid and electrolytes that are lost from various body fluids. Replacement fluids are administered based on measured losses and in amounts required to maintain an adequate urine output. We have developed a number of oral rehydration recipes that are used depending on the patients' fluid and electrolyte requirements and GI anatomy.

Almost all of the patients require vitamin and mineral supplementation, especially for patients not receiving parenteral nutrition (Chapter 7). Since absorption is impaired, these patients may require doses that are several times greater than the recommended dietary allowance to maintain adequate tissue and functional levels. In some instances it may be beneficial to provide the vitamin in a liquid or chewable form in order to maximize absorption (Chapter 20). Vitamin B_{12} injections should be started after surgical resection of more than 100 cm of terminal ileum to avoid the development of hematologic and neurologic consequences of vitamin deficiency.[10]

Specialized enteral nutrition by the oral route or by tube may be required to provide total or partial nutrition support either short term during the rehabilitation process or permanently (Chapter 14). Care must be taken in the appropriate selection of an enteral feeding product that will maximize absorption and minimize gastrointestinal symptoms. As with diet, the choice of enteral formula is dependent on the anatomy and functional capacity of the GI tract.

Many of these patients will require intravenous hydration or parenteral nutrition temporarily until they can be rehabilitated or become a candidate for a transplant (Chapter 15). In some circumstances it may be determined that long-term intravenous support is the best option for the patient. Patients with short

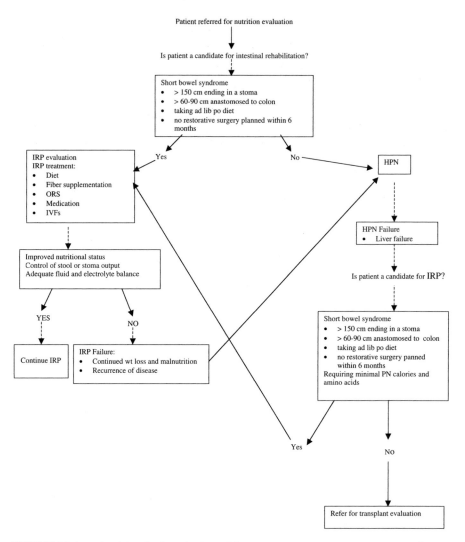

FIGURE 23.15 Algorithm for intestinal rehabilitation, HPN, and intestinal transplant[7]

bowel syndrome and continued symptoms of malabsorption or other intestinal dysfunction may be candidates for nontransplant surgical procedures to improve intestinal function (Chapters 17 and 18).[11–13] These procedures are referred to as Surgical Intestinal Rehabilitation (SIR) or Autologous Gastro-Intestinal Reconstruction (AGIR) and can be effective in allowing freedom from HPN and its potential complications. With improvements in surgical techniques and refinement of antirejection medications, intestinal and multivisceral transplantation has become an option for those individuals who cannot adapt or have failed attempts to utilize these other therapies (Chapter 19).[14]

MONITORING

It is important to make certain that the patient being followed by the IRP is able to maintain nutritional status and fluid and electrolyte balance. This may require periodic office visits, phone calls, and laboratory studies. Additionally, the goal should always be to transition the patient to the most benign therapy possible that will enhance physiologic functioning and quality of life (Chapters 21 and 22). These patients are chronically ill and tend to have very complicated medical conditions that change frequently. Communicating recommendations and the results of these evaluation to their primary or referring physicians will help to maintain the continuum of care necessary to optimize good outcomes.

CONCLUSION

The management of patients with intestinal failure is complex and requires a comprehensive multidisciplinary approach. The goal is to provide the safest most efficacious therapy to improve the nutritional status and quality of life of these patients. Appropriate patient selection is imperative. Not all patients are suitable candidates for intestinal rehabilitation therapy. It is important to identify those patients who are most likely to respond. Patients who fail the rehabilitation process are candidates for long-term parenteral nutrition or small bowel transplant. These are interrelated services, and it is important that the patient receive a thorough evaluation so that the most effective therapy can be provided. The goal is to provide the safest most effective therapy to improve nutritional status and the quality of life.

With each of these therapies, the programs need to be patient-focused and provide intensive education, training, and monitoring. Successful management depends on a multidisciplinary approach at a center that can offer a variety of diagnostic and therapeutic options.

REFERENCES

1. Howard, L. et al., Current use and clinical outcomes of home parenteral and enteral nutrition therapies in the United States, *Gastroenterology,* 109, 355, 1995.
2. Dudrick, S.J. et al., Long-term total parenteral nutrition with growth, development and positive nitrogen balance, *Surgery,* 62, 134, 1968.
3. Starzl, T.E. et al., Transplantation of multiple abdominal viscera, *JAMA,* 261,1 449, 1989.
4. Byrne, T.A. et al., Growth hormone, glutamine, and a modified diet enhance nutrient absorption in patients with severe short bowel syndrome, *J. Parent. Enter. Nutr.,* 19, 296, 1995.
5. Irving, M., An intestinal failure unit, in *Intestinal Failure,* Nightingale, J., Ed., Greenwich Medical Media Limited, London, 2001, chap. 30.
6. Nightingale, J.M.D., Introduction: definition and classification of intestinal failure, in *Intestinal Failure,* Nightingale J., Ed., Greenwich Medical Media Limited, London, 2001, xix.

7. Matarese, L.E., Seidner, D.L., and Steiger, E., Intestinal rehabilitation program. Clinical pathways and algorithms, the Cleveland Clinic Foundation, Cleveland, OH, 2002.

8. Scolapio, J.S. and Fleming, C.R., Short bowel syndrome, *Gastro. Clin. N. Amer.*, 27, 467, 1998.

9. Sladen, G.E. and Dawson, A.M., Interrelationships between the absorption of glucose, sodium and water by the normal human jejunum, *Clin. Sci.*, 36, 119, 1969.

10. Booth, C.C., The metabolic effects of intestinal resection in man, *Postgrad. Med. J.*, 37, 725, 1961.

11. Thompson, J.S., Reoperation in patients with the short bowel syndrome, *Am. J. Surg.*, 164, 453, 1992.

12. Devine, R.M. and Kelly, K.A., Surgical therapy of the short bowel syndrome, *Gastro. Clin. N. Amer.*, 18, 603, 1989.

13. Bianchi, A., Intestinal loop lengthening: A technique for increasing small intestinal length, *J. Pediatr. Surg.*, 15, 145, 1980.

14. Abu-Elmagd, K. et al., Clinical intestinal transplantation: A decade of experience at a single center, *Ann. Surg.* 234, 404, 2001.

Index